REVIEW OF CARDIOLOGY FOR DM ENTRANCE

Nitin Parashar
MBBS, MD, DM (Fellow)
All India Institute of Medical Sciences
New Delhi

Mumun Sinha
MBBS, MD, DM (Fellow)
All India Institute of Medical Sciences
New Delhi

Peepee Publishers and Distributors (P) Ltd.®

Review of Cardiology for DM Entrance

Published by
Pawaninder P. Vij and Anupam Vij

Peepee Publishers and Distributors (P) Ltd.
Head Office: 160, Shakti Vihar, Pitam Pura
Delhi-110034 (India)

Correspondence Address:
7/31, First Floor, Ansari Road, Daryaganj
New Delhi-110002 (India)

Ph: 41512412, 23246245, 9811156083

e-mail: peepee160@yahoo.co.in

e-mail: peepee160@gmail.com

www.peepeepub.com

First Edition: 2019

ISBN : 978-81-8445-262-4

Dedication

To Lobia, who was my constant companion and support through many long nights of writing and editing this book, to my parents due to whom I could become what I am today, and to my sweet brother with whom my childhood and adolescence could become everlastingly memorable.

PREFACE

This book is a very comprehensive review of all major topics in cardiology with an intent to help those preparing for entrance examination in cardiology and for medicine residents who want to review cardiology in a short span of time. The book is organized in a multiple-choice-question and answer format and has explanation along with detailed topic review of those questions. This book encompasses all topics in cardiology and is divided into easy-to-follow chapters related to different areas of cardiovascular medicine. The questions included in this book were recently asked in various entrance examinations. The explanations are clear and evidence-based. The book highlights a special section on images in cardiology which are of high resolution. The detailed topic review will allow students to prepare for and write exam with greater confidence.

Nitin Kumar Parashar
Mumun Sinha

ACKNOWLEDGEMENTS

I am indebted to all the contributors and co-authors of this book who have taken time from their clinical and academic responsibilities to contribute to this book.

I would like to extend my deep thanks to Mr. Pawaninder P. Vij and whole Peepee Publishers and Distributors (P) Ltd. team for outstanding support in the publication of this book without which this book could never have come to fruition.

I would like to extend a deep personal thanks to the following:

- To Dr. S. Ramakrishnan, Dr. Sandeep Seth, Dr. Sandeep Singh, Dr. S. S. Kothari, Dr. Pankaj Malhotra, Dr. Subhash Varma, Dr. Sanjay Jain, Sushil Khanna Sir who have been my professional and academic mentors and role models.
- To my parents, who have always been supportive of my medical education, training, career and aspirations.

CONTRIBUTORS

Dr. Anupam Kumar Singh (MBBS, MD, DM)
Post Graduate Institute of Medical Sciences
Chandigarh

Dr. Shardool Vikram Gupta (MBBS, MS, MCh)
All India Institute of Medical Sciences
New Delhi

Dr. Nitin Arora (MBBS, MD)
Maulana Azad Medical College
New Delhi

Dr. Faraz Ahmad Farooqi (MBBS, MD, DM)
All India Institute of Medical Sciences
New Delhi

Dr. Suraj Maratrao Patil (MBBS, MD, DM)
All India Institute of Medical Sciences
New Delhi

Dr. Jay Relan (MBBS, MD, DM)
All India Institute of Medical Sciences
New Delhi

Dr. Bharathraj Kidambi (MBBS, MD, DM)
All India Institute of Medical Sciences
New Delhi

Dr. Venkatakrishnan (MBBS, MD, DM)
All India Institute of Medical Sciences
New Delhi

Dr. Sai Krishna Reddy (MBBS, MD, DM)
All India Institute of Medical Sciences
New Delhi

Dr. Aseem Basha (MBBS, MD, DM)
All India Institute of Medical Sciences
New Delhi

Dr. Ayush Singhal (MBBS, MD, DM)
All India Institute of Medical Sciences
New Delhi

Dr. Nitish Rai (MBB, MD, DM)
All India Institute of Medical Sciences
New Delhi

Dr. Jaskaran Singh (MBBS, MD, DM)
All India Institute of Medical Sciences
New Delhi

Dr. Shanmugam Krishnan (MBBS, MD, DM)
All India Institute of Medical Sciences
New Delhi

Dr. Pruthvi CR (MBBS, MD, DM)
Post Graduate Institute of Medical Sciences
Chandigarh

Dr. Krishna Santosh (MBBS, MD, DM)
Post Graduate Institute of Medical Sciences
Chandigarh

Dr. Mohit Garg (MBBS, MD)
All India Institute of Medical Sciences
Rishikesh

Dr. Niraj Nirmal Pandey (MBBS, MD, DM)
All India Institute of Medical Sciences
New Delhi

Dr. Rengarajan Rajagopal (MBBS, MD, DM)
All India Institute of Medical Sciences
New Delhi

CONTENTS

1 Clinical Examination

Clubbing

1. **All are involved in the pathogenesis of clubbing except:**
   A. Prostaglandin dehydrogenase gene mutation
   B. Hypoxia
   C. Vagal stimulation
   D. Vascular endothelial growth factor

2. **Clubbing and cyanosis in lower limbs, but not upper limbs, may be seen in which of the following?**
   A. PDA with coarctation of aorta
   B. PDA with pulmonary hypertension
   C. Ventricular septal defect Eisenmenger's
   D. ASD Eisenmenger's with coarctation of aorta

3. **An abnormal Schamroth's test may be found in all of the following except:**
   A. Tetralogy of Fallot
   B. Subacute bacterial endocarditis
   C. Left atrial myxoma
   D. Aortic stenosis

Blood Pressure

4. **Tamponade may not be associated with pulsus paradoxus in which of the following:**
   A. ASD
   B. Aortic stenosis
   C. Mitral stenosis
   D. Old age

5. **All of the following may be associated with pulsus paradoxus except;**
   A. Tamponade
   B. Status asthmaticus
   C. Pulmonary embolism
   D. Aortic stenosis

Valsalva Maneuver

6. **Square-wave response in Valsalva maneuver indicates:**
   A. LV systolic dysfunction
   B. Elevated filling pressures
   C. Normal LV systolic function
   D. Normal LV diastolic function

7. **All of the following are physiological responses during the Phase 2 (Maintenance Phase) of Valsalva maneuver in a normal person except:**
   A. Decrease in pulse rate
   B. Decrease in aortic systolic pressure
   C. Decrease in pulse pressure
   D. Decrease in left ventricular filling

8. **Square sign during Valsalva maneuver is seen in which of the following?**
   A. HOCM
   B. MVP
   C. Aortic stenosis
   D. Congestive heart failure

9. **All are true regarding auscultatory gap, except:**

A. More likely to occur in older hypertensives with target end organ damage
B. It may over estimate systolic pressure
C. It may over estimate diastolic pressure
D. It should be distinguished from pulsus paradoxus

10. Pulsus paradoxus is seen in:
A. Pulmonary embolism
B. Marked obesity
C. Acute severe asthma
D. All of the above

11. Pulsus paradoxus without pericardial effusion is seen in all except:
A. Pulmonary embolism
B. CRF
C. RVMI
D. Tension pneumothorax

Jugular Venous Pressure

12. "Ventricularization" of Jugular venous waveform is seen in
A. Severe tricuspid regurgitation
B. Severe pulmonary stenosis
C. Severe mitral regurgitation
D. Severe aortic stenosis

13. Prominent x descent is seen in:
A. Tricuspid stenosis
B. Cardiac tamponade
C. Both of the above
D. None of the above

14. Loss of y descent in jugular venous pulse is a characteristic feature of:
A. Constrictive pericarditis
B. Cardiac tamponade
C. Restrictive cardiomyopathy
D. Tricuspid stenosis

15. Causes of prominent "a" wave in jugular venous pulsations include all of the following except?
A. PS
B. Pulmonary hypertension
C. Tricuspid stenosis
D. ASD

16. In JVP, Kussumaul's sign may be a feature in:
A. Mitral stenosis
B. Right ventricular MI
C. Severe LV failure
D. HOCM

17. The Y descent in JVP is absent in:
A. Cardiac tamponade
B. Constrictive pericarditis
C. Effusive constrictive pericarditis
D. Restrictive cardiomyopathy

18. Which of the following is false statement about arterial pulse?
A. In pulsus paradoxus, rate slows during inspiration
B. Tachycardia > 150/min at rest implies underlying cardiac arrhythmia
C. Pulsus alternans indicates poor function of LV
D. Collapsing pulse is seen in thyrotoxicosis

Pulse

19. Each of the following statements regarding pulsus alternans in patients with marked LV dysfunction is true except:
A. It is usually associated with electrical alternans of the QRS complex
B. It is more readily detected in the femoral as compared with radial arteries
C. It can be detected by sphygmomanometry
D. It can be elicited by the assumption of erect posture

20. Bifid pulse is not seen in:
A. Chronic severe AR
B. HOCM

C. IABP (Intra-aortic balloon pump)
D. Severe MR

Cardiac Sounds

21. Paradoxically split S2 is heard in:
A. VSD
B. MR
C. Severe AS
D. All the above

22. In a patient with chronic left ventricular disease, the patient having predominant S4 gallop (as compared to having S3 gallop) will have:
A. Higher mean left atrial pressure
B. Higher left ventricular filling pressure in early diastole
C. Higher atrial contractile function
D. Higher atrial volume

23. S1 (First heart sound) is likely to be loud in:
A. PR interval of 100 msec
B. LV EF of 30%
C. Calcified mitral stenosis
D. Patients on B-blockers

24. Reverse splitting of 2nd heart sound is not a feature in:
A. LBBB
B. Severe aortic stenosis
C. Left ventricular pacing
D. Acute myocardial ischemia

25. Ejection click may be heard in all except:
A. Valvar pulmonary stenosis
B. Dilated pulmonary artery in PH
C. Aortic root dilatation
D. Supravalvar aortic stenosis

26. Decrease in intensity of S1 is seen in:
A. RBBB
B. Left atrial myxoma
C. Acute AR
D. Atrial septal defect

27. 38 year old female with history of smoking of 20 pack years with childhood RF presents with fatigue and wide split S2 that persists throughout the respiratory cycle. Diagnosis is:
A. ASD B. LBBB
C. PS D. MS

Murmurs

28. Which of the following is an incorrect description for dynamic auscultation?
A. Systolic murmur of HOCM becomes louder with Valsalva
B. Murmur of AR decreases with handgrip exercise
C. With squatting, murmur of MVP softens
D. Left sided murmurs are louder during expiration

29. In the beat after long cycle length in atrial fibrillation, which of the following murmur increases in intensity?
A. Pulmonary Stenosis
B. Rheumatic mitral regurgitation
C. Mitral regurgitation due to papillary muscle dysfunction
D. Mitral regurgitation due to mitral valve prolapse

30. All are causes of Pansystolic murmur except:
A. Mitral valve prolapse
B. Primary pulmonary hypertension
C. Post MI VSD
D. Acute AR

31. Pansystolic murmur can be seen in all except:
A. Traumatic TR B. Post MI VSD
C. MVP D Pulmonary HTN

32. All are causes of early systolic murmur except?
A. Acute MR

B. Infundibular pulmonary stenosis
C. Acute TR with normal PA pressure
D. Muscular VSD

33. Intensity of HOCM murmur decreases during:
A. Valsalva strain phase
B. Standing
C. Squatting
D. Exercise

34. All of the following are true about Carey Coomb's murmur except:
A. Associated with mitral valvulitis
B. Associated with rapid ventricular filling in early diastole followed by obstruction to flow
C. Usually disappears over time
D. Typically begins with S3

Others

35. Branham's sign is seen in:
A. Pulmonary AV fistula
B. Systemic AV fistula
C. Pulmonary Embolism
D. Cardiac tamponade

36. Hereditary telangiectasia is associated with:
A. ASD
B. VSD
C. TOF
D. Pulmonary AV fistula

37. Fingerized thumb and hypoplastic radial side of the forearm can be seen in association with:
A. ASD B. PDA
C. TOF D. CoA

38. Which of the following is not associated with Coarctation of aorta?
A. Pistol shot sounds on femoral arteries
B. A continuous murmur on the back
C. Lower blood pressure in legs compared with arm
D. Radiofemoral delay

ANSWERS

Clubbing:

Answer: 1. C. Vagal stimulation

Answer: 2. B. PDA with pulmonary hypertension.

Answer: 3. D. Aortic stenosis.

Proposed mechanisms of clubbing: Vasodilation (i.e., distended blood vessels), Hypoxia causing secretion of growth factors (e.g., platelet-derived growth factor and hepatocyte growth factor) from the lungs, overproduction of PGE2 by other tissues.

Schamroth's test: In the absence of clubbing, nail-to-nail opposition creates a diamond-shaped window. In clubbed fingers, the loss of the profile angle with the increase in tissue at the nailbed causes obliteration of this space.

Causes of clubbing:

Cardiac: Cyanotic heart diseases, Subacute bacterial endocarditis, Atrial myxoma.

Pulmonary: Lung cancer, ILD, Suppurative lung disease (Lung abscess, Empyema, Bronchiectasis), Pleural mesothelioma, Pulmonary AV fistula.

Gastrointestinal: Crohn's and ulcerative colitis, primary biliary cirrhosis, hepatopulmonary syndrome.

Differential clubbing and cyanosis:

Differential lower limb clubbing: 1. PDA with Eisenmenger causes reversal of shunt through PDA causing desaturation in lower limb only, and results in cyanosis and clubbing in lower limbs not in upper limbs. 2. Interruption of aortic arch and a PDA

Differential upper limb clubbing: 1. Complete TGA with preductal CoA

Blood Pressure:

Answer: 4. A. ASD.

Answer: 5. D. Aortic stenosis.

Answer: 6. B. Elevated filling pressures

Answer: 7. A. Decrease in pulse rate

Answer: 8. D. Congestive heart failure.

Answer: 9. B. It may over estimate systolic pressure

Answer: 10. D. All of the above

Answer: 11. B. CRF

Cuff length/ width: 80%/40% of arm circumference.

Significant difference in pulses and BP in arms: >20 mmHg in BP is associated with aortic coarctation or dissection, subclavian artery disease, supravalvular (right > left in BP) and aortic stenosis (AS)

Pressure in UL>LL: CoA, PAD

Pressure LL>UL: Severe AR (Hill sign)

Wide pulse pressure (systolic – diastolic pressure): AR, Old age, atherosclerosis

Narrow pulse pressure: HF, AS, HCM

Orthostatic hypotension: a drop in systolic BP >20 mmHg, a drop in diastolic BP >10 mmHg or HR rise >10 bpm

Valsalva Maneuver:

The Valsalva maneuver involves expiration against a closed glottis, increasing the intrathoracic pressure. There are four phases of heart rate and BP response. Normal response includes the following:

- Phase 1: Early during the Valsalva maneuver, pressure on the intrathoracic aorta and pulmonary veins emptying into left heart transiently increases ventricular filling, stroke volume, and BP with reflex slowing of heart.
- Phase 2: With a continued Valsalva maneuver, LV filling diminishes and lowers stroke volume and BP, resulting in compensatory tachycardia. Reflex peripheral vasoconstriction slowly increases BP and lowers heart rate.
- Phase 3: With release of the Valsalva maneuver, pressure on the aorta drops, and BP drops with some increase in heart rate.

- Phase 4: Left ventricle fills, with increase in stroke volume with continued peripheral vasoconstriction causing BP to overshoot the baseline value. This will reflexly reduce heart rate below baseline.

Phase 2 is used in dynamic auscultation.

Except for the murmurs of HOCM and MVP, rest all the murmurs decrease in intensity with Valsalva.

In HOCM, the Valsalva maneuver results in smaller left ventricle size causing increased LVOT obstruction and an increase in murmur intensity.

In MVP, reduced LV volume with phase 2 Valsalva results in earlier and greater prolapse and the MR murmur lengthens.

Absent overshoot response: No phase 4 rise in systolic BP, associated with moderately decreased left ventricular ejection fraction (LVEF)

Square wave response: Presence of Korotkoff sounds during the entire straining phase and no Phase 4 rise in systolic BP, associated with CHF, severely decreased LVEF

Pulsus paradoxus

Exaggerated fall in systolic BP >10 mmHg with inspiration, seen in cardiac tamponade.

Other causes: Constrictive pericarditis, pulmonary embolism, chronic lung disease, severe emphysema, severe asthma, morbid obesity.

Causes of no pulsus paradoxus in tamponade: Low pressure tamponade, ASD, severe AR or MR.

Auscultatory gap

A transient disappearance of Korotkoff sounds between systolic and diastolic pressures during blood pressure cuff deflation

It is related to carotid atherosclerosis and to increased arterial stiffness in hypertensive patients, independent of age

The improper interpretation of this gap may lead to blood pressure monitoring errors:

- Underestimation of systolic blood pressure
- Overestimation of diastolic blood pressure

Jugular Venous Pressure:

Answer: 12. A. Severe tricuspid regurgitation

Answer: 13. B. Cardiac tamponade

Answer: 14. B. Cardiac tamponade

Answer: 15. E. ASD.

Answer: 16. B. Right ventricular MI

Answer: 17. A. Cardiac tamponade

Answer: 18. A. In pulsus paradoxus, rate slows during inspiration

Calculation of jugular venous pressure (JVP) in mmHg

1. Determine vertical distance above the sternal angle to the top of the venous pulsation (in cm water)
2. Add to above, 5 cm if incline is at 0–45° or 10 cm if incline is at 45+°
3. Divide by 1.36

Normal RA pressure is <8 mmHg

Prominent a wave: Obstruction to RA emptying

TV abnormalities: TS, RA myxoma, carcinoid heart disease, lupus endocarditis, RA thrombus, tricuspid atresia

Distal to tricuspid valve: decreased RV compliance such as in RVH, RV outflow obstruction such as in PS

PH

Uncommon in conditions with VSD or ASD

Cannon a wave: RA contraction against a closed TV.

Irregular cannon a wave: atrial, ventricular, or junctional premature beats, ventricular tachycardia, first-degree atrioventricular block with a markedly prolonged PR interval, high-grade atrioventricular block, ventricular pacing, and atrioventricular dissociation.

Regular cannon a waves: Junctional rhythm and isorhythmic atrioventricular dissociation.

Absent a wave: No effective atrial contraction

Atrial fibrillation

Ebstein's anomaly

Equal a wave and v wave

ASD

TR

Prominent C or CV wave

TR (Venricularization of JVP)

Prominent × descent

ASD

Early cardiac tamponade

Blunted or absent y descent

Late pericardial tamponade

TS

Severe RVH

Steep y descent

Constrictive pericarditis (classic M or W contour with prominent x and y descents)

Restrictive cardiomyopathy

Severe right side HF

TR

Hepatojugular (Abdominojugular) Reflux

When neck veins distend (≥4 cm H_2O) with steady (>10 seconds) upper abdominal compression while the patient continues to breathe normally without straining.

Positive in LV failure with pulmonary hypertension.

Kussumaul's sign

Kussmaul's sign is the paradoxical rise in jugular venous pressure with inspiration.

Causes of Kussmaul's sign include:

1. Right ventricular infarction
2. Severe right ventricular failure
3. Restrictive cardiomyopathy
4. Constrictive pericarditis
5. Tricuspid stenosis.

PULSE

Answer: 19. A. It is usually associated with electrical alternans of the QRS complex

Answer: 20. D. Severe MR

Unequal or delayed pulses: PVD, aortic disease (dissection, aneurysm, coarctation), Takayasu disease, supravalvular aortic stenosis (right > left upper extremity pulses)

Pulsus alternans: associated with cardiac tamponade, severe LV systolic HF, severe AR, HTN and hypovolemic state, ectopy.

Bounding: AR, AV fistula, hyperkinetic states such as fever, anemia, thyrotoxicosis

Bifid

1. Pulsus bisferiens (both peaks during systole): Significant AR, HCM, AV fistula, large PDA
2. Dicrotic pulse (one peak in systole and one peak in diastole): Severe HF, cardiac tamponade, intra-aortic balloon counterpulsation, immediate post-operative aortic valve replacement, hypovolemic shock, hyperkinetic states

Weak and delayed: Severe AS

Abrupt carotid upstroke with a rapid fall-off: Severe AR (water-hammer or Corrigan pulse), PDA, large AV fistula, hyperkinetic states, older patients with HTN and wide pulse pressures

Cardiac Sounds:

Answer: 21. C. Severe AS

Answer: 22. C. Higher atrial contractile function

Answer: 23. A. PR interval of 100 msec

Answer: 24. C. Left ventricular pacing

Answer: 25. D. Supravalvar aortic stenosis

Answer: 26. C. Acute AR

Answer: 27. A. ASD

Patient has wide and fixed split of S2 which is a feature of ASD.

Accentuated S1

MS, TS, Atrial myxoma, hyperkinetic states (PDA, VSD, ASD, high output states), Short PR interval (Pre-excitation, tachycardia)

Soft S1

Calcific MS, MR, TR, Presystolic semiclosure of AV valve (Severe acute AR), Bradycardia

Wide splitting of S1: RBBB, LV pacing, pre-excitation syndrome, Ebstein's anomaly, TS, ASD

Reverse splitting of S1: LBBB, RV pacing, RV ectopy, severe MS and left atrial (LA) myxoma

Normal S2

Best heard over the left and right upper sternal border with S2 > S1 in intensity

Normal (physiologic) S2 splitting: A2 and P2 are coincident during expiration; during inspiration, P2 is relatively delayed due to delayed closure of pulmonary valve, resulting in physiologic splitting.

Accentuated P2: P2 > A2 at the left upper sternal border or P2 can be heard at the apex

Pulmonary hypertension (PH), ASD (not necessarily with PH), Soft A2 (relative intensity)

Wide and variable S2 splitting

Delayed activation of RV: RBBB, ectopy/arrhythmia originating from LV such as Wolff-Parkinson White syndrome

PH with RV failure, RV outflow obstruction (pulmonic stenosis [PS], pulmonary embolism)

Severe MR (due to premature AV closure), VSD, constrictive pericarditis

Wide and Fixed splitting of S2

Ostium secundum ASD

PAPVC

Severe RV failure

Reversed or paradoxical, splitting of S2 due to a pathologic delay in AV closure

Delay in LV activation: complete LBBB and ectopy/arrhythmia from RV, RV pacing

Delayed LV ejection: severe AS, HCM, AR, PDA, myocardial ischemia

Single S2: AV or pulmonic valve (PV) abnormalities or fused A2 and P2 (Eisenmenger's VSD, common ventricle)

S3

Normal in healthy people <40 years of age or in high output states (pregnancy, thyrotoxicosis)

A low-pitched sound best heard over the LV apex/PMI in the left lateral decubitus position with the bell; a right-sided S3 is best heard at the lower left sternal border (LLSB) or subxiphoid position with the patient supine, and may become louder with inspiration

Associated with HF: elevated LVEDP, reduced LVEF, or elevated B-type natriuretic peptide (BNP)

Associated with MR, not necessarily indicative of HF

S4

Low-pitched sound best heard over the LV apex in the left lateral decubitus position with the bell

Common in patients with **accentuated atrial contribution** to ventricular filling such as LVH

Associated with abnormal LV compliance: hypertensive heart disease, AS, HCM, acute MI, MR, AR

Aortic ejection sound or click:

A high-pitched early to mid systolic sound widely transmitted, best heard at the LLSB > base of the heart

Congenital bicuspid AV (including in the absence of stenosis) or aortic root dilation with a normal AV

Absent in subvalvular and supravalvular AS

Pulmonary ejection sound or click:

Similar in quality to the aortic ejection sound, but best heard at the left upper and lower sternal border and decreases with inspiration

Congenital bicuspid PV or pulmonic root dilation with a normal PV

Only right-sided sound/murmur that is attenuated by inspiration is pulmonary ejection click of valvular PS

Midsystolic click

A systolic click best heard over right or left upper sternal border from MVP

Opening snap (OS)

A high-pitched diastolic opening snap of MV in MS, best heard over left upper and lower sternal border

Pericardial knock

A high-pitched early diastolic sound (between S2 and S3) best heard at the lower right sternal border

Results from abrupt cessation of ventricular expansion after atrioventricular valve opening in constrictive pericarditis-prominent y descent seen in JVP waveform

Tumor plop

A low-pitched diastolic sound caused by prolapse of tumor (usually atrial myxoma) across the MV

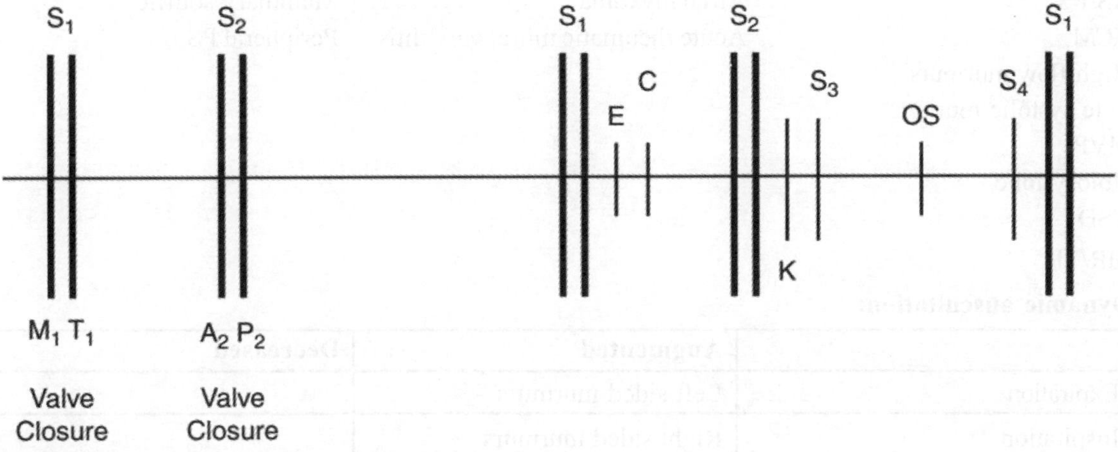

Murmurs

Answer: 28. B. Murmur of AR decreases with handgrip exercise

Answer: 29. A. Pulmonary Stenosis

Answer: 30. D. Acute AR

Answer: 31. A. Traumatic TR

Answer: 32. B. Infundibular pulmonary stenosis

Answer: 33. C. Squatting

Answer: 34. B. Associated with rapid ventricular filling in early diastole followed by obstruction to flow

All diastolic murmurs are pathologic.

Findings that suggest that a systolic murmur is pathologic:

- Loud (grade 3 or more)
- Long duration
- Associated with ejection or nonejection click
- Loud S1, A2, or P2
- Presence of an opening snap
- Presence of left or right ventricular hypertrophy or heave
- Fixed or expiratory splitting of S2

Classification of murmurs

SYSTOLIC	**DIASTOLIC**	**CONTINUOUS**
Early	**Early**	PDA
Acute MR or TR	AR/PR	RSOV
VSD	**Mid to late**	AV fistula
Midsystolic ejection	MS/TS	Cervical venous hum

AS/PS
HCM
High flow murmurs
Late systolic murmur
MVP
Holosystolic
VSD
MR/TR

Atrial myxoma
Acute rheumatic mitral valvulitis

Mammary souffle
Peripheral PS

Dynamic auscultation:

	Augmented	**Decreased**
Expiration	Left sided murmurs	
Inspiration	Right sided murmurs	
Standing	HOCM MV prolapse	AS PS
Squatting	AR, MR, VSD	HOCM MV prolapse
Handgrip	AR, MR, VSD, MS	HOCM
Valsalva maneuver	HOCM MV prolapse	AS PS
Long cardiac cycle length (e.g., atrial fibrillation, premature ventricular contraction)	AS PS HOCM	MR AR
Amyl nitrite	HOCM AS, PS Innocent SM MS, TS	MR VSD AR Austin Flint

Other important murmurs:

Gibsons murmur: Continuous machinery murmur in PDA due to flow from the descending thoracic aorta to the pulmonary artery, with maximal intensity at S2.

Carey Coombs murmur: Mid-diastolic mitral murmur due to mitral valvulitis in rheumatic fever. There is no mitral stenosis and it usually disappears over time as the valvulitis improves. It is usually associated with S3. It occurs because of increased blood flow across thickened mitral valve.

Austin Flint murmur: Mitral mid-diastolic murmur heard in severe AR

Graham Steel murmur: Early diastolic murmur of PR seen in severe pulmonary hypertension

Gallavardin phenomenon: A loud, harsh, blowing murmur at the apex associated with AS (easily confused with MR or HCM often and can be differentiated by maneuvers)

Cabot–Locke Murmur: Early diastolic murmur seen in severe anemia, best heard at left sternal border.

Dock's murmur: Continuous diastolic murmur seen in stenosis of left anterior descending artery.

Key–Hodgkin Murmur: Diastolic murmur of AR due to retroversion of aortic valve leaflets in syphilitic aortitis.

Roger's Murmur: Harsh holosystolic murmur of small VSD, best heard at left upper sternal border.

Still's murmur: Musical systolic ejection murmur seen in children which increases with fever, anxiety, or exercise. Exact cause is unknown, however, source may be vibration of chordae tendineae in left ventricle or sound of blood gushing into the aorta.

Answer: 35. B. Systemic AV fistula

Branham-Nicoladoni sign:

If pressure is applied to artery proximal to an arteriovenous fistula, swelling of fistula reduces in size and there is reflex bradycardia. Bruit and thrill also disappear.

Answer: 36. D. Pulmonary AV fistula

Answer: 37. ASD

Answer: 38. D. Pistol shot sounds on femoral arteries.

Pistol shot sounds occur in severe aortic regurgitation (AR). Others are features of aortic coarctation.

Aortic regurgitation peripheral signs:

Austin Flint murmur	A mid-diastolic to late diastolic or presystolic mitral murmur best heard at the apex that is low-pitched and rumbling inthe presence of aortic regurgitation with no underlying mitral pathology
Becker sign	Increased retinal arteriole and pupillary pulsation
Bozzolo sign	Pulsatile nasal mucosa
Cole-Cecil murmur	Early diastolic murmur radiated to the apex and left axilla first described in the context ofsyphilitic aortitis
Corrigan pulse/sign	Initially described as a visible pulsation now tactile test in carotid or larger arteries wherea jumpy pulse that fully expands appears to suddenly collapse and be completely empty between beats. Associated with a widenedpulse pressure. Also called cannonball, collapsing, pistol-shot, pulsus celer et altus, trip-hammer or water-hammer pulse

de Musset sign	Pulsatile, rhythmic nodding of the head in synchrony with the regurgitant heart beat.
Dennison sign/ Shelley sign	Pulsatile cervix
Drummond sign	Pulsatile systolic expulsion of air from nostrils when mouth is closed
Duroziez sign	Double intermittent, systolic diastolic (antegrade-retrograde) murmur produced bycompression of femoral artery with a stethoscope by altering proximal and distal stethoscope bell pressure.
Gerhardt sign	Pulsatile spleen
Hill sign	An exaggerated increase of systolic arterial pressure in lower compared to upper limbs.
Landolfi sign	Pulsatile pupils
Mayne sign	Drop of more than 15 mm Hg in diastolic BP when arm is raised
Morton and Mahon sign	Facial flushing and blanching corresponding to head and neck arterial pulsations
Muller sign	Pulsating uvula
Penny sign	Flashing wheal-exaggerated pulsatility noted in an urticarial skin reaction in patients withaortic regurgitation.
Pulsus Bisferiens	Double systolic arterial wave separated by a midsystolic dip
Quincke sign	Exaggerated visible pulsation in nail beds
Rosenbach sign	Pulsatile liver
Sherman sign	An unexpectedly prominent and quickly found dorsalis pedis pulse (1–2 s) in patients aged 75 or older.
Traube sign	On auscultation of the femoral artery, the presence of a booming double sound orpistol shot

Important findings and associations:

Finding	Association
Bronze discolouration of skin, HF	Hemochromatosis
Leathery, cobblestone, plucked-chicken appearance of skin in axilla, premature CAD	Pseudoxanthoma elasticum
High arched palate	Marfan syndrome

Large protruding tongue with parotid enlargement, raccoon eyes	Amyloidosis
Bifid uvula	Loeys-Dietz syndrome
Orange tonsils	Tangier disease
Elfin facies	William syndrome with supravalvular AS, branch PS
Moon facies	Down syndrome with AV canal defects, ASD, VSD
Macroglossia	Amyloidosis; Down syndrome, Myxedema
Roth spots, conjunctival petechiae	Endocarditis
Xanthelasmas	Dyslipidemia (Familial hypercholesterolemia
Blue sclerae	Osteogenesis imperfecta with aortic disease, AR, MVP
Icteric sclerae	Cardiac cirrhosis
Ectopia lentis (upward displacement)	Marfan syndrome
Ectopia lentis (downward displacement)	Homocystinuria and premature CAD, stroke, PVD
Straight back syndrome	MVP; Ankylosing spondylitis with AR
Rudimentary or absent thumbs	Holt-Oram syndrome with ASD
Osler nodes, Janeway lesions, splinter hemorrhage	Endocarditis
Hyperextensible joints	Ehlers-Danlos syndrome
Central Cyanosis	Right-to-left shunts (Eisenmenger syndrome); Methemoglobinemia
Differential Cyanosis	Right-to-left shunt with (PDA)
Peripheral Cyanosis	Cardiogenic shock, severe peripheral vascular disease
Telangiectasias (dilated blood vessels)	Hereditary hemorrhagic telangiectasias with pulmonary AV fistula; Scleroderma
Lentigines (brown skin lesions)	LEOPARD syndrome; Carney syndrome with atrial myxomas
Angiofibromas (shiny papules-on face-adenoma sebaceum)	Tuberous sclerosis with rhabdomyomas
Erythema marginatum	Acute rheumatic fever

2 Investigations in Cardiology

Electrocardiography

1. **ST segment elevation is seen in:**
   A. Acute myocardial infarction
   B. Prinzmetal angina
   C. Acute pericarditis
   D. All of the above
2. **Tall R wave in V1 present in all except:**
   A. HCM
   B. RBBB
   C. Duchenne muscular dystrophy
   D. Accessory right sided pathway WPW
3. **RAE finding on ECG all except:**
   A. P wave in II > 0.25 mV
   B. P wave amplitude duration ratio > 1.6
   C. qR in right precordial lead in absence of MI
   D. P wave initial phase > 0. 15 seen in V1
4. **The following criteria is not applicable for left ventricular hypertrophy:**
   A. Sokolow-Lyon B. Romhilt-Estes
   C. Schamroth D. Cornell
5. **SV3 + RaVL > 2.8 mV (for men) & 2.0 mV (for women) is a diagnostic criteria for diagnosing left ventricular hypertrophy. This ECG criteria is known as:**
   A. Romhilt Estes score system
   B. Sokolow- Lyon Index
   C. Cornell voltage criteria
   D. None of the above
6. **SV1 + RV5 > 3.5 mV is defined as LVH by which criteria?**
   A. Romhilt-Estes criteria
   B. Sokolow-Lyon index
   C. Cornell voltage criteria
   D. Cornell regression equation
7. **Which one of following ECG pattern is not true for left anterior fascicular block?**
   A. rS pattern in leads I and aVL
   B. qR pattern in lead aVL
   C. Time to peak r wave in aVL 45 msec
   D. Frontal plane mean QRS axis is - 45 to - 90 degrees
8. **Left anterior hemiblock is characterized by?**
   A. Q waves in II, III, aVF
   B. QRS > 120 msec
   C. qR in aVL
   D. Right axis deviation
9. **Which one of following is not true for left posterior hemiblock in ECG?**
   A. North west axis deviation
   B. Small q in 2,3 & aVF
   C. Increased QRS voltage in limb leads
   D. No evidence of right ventricular hypertrophy
10. **Which one of following is not true for ECG in hypokalemia?**
    A. Depression of ST segment
    B. Prominent U wave

C. P wave becomes small & narrow
D. T wave becomes small or inverted

11. Which one of following is not true for sino-ventricular rhythm in ECG?
A. It is seen in hyperkalemia
B. Absent P wave
C. It is common after heart transplant
D. Conduction between SA node & AV node persists

12. Which one of following is true for electrical alternans in ECG?
A. It is common in patients with cardiac tamponade
B. It is ventricular bigeminy pattern
C. It is atrial bigeminy pattern
D. It is common in patients with rheumatic heart disease

13. Which of the following ECG feature is typical of LAHB?
A. Q wave in inferior leads
B. Mean QRS axis between 0 and —30 degree
C. rS pattern in inferior leads and qR pattern in lateral leads
D. Marked right axis deviation

14. All of the following are true regarding the acquisition of ECG, except:
A. A band width limitation to 50 Hz is recommended by the American Heart Association for electrocardiography in children
B. The standard amplifier gain for routine electrocardiography is 1000
C. Time is usually represented as 400 milliseconds/cm on the horizontal scale on an ECG
D. The bandwidth recommended for ECG in adults is 0.05 to 150 Hz

15. Macruz index is:
A. 'P' duration/PR segment in L-II is >1.6
B. Duration X depth of 'P'terminal force in V1 is >0.04mm.sec
C. Bifid 'P' waves
D. P duration >120 m.sec

16. Which one of following is not true Osborn waves in ECG?
A. It is seen in hypothermia
B. It is an elevated J waves
C. It represents distortion of the earliest stage of repolarisation
D. QT interval shortens

17. Following statement are true about early repolarization pattern except:
A. Prevalence of 1-13% in general population
B. Phase 2 re-entry can be initiated with trigger VT
C. Characterized by J point elevation with or without ST elevation in inferior limb and lateral precordial leads
D. Early repolarization with ascending ST segment is predictor of sudden cardiac death

18. Which of these suggest RV Hypertrophy in the ECG of a neonate 7 days old?
A. R/S ratio in VI > 1
B. Right axis deviation
C. S waves in V6
D. Upright T wave in V1

19. All of the following are expected to occur in ECG during exercise, except:
A. PR interval shortens
B. QT Interval shortens
C. R amplitude decreases
D. QRS duration shortens

20. Identify the correct statement regarding metabolic and drug effects on ECG:
A. Digitalis glycosides prolong QT interval
B. Hypercalcemia shortens QT interval
C. Prominent U waves are a feature of Hyperkalemia
D. "Sino ventricular rhythm" may be seen in hypokalemia

Treadmill Testing (TMT)

21. Mason-Likar modification is useful during:
A. Holter analysis
B. Coronary angiography
C. Ambulatory blood pressure recording
D. Treadmill test

22. Mason Likar modification of standard 12 lead ECG requires that extremity electrodes be moved to torso to reduce motion artefact. This modification results in:
A. New q waves in inferior leads
B. Loss of q waves in aVL
C. Right axis shift
D. Decreased voltage in inferior leads

23. All occur in ECG with exercise except:
A. QT interval decreases
B. PR interval decreases
C. QRS interval decreases
D. P wave amplitude decreases

24. Regarding Duke Treadmill Score, choose the wrong statement:
A. Calculated as Exercise time - (5 × ST deviation) - (4 X TM Angina Index)
B. TM Score of -11 or less had a 5 year survival rate of 72%
C. TM Score of + 5 or more had a 5 year survival rate of 97%
D. Duke TM score is as effective in elderly more than 75 years of age as in young individuals

25. Stage 6 of Bruce protocol is equivalent to:
A. 15.8 METs B. 16.5 METs
C. 16.9 METs D. 17.1 METs

26. Duke treadmill score is calculated using all of the following parameters except:
A. Exercise duration
B. Angina
C. ST depression
D. Double product

27. The strongest prognostic variable during treadmill testing is?
A. Ventricular ectopics during exercise
B. LBBB during exercise
C. Exercise duration
D. 3 mm ST segment depression during exercise

28. A 55-year-old male patient has exercised on treadmill for 6 minutes using standard Bruce protocol. He developed 2 mm maximum ST segment depression and non-limiting angina at peak exercise. The Duke Treadmill score will be:
A. -8 B. -6
C. -4 D. -10

29. All of the following are absolute contra indications for exercise testing except:
A. Acute MI (< 2 days)
B. Acute systemic infection accompanied by fever
C. High grade AV block
D. Acute myocarditis

30. 1 MET =
A. 2 ml O2/kg/min of body weight
B. 3.5 ml O2/kg/min of body weight
C. 5 ml O2/kg/min of body weight
D. 7.5 ml O2/kg/min of body weight

31. ST segment elevation was seen in abnormal q wave leads on TMT. All of the following are true except:
A. It is suggestive of ischemia
B. It is suggestive of poor prognosis
C. More common in anterior wall MI
D. It is suggestive of severity of Regional wall motion abnormality

32. 48 year old male with history of anterior wall MI 2 years back with EF 45%, ECG shows QS waves in V1 – V3 presents with complaints of chest pain on exertion for past 2 months. Stress test done shows ST

elevation in V1 – V3 after 8 METS, 85% THR achieved. Likely diagnosis?
A. Inducible ischemia in LAD territory
B. Inducible ischemia in RCA territory
C. Inducible ischemia present but territory cannot be defined
D. Not suggestive of ischemia

33. All of the following are beneficial effect of regular exercise except:
A. Favorable changes in fibrinolytic pathway
B. Decreased heart rate variability
C. Increased of expression of nitric oxide synthetase
D. Decreased systolic and diastolic blood pressure

34. 60 year old male with typical class 2 angina is referred for exercise ECG. His pre-test probability is:
A. Intermediate B. High
C. Low D. Very low

35. In which of the following clinical scenario, ST depression during TMT increases diagnostic probability of significant CAD?
A. 65 years old diabetic female with recent onset exertional dyspnea and normal LV function
B. 45 years old premenopausal women with atypical chest pain
C. 60 years old male with HTN, angina and LVH on ECG
D. 55 years old male diabetic with pre-excitation

Echocardiography

36. Which of the following is associated with continuous-wave Doppler (CWD) compared with pulsed-wave Doppler (PWD)?
A. Aliasing
B. Range specificity
C. Ability to record higher velocities
D. All of the above

37. LV Ejection Fraction (LVEF) is calculated by all of the following methods except:
A. [(LVEDV-LVESV)/LVEDV] × 100
B. [(LVEDD2-LVESD2)/LVEDD2] × 100
C. (S.V/LVEDV) × 100
D. (LVEDD-LVESD)/LVEDD

38. False statement about Tei index:
A. (IVCT + IVRT)/LVET
B. Myocardial performance index
C. (IVCT-IVRT)/LVET
D. Global ventricular function

39. Incorrect about normal diastolic filling pattern:
A. E/A > 1.5
B. DT (septal) = 160-240 ms
C. Septal e'> 10 cm/sec
D. E/e' > 8

40. Inverted Mercedes - Benz sign on echocardiography is used for following valve:
A. Tricuspid B. Aortic
C. Pulmonary D. Mitral

41. Which one of the following is more specific view to diagnose MVP?
A. Short axis view
B. Apical four chamber view
C. Subcostal view
D. Parasternal long axis view

42. Which one of the following is not true for echo finding in patients with severe diastolic dysfunction?
A. E/A > 2
B. Deceleration time of E wave >220 msec
C. E/e' >15
D. e' < 8 cm /sec

43. TAPSE (tricuspid annular plane systolic excursion) is determined by:
A. M-mode echo
B. 2-dimension echo

C. 3-dimension echo
D. Doppler

44. If inferior vena cava diameter is <2.1 cm & show >50% collapse with inspiration, then estimated RA pressure is:
A. 5 mm of Hg
B. 10 mm of Hg
C. 15 mm of Hg
D. 20 mm of Hg

45. All of the following are true about MPI (Myocardial performance index) except:
A. Measured by the formula (IVRT + IVCT) / LVET
B. Done for both ventricles
C. Denotes both systolic and diastolic dysfunction
D. Decreases in LV systolic dysfunction

46. All of the following are true about doppler echocardiography except?
A. PAEDP = 4 × (pulmonary end regurgitation velocity)^2 + RAP
B. LAP= Aortic systolic pressure - 4 × (Peak mitral regurgitant velocity)^2
C. Pulmonary artery systolic pressure = Aortic systolic pressure – peak gradient across PDA
D. RV Systolic Pressure = 4 (TR Systolic Velocity)2 - RA Pressure

47. Pressure half time of mitral valve is 250 msec. Area of mitral valve is?
A. 0.48 cm^2
B. 0.88 cm^2
C. 1.26 cm^2
D. 1.40 cm^2

48. Aortic pressure in a patient with AS is 116/90 mmHg. Echo showed peak aortic valve velocity of 4 m/s. The peak LV systolic pressure is?
A. 180 B. 186
C. 190 D. 196

Cardiac CT

49. Which of the following attenuation values is correct for non-contrast CT?
A. Air : 0-10 B. Bone : -1000
C. Water : 3000 D. Blood : 35-65

50. Coronary calcification on computerised tomography is helpful in predicting obstructive CAD. Which one of the following is true?
A. Sensitivity-90%
B. Sensitivity-50%
C. Sensitivity-60%
D. Sensitivity-80%

51. Which of the following organs gets the highest radiation dose during cardiac CTA?
A. Heart B. Lungs
C. Esophagus D. Breast

52. Which of the following affects radiation dose?
A. Tube voltage
B. Tube current
C. Pitch
D. All of the above

53. Which of the following agents may be used to slow the heart rate for coronary CTA?
A. Beta blockers
B. Nondihydropyridine calcium channel blocker (e.g., diltiazem)
C. Ivabradine
D. All of the above

54. Maximum limit for radiation dose to a pregnant woman for the entire length of pregnancy is?
A. 0.05 mSv B. 0.5 mSv
C. 5 mSv D. 50 mSv

55. The typical HU value for fat is?
A. -1000 HU B. -50 HU
C. 0 HU D. 1000 HU

56. Typical HU threshold of calcium for calculation of calcium score is:

A. 100 B. 130
C. 0 D. 400

57. Which of the following characteristics is associated with a potentially severe coronary artery stenosis?

A. Spotty calcification
B. Positive remodelling
C. Low-attenuation plaque <30 HU
D. All of the above

Cardiac MRI

58. Which of the following is not a limitation of cardiac MRI?

A. Need for iodinated contrast agents
B. Risk of developing nephrogenic systemic fibrosis (NSF) in patients with renal disease receiving gadolinium
C. Long acquisition time
D. Cerebral aneurysm clips

59. Which one of following is not true for MRI in acute myocardial infarction?

A. It assesses perfusion in infarcted & non-infarcted myocardium
B. Reperfused myocardium
C. Assess coronary anatomy precisely
D. Identify myocardial fibrosis, wall thinning

60. Cardiac MRI differentiates ischemic cardiomyopathy from non-ischemic cardiomyopathy by?

A. Epicardial enhancement
B. No enhancement
C. Midmyocardial enhancement
D. Subendocardial enhancement

61. Cardiac Magnetic resonance imaging is useful for the diagnosis of:

A. ARVD B. Sarcoidosis
C. Amyloidosis D. All of the above

62. Global myocardial enhancement on MRI is seen in all except:

A. Idiopathic Dilated Cardiomyopathy
B. Post cardiac transplant
C. Amyloidosis
D. Systemic sclerosis

63. Which of the following modality is best useful to detect infiltrative cardiomyopathy related to Hemochromatosis?

A. Multi-slice CT
B. 3D echo
C. Cardiac MRI
D. Radionuclide angiography

64. Cardiac MRI is not advisable with which of the following?

A. Automated implantable cardioverter defibrillator
B. Cerebral aneurysm clips
C. Iron-containing foreign body in the eye that has been there for 6 years
D. All of the above

65. What may be the effects of a strong magnetic field in a patient with a pacer or implantable cardioverter-defibrillator?

A. May burn the circuits
B. Heat generation at lead tip and tissue coagulation and rise in threshold
C. Reset device
D. All of the above

66. Which of the following is done by gadolinium?

A. Shortens T1 and increases signal on T1-weighted images
B. Lengthens T1 and increases signal on T1-weighted images
C. Shortens T1 and reduces signal on T1-weighted images
D. Lengthens T1 and reduces signal on T1-weighted images

Cardiac Nuclear Imaging

67. Drug used in pharmacological stress testing except:

A. Adenosine B. Dipyridamole
C. Aminophylline D. Regadenoson

68. Physical half-life of Thallium 201 is:

A. 6 hours B. 8 hours
C. 36 hours D. 73 hours

69. One of the following SPECT tracers has long half life:

A. 99Tc-Sestamibi
B. Thallium - 201
C. 99Tc-Tetrafosmin
D. 99Tc-Teboroxime

70. One of the following is metabolism tracer in PET imaging:

A. Fluorine - 18
B. Oxygen - 15
C. Nitrogen - 13
D. Rubidium - 82

71. Not true regarding the properties of SPECT tracers:

A. Half-life of Thallium-201 is 73 hours
B. Differential washout is minimal for Thallium-201 &Tc 99m teboroxime
C. Half- life of Tc 99m sestamibi is 6 hours
D. Uptake for Thallium is active while that for Technetium tracers is passive

72. Which is not a perfusion tracer for cardiac imaging?

A. Nitrogen - 13 B. Rubidium - 82
C. Fluorine - 18 D. Oxygen - 15

73. Hibernating myocardium on PET testing is demonstrated by?

A. Preserved perfusion and preserved glucose metabolism
B. Reduced perfusion and reduced glucose metabolism
C. Reduced perfusion and preserved glucose metabolism
D. Preserved perfusion and reduced glucose metabolism

ANSWERS

Electrocardiography

Answer: 1. D. All of the above

Answer: 2. D. Accessory right sided pathway WPW

Answer: 3. B. P wave amplitude duration ratio > 1.6

Answer: 4. C. Schamroth

Answer: 5. C. Cornell voltage criteria

Answer: 6. B. Sokolow-Lyon index

Answer: 7. A. rS pattern in leads I and aVL

Answer: 8. C. qR in aVL

Answer: 9. A. North west axis deviation

Answer: 10. C. P wave becomes small & narrow

Answer: 11. C. It is common after heart transplant

Answer: 12. A. It is common in patients with cardiac tamponade

Answer: 13. C. rS pattern in inferior leads and qR pattern in lateral leads

Answer: 14. A. A band width limitation to 50 Hz is recommended by the American Heart Association for electrocardiography in children

AHA recommends a minimum bandwidth of 250 Hz to record pediatric ECGs.

ECG Diagnostic Criteria

Normal sinus P wave

P wave duration <120 ms

Amplitude ≤2.5 mm

P wave axis between 45° and 75° in frontal plane

Criteria for left atrial enlargement

P wave duration >120 ms in lead II

Notched P wave in lead II with inter-notch distance >40 ms (P mitrale)

P-terminale in V1 (Terminal negative deflection) > 1 mm

P wave axis between +45° and -30° in frontal plane (left axis deviation)

Criteria for right atrial enlargement

P wave amplitude >2.5 mm in lead II (P-pulmonale)

Positive deflection of P-wave in V1 > 1.5 mm

Area under initial positive part of P wave in V1 >0.06 mm

P wave axis >75° in frontal plane (right axis deviation)

Detection of RAE in the presence of Atrial fibrillation:

qR complex in lead V1 in the absence of evidence of CAD

Diminution of height of QRS complex in V1 with marked increase in its height in lead V2

Criteria for LVH

Sokolow criteria: S in V1 plus R in V5 or V6 >35 mm; R in aVL >11 mm

Cornell criteria: S in V3 plus S in V1 ≥28 mm for men and ≥20 mm for women

Romhilt–Estes criteria (LVH if 5 points): R wave in any limb lead ≥20 mm, or S in V1 or V2 ≥30 mm, or R in V5 or V6 ≥30 mm (3 points); left atrial abnormality (3 points); ST–T changes without digoxin (3 points) or with digoxin (1 point); QRS axis <-30° (2 points); QRS duration >90 ms (1 point); intrinsicoid deflection in V5 or V6 >50 ms (1 point)

Criteria for RVH

R in V1 ≥7 mm

QR in V1

R/S in V1 >1 with R at least 5 mm

R/S in V5 or V6 <1

S1Q3T3 pattern (pulmonary embolism)

S1S2S3 pattern

Criteria for biventricular hypertrophy

Tall R in both left and right chest leads

LVH with right axis deviation

LVH with deep S in V5 or V6

LVH with shift of precordial transition (R/S = 1) to the left of V4

Criteria for LAFB

QRS axis <-45° (LAD) with rS in inferior leads (II, III, aVF) and qR in high lateral leads (I, aVL) plus QRS duration <120 ms

Criteria for left posterior fascicular block

QRS axis >120° (RAD) with rS in high lateral leads (I, aVL) and qR in inferior leads (II, III, Avf) plus QRS duration <120 ms

Criteria for LBBB

Broad notched R wave in lateral leads, absent q in left-sided leads (septal activation will be right to left), QRSd ≥120 ms

Criteria for RBBB

Broad notched R wave in V1 and V2 with right rabbit ear, deep slurred S in left-sided leads (reciprocal of R2), QRSd ≥120 ms

Causes of tall R wave in V1

RVH (generally with right axis deviation and secondary ST–T changes or right atrial enlargement)

True posterior infarct (generally with upright T, inferior or lateral Q)

Hypertrophic obstructive cardiomyopathy (due to septal depolarization)

Duchenne muscular dystrophy

RBBB

WPW syndrome with posterior or lateral pathways

Heart shifted to right

Causes of Q waves

Normal in V1/V2 and III (in lead III will disappear with deep breath which makes heart vertical)

Myocardial infarction

Myocardial infiltration (sarcoid, amyloid)

Myocarditis

WPW syndrome

LBBB results in Q in V1/V2

Hypertrophic obstructive cardiomyopathy (septal hypertrophy causing Q in lateral leads)

Causes of ST elevation

Normal variant (early repolarization, generally V1–V4)

Myocardial injury (convex up)

LV aneurysm (persistent beyond 6 months)

Pericarditis (concave up, diffuse, ST and PR elevation in aVR, PR depression)

Brugada syndrome

Hyperkalemia ("dialyzable current of injury")

Type IC antiarrhythmic agents

LVH and LBBB (in right chest leads as reciprocal of ST depression on left chest leads)

Hyperkalemia

Peaked T wave (early sign)

PR prolongation

Increased QRS duration

Absent P wave

Sine wave morphology in late stage (Sinoventricular rhythm: P wave disappears and QRS becomes wide in morphology)

Hypercalcemia

Shortened QT interval

ST segment depression

Hypocalcemia

QT lengthening (especially ST segment lengthening)

U waves

Digoxin effect

Downsloping ST segment (reverse tick shape)

T wave inversion

Digoxin toxicity

AV block

Atrial tachycardia with block

Ventricular arrhythmias

Answer: 15. A. 'P' duration/PR segment in L-II is >1.6

Macruz index

Macruz Index is a ratio of the P wave duration and PR segment (not PR interval) (P/PR).

Normal reference range between 1 and 1.6

Macruz index >1.6 indicates P mitrale

while <1 indicates P pulmonale

Answer: 16. D. QT interval shortens

Osborn waves

The Osborn wave (Elevated J wave: occurs at RS-T junction also known as J point) is a positive deflection at the J point (negative in aVR and V1)

Causes:

Characteristically seen in hypothermia, but they are not pathognomonic.

Normal variant

Hypercalcaemia

Medications

Subarachnoid haemorrhage

Le syndrome d'Haïssaguerre (idiopathic VF)

Mechanism: Distortion in early repolarization stage

Answer: 17. D. Early repolarization with ascending ST segment is predictor of sudden cardiac death

Early repolarization pattern (ERP):

Widespread concave ST elevation, most prominent in the mid- to left precordial leads (V2-5).

Notching or slurring at the J-point.

Prominent, slightly asymmetrical T-waves that are concordant with the QRS complexes (pointing in the same direction).

The degree of ST elevation is modest in comparison to the T-wave amplitude (less than 25% of the T wave height in V6)

No reciprocal ST depression to suggest STEMI (except in aVR).

ST changes are relatively stable over time (no progression on serial ECG tracings).

Usually ERP is benign, however in some patients be associated with ventricular fibrillation.

Prevalence: 2 to 24% in various population based studies

Benign Early Repolarisation vs Pericarditis

- Both conditions are associated with concave ST elevation.
- ST segment / T wave ratio:
  - A ratio of > 0.25 suggests pericarditis
  - A ratio of < 0.25 suggests ERP

High risk features in ERP

- Male gender
- Family history of sudden death

- H/o idiopathic VF
- Horizontal or descending ST segment

NB: Upsloping ST segment is essentially benign

Answer: 18. D. Upright T wave in V1

ECG in neonates:

At birth, the right ventricle is larger and thicker than the left ventricle. This produces an normal ECG picture reminiscent of right ventricular hypertrophy in the adult: marked rightward axis, dominant R wave in V1 and T-wave inversions in V1-3

Conduction intervals (PR interval, QRS duration) are shorter than adults due to the smaller cardiac size. Heart rates are much faster in neonates and infants, decreasing as the child grows older.

Normal ECG findings in neonates:

- Heart rate >100 beats/min
- Rightward QRS axis > +90°
- T wave inversions in V1-3 ("juvenile T-wave pattern")
- Dominant R wave in V1
- RSR' pattern in V1
- Short PR interval (< 120ms) and QRS duration (< 80ms)
- Slightly peaked P waves (< 3mm in height is normal if ≤ 6 months)
- Slightly long QTc (≤ 490ms in infants ≤ 6 months)
- Q waves in the inferior and left precordial leads.

RV hypertrophy in neonates and children:

Neonates and infants should have inverted T waves in the right precordial leads. These findings persist throughout childhood with inversion to V4 being accepted as normal. Until 8 years of age an **upright T wave in V1** is considered a sign of right ventricular hypertrophy.

Answer: 19. C. R amplitude decreases

ECG changes during exercise:

- PR, QRS, QT and RR intervals decrease
- P-wave amplitude and morphology don't undergo major changes
- Septal Q-wave amplitude increases
- R-wave height increases from rest to submaximal exercise and then reduces to a minimum at maximal exercise
- J-point depression occurs
- Tall, peaked T waves occur (high interindividual variability)
- ST segment becomes upsloping
- Superimposition of P waves and T waves on successive beats may be observed

Answer: 20. B. Hypercalcemia shortens QT interval

Digoxin does not affect QT interval; U waves are feature of hypokalemia; Sino-ventricular rhythm is a feature of hyperkalemia.

Treadmill Testing (TMT)

Answer: 21. D. Treadmill test

Answer: 22. C. Right axis shift

Answer: 23. D. P wave amplitude decreases

Answer: 24. D. Duke TM score is as effective in elderly more than 75 years of age as in young individuals

Answer: 25. C. 16.9 METs

Answer: 26. D. Double product

Answer: 27. C. Exercise duration

Answer: 28. A. -8

Answer: 29. C. High grade AV block

High grade AV block is relative contraindication for TMT.

Answer: 30. B. 3.5 ml O2/kg/min of body weight

Answer: 31. A. It is suggestive of ischemia

Answer: 32. D. Not suggestive of ischemia

Indications of electrocardiographic stress testing or Treadmill testing (TMT)

1. Diagnosis of obstructive or flow-limiting CAD

   Most useful in patients with an intermediate pretest probability

   Patients must also have a baseline ECG in which ST segments and subsequent changes are interpretable

   Patients with left bundle branch block, paced rhythms, >l mm of resting ST depression (e.g. digoxin therapy or left ventricular hypertrophy with strain pattern), and Wolû-Parkinson-White syndrome are therefore not recommended

   In patients with underlying left bundle branch block on ECG, pharmacologic stress is preferred over exercise stress due to the risk of diagnosing false positive septal ischemia.
2. Stress testing can also be used to assess prognosis in patients with known or suspected CAD
3. In patients with valvular heart disease, stress testing is used for evaluation of exercise capacity and may be very useful in determining the appropriate timing of surgery
4. Assessment of suspected exercise induced arrhythmias, and evaluation of therapy in patients with suspected exercise-induced arrhythmias.

Baseline ECG abnormalities unsuitable for TMT:

- Complete LBBB
- Preexcitation syndrome
- Left ventricular hypertrophy (LVH)
- Digoxin therapy
- Greater than 1 mm of resting ST-segment depression
- Electronically paced ventricular rhythm

Most commonly **Bruce protocol** is used for exercise.

Modified Bruce protocol is used soon after MI or in elderly patients, in which two stages prior to stage 1 are added.

Other protocols include Cornell, Naughton, and Balke protocols

Bruce protocol for TMT

Stage	Speed (mph)	METs
Rest	0	1
1	1.7	4.6
2	2.5	7.0
3	3.4	10.1
4	4.2	12.9
5	5.0	15.1
6	5.5	16.9
7	6.8	19.2

Placement of electrodes for ECG measurement differs in exercise testing compared to standard 12-lead ECG. **Mason-Likar modification** is used in which arm electrodes are placed on chest to reduce interference because of physical activity. It results in **rightward axis shift** and false positive or negative inferior Q waves.

ECG exercise stress testing, are less sensitive and specific in women.

The test is completed when the patient attains 85% of the age predicted maximum heart rate or cannot proceed because of symptoms.

The age-predicted maximum heart rate:

- HRmax= 220 – Age in years
- HRmax (when on beta blockers) = 164 – (0.7 × age)

Non-diagnostic study is said when HR could not be reached to predefined goal.

Contraindications and indications to terminate TMT:

Absolute contraindications for TMT	Absolute indications for termination
Recent MI <2 days	SBP drop of ≥10 mm Hg in the presence of other signs of ischemia
Unstable angina not medically controlled	Moderate to severe angina
Uncontrolled arrhythmia causing hemodynamic compromise	Increasing ataxia, dizziness, and near-syncope Technical difficulties with ECG or blood pressure monitoring
Uncontrolled heart failure	Subject request
Severe symptomatic aortic stenosis	Sustained VT
Acute pulmonary embolism	ST elevation ≥l mm in leads without pathologic Q waves
Acute myocarditis or pericarditis	
Suspected or known aortic dissection	
Acute systemic infection	

Diagnostic interpretation:

ST segment depression:

Most common manifestation of myocardial ischemia on TMT.

P-R segment is isoelectric baseline for practical purposes (True isoelectric line is T-P segment).

At least 3 consecutive beats should be assessed.

The classic positive finding is ≥l mm of horizontal or down-sloping ST-segment depression 80 ms (ST80) after the J point.

Upsloping ST depression is not considered positive response.

More widespread the ECG changes, usually the more severe the disease.

ST segment elevation:

In leads with Q waves- **Not** marker of new ischemia; suggestive of old AWMI and marker of poor prognosis.

In leads without Q waves- Suggestive of transmural ischemia

ST elevation in aVR is may be marker of LM or proximal LAD disease.

ST-segment depression does not localize ischemia; however, ST-segment elevation in leads without Q waves does localize the distribution of ischemia and is an absolute indication for termination of the test.

U wave inversion:

Uncommon, observed in recovery phase and associated with LAD or LMCA disease.

Intraventricular block:

Rate related intraventricular blocks are common and may not be marker of ischemia.

Exercise induced RBBB- Benign finding

Exercise induced LBBB- Increased risk of mortality and future cardiac events.

Arrhythmia:

Exercise induced ventricular ectopics and VT after MI associated with increased mortality. Atrial arrhythmias not associated with worse prognosis.

Blood pressure response:

SBP normally rises, while DBP decreases during exercise.

A lack of rise in SBP or fall in DBP with exercise is suggestive of significant underlying ischemia.

High risk markers of severe CAD: Drop in systolic blood pressure of more than 10 mmHg from rest, exercise-limiting angina, poor exercise capacity <5 METs, down-sloping ST depression in recovery, and ST depression at low work load, HR recovery less than 12 beats/min after 1 minute of recovery, DTS of ≤-11 and presence of ventricular arrhythmias.

Exercise capacity is the most important prognostic variable.

Duke treadmill score (DTS)

DTS = Exercise minutes – (5 × ST deviation) – (4 × Angina index)

where the angina index is 0 = no angina, 1 = angina, but not test limiting, and 2 = test-limiting angina

Low risk (Score ≥+ 5): Mortality risk <1 % per year

Intermediate risk (Score -10 to +4): Mortality risk 1 to 3% per year

High risk (Score ≤-11): Mortality risk >3% per year

Metabolic Gas-Exchange Analyses

Metabolic stress testing is indicated for the evaluation of exercise capacity and response to therapy in patients with heart failure being considered for heart transplantation.

The peak Vo2 (oxygen uptake) defines the patient's aerobic capacity and is proportional to the cardiac output.

A peak Vo2 of <14 mL/kg/min identifies high-risk patients who are reasonable candidates for cardiac transplant despite ambulatory status.

Vo2 is easily expressed in multiples of resting oxygen requirements (metabolic equivalents [METs])

1MET= Resting energy expenditure = 3.5 ml O_2/kg/min of body weight

VO2max is the peak oxygen uptake achieved during performance of the highest level of dynamic exercise

Cardiac output during exercise can increase as much as **four to six times resting levels.**

Maximum cardiac output is the result of a **twofold to threefold increase in heart rate** from resting levels and **twice increase in stroke volume.**

Oxygen extraction at the periphery can increase as much as **threefold,** and the maximum arteriovenous O_2 difference has a physiologic limit of 15 to 17 mL O_2/100 mL blood.

Myocardial Oxygen Demand:

Depends upon HR, BP, LV contractility and LV wall stress. LV wall stress is related to LV pressure, wall thickness and cavity size.

Rate pressure product= HR × BP

Answer: 33. B. Decreased heart rate variability

Increased HR variability is seen with exercise which is a good prognostic marker. Whereas, decreased HR variability is associated with increased risk for cardiac events.

Answer: 34. B. High

Pretest probability of CAD by age, sex and symptoms

Age	Typical/ definite angina	Atypical/ probable angina	Non-anginal chest pain	Asymptomatic
30-39	Intermediate	Very low	Very low	Very low
40-49	Intermediate	Low	Very low	Very low
50-59	Intermediate	Intermediate	Low	Very low
60-69	High	Intermediate	Intermediate	Low
>70	High	Intermediate	Intermediate	Low

Answer: 35. A. 65 years old diabetic female with recent onset exertional dyspnea and normal LV function

Atypical chest pain has low likelihood for true positive TMT; LVH and pre-excitation make TMT unsuitable for the person.

Echocardiography

Answer: 36. C. Ability to record higher velocities.

Answer: 37. D. (LVEDD-LVESD)/LVEDD

Answer: 38. C. (IVCT-IVRT)/LVET

Answer: 39. D. E/Ea > 8

Answer: 40. B. Aortic

Answer: 41. D. Parasternal long axis view

Answer: 42. B. Deceleration time of E wave >220 msec

Answer: 43. A. M-mode echo

Answer: 44. A. 5 mm of Hg

Answer: 45. D. Decreases in LV systolic dysfunction

Lower Tei index is associated with better ventricular function.

Answer: 46. D. RV Systolic Pressure = 4(TR Systolic Velocity)2 - RA Pressure

Answer: 47. B. 0.88 cm2

Mitral valve area = 220/ PHT

Various modes of Echocardiography:

Continuous wave Doppler echocardiography

It measures all velocities in the path of the ultrasound beam hence it is not site specific.

It is not limited by aliasing at high velocities.

The disadvantage is that specific site of highest velocity can't be localized.

Continuous wave Doppler echocardiography is typically used to measure high-velocity jets and gradients.

Pulsed wave Doppler echocardiography

It is "site specific," allowing the measurement of blood velocities at a particular region of interest.

The disadvantage is aliasing of the signal when velocities reach one-half of the pulse repetition frequency, also called as the Nyquist limit.

This property limits the maximal velocity that can be measured with pulsed wave Doppler echocardiography

Colour flow imaging

A type of computer-enhanced pulsed wave

Doppler echocardiography that displays the velocity and directional information of blood flow

Red colour depicts blood flow toward the transducer and blue, away from the transducer.

Colour flow imaging, like pulsed wave Doppler imaging, has a Nyquist limit and displays aliasing.

Tissue Doppler imaging

Mainly used for diastolic function assessment

Velocity of the mitral annulus motion represents the velocity of changes in the LV long-axis dimensions.

The E/e' ratio provides an excellent assessment of LV diastolic filling pressures in sinus rhythm and in atrial fibrillation

E/e' is considered elevated if it is more than 15 and low or normal if it is less than 8.

Global Systolic Function Assessment

Stroke volume (SV) = LVEDV – LVESV

Cardiac output= Stroke volume × Heart rate

Cardiac index = Cardiac output / Body surface area

EF = (LVEDV – LVESV) / LVEDV × 100

EF= ($LVEDD^2$ – $LVESD^2$) / $LVEDD^2$ × 100

Fractional shortening (FS)= (LVEDD – LVESD) / LVEDD × 100

Where,

LVEDV= Left ventricular end diastolic volume

LVESV= Left ventricular end systolic volume

LVEDD= Left ventricular end diastolic diameter

LVESD= Left ventricular end systolic diameter

TAPSE:

Tricuspid annular plane systolic excursion

Determined by M-mode echo and tells about RV longitudinal function

It is vertical distance between maximum and minimum excursion at the lateral tricuspid annulus.

Normal value- More than 16 mm.

Tei index (Myocardial performance index)

Index that incorporates both systolic and diastolic time intervals in expressing global systolic and diastolic ventricular function.

Can be used for both right and left ventricle.

Tei index, is defined as the sum of isovolumic relaxation time and isovolumic contraction time divided by ejection time.

MPI= (IVCT + IVRT) / ET

OR

MPI= (MCT – ET) / ET

Where,

IVCT = Isovolumetric contraction time

IVRT = Isovolumetric relaxation time

MCT = Myocardial contraction time

ET = Ejection time

Normal value for LV is less than 0.40. More than this is suggestive of LV dysfunction.

Normal value for RV is less than 0.30. More than this suggestive of RV dysfunction.

Diastolic Function Assessment

Impaired relaxation (grade 1 diastolic dysfunction), pseudonormal filling (grade 2 diastolic dysfunction), and restrictive filling (grade 3 [reversible] and grade 4 [irreversible]

Parameter	Normal	Grade 1	Grade 2	Grade 3	Grade 4
E/A ratio	More than 1	Less than 1	More than 1	More than 2	More than 2
Deceleration Time (DT)	160 to 200 ms	More than 200	160-200	Less than 160	Less than 160

IVRT	70 +/- 12 ms	More than 110	Less than 60	Less than 60	Less than 60
Septal e'	More than equal to 10 cm/sec	Less than 8 cm/sec	Less than 8	Less than 8	Less than 8
Lateral e'	More than 12 cm/sec	Less than 10	Less than 10	Less than 10	Less than 10
E/e'	Less than 8	Equal or more than 8-15	More than 15	More than 15	More than 15
Valsalva manoeuvre (strain phase)			E/A Revert to grade 1	E/A Revert to grade 2	Does not Revert

Pressure Gradient (△P), mm Hg

$\triangle P = P_2 - P_1 = 4(V)^2$

With this equation, various pressures can be estimated across any gradient.

1. RV or PA Systolic Pressure = 4(TR Systolic Velocity)^2 + RA Pressure
2. PA Diastolic Pressure = 4(PR End-Diastolic Velocity)^2 + RA Pressure
3. LA Pressure = Systolic BP – 4(MR Systolic Velocity)^2
4. RV Systolic Pressure = Systolic BP – 4(VSD Velocity)^2
5. Pulmonary artery systolic pressure = Aortic systolic pressure – Peak gradient across PDA
6. Pulmonary artery diastolic pressure = Aortic diastolic pressure – Least gradient across PDA

Mitral Valve Area (MVA) by Pressure Half time Measurement

MVA = 220/ PHT

Right atrial pressure

IVC size	% Collapse with inspiration	RA pressure
< 2.1 cm	> 50%	5 mmHg
< 2.1 cm	< 50%	10 mmHg
> 2.1 cm	> 50%	10 mmHg
> 2.1 cm	< 50%	>15 mmHg

Answer: 48. A. 180

Aortic systolic pressure = 160; Aortic diastolic pressure = 90 mmHg

Peak LV systolic pressure = Aortic systolic pressure + 4 × (Peak aortic valve velocity)^2

Peak LV systolic pressure = 116 + 4 × (4)^2

Peak LV systolic pressure = 180 mmHg

Cardiac commuted tomography (CT)

Answer: 49. D. Blood : 35-65

Answer: 50. A. Sensitivity-90%

Answer: 51. D. Breast.

Breast and skin get the highest radiation dose, and then lung, heart, and esophagus in descending order.

Answer: 52. D. All of the above

Answer: 53. D. All of the above.

Answer: 54. C. 5 mSv. mSv is for adult radiation workers.

Answer: 55. B. -50 HU. Water is 0 HU, air is -1000 HU.

Answer: 56. B. 130.

Answer: 57. D. All of the above.

Advantages of CT:

Rapid acquisition

Compatible with metal devices

Disadvantages:

Ionizing radiation

Iodinated contrast complications

Diagnostic accuracy reduced by HR > 70 b/m, irregular rhythm, severe coronary calcification, inability to hold breath for 5-10 seconds

Less accuracy in assessment of coronary stent with diameter <3 mm.

HR control:

Beta blockers, CCBs, Ivabradine.

Indications:

Detection of CAD in high risk asymptomatic patients, symptomatic low risk patients.

- High negative predictive value (98%)
- Detection of obstructive CAD with sensitivity of 98% and specificity of 88%.
- Functional assessment of CAD by FFR_{CT}

Assessment of congenital heart disease

Assessment of coronary anomalies

Adverse plaque characteristics on CT:

1. Positive arterial remodelling
2. Spotty calcifications
3. Low attenuation plaque <30 Hounsfield units- correlate with lipid laden necrotic core

CT densities:

CT densities are expressed as Hounsfield units (HU), which range in value from -1,024 to +3,071 HU.

Air: -1000

Fat: -50

Water: 0

CSF: +8

Blood: +40 to 70

Bone/calcification: +1000

Coronary Artery Calcium Scoring

Agatston score is used for quantification of coronary artery calcium.

Only areas of calcification ≥1 mm2 and >130 HU are included in this algorithm

CAC score of 0 indicates the absence of calcified plaque and that scores of 1 to 10, 11 to 100, 101 to 400, and greater than 400 indicate minimal, mildly elevated, moderately elevated, and severely elevated CAC level, respectively.

Effective radiation dose

Radiation dose is proportional to tube current and square of tube voltage. It is inversely proportional to pitch.

Study	Radiation dose (mSv)
Natural background	3-4 (in one year)
CXR	0.04
CT head	2
CT abdomen/pelvis	15
Coronary artery calcium scoring	1-3
Coronary CT angiography	15
Tc 99m sestamibi	12
FDG PET for viability	14
Diagnostic catheterization	4-7
Coronary angioplasty	15

Methods to reduce radiation dose:

Decrease current (mA), increase tube potential (Kv), increase pitch

Increase slice width

Apply filter

Prospective ECG gating

Tube current modulation

Iterative reconstruction

Measures of ionizing radiation:

Measure	Definition	Unit	SI unit
Exposure	No of ions produced by X-ray or gamma radiation per kg of air	Roentgen ®	C/kg
Dose	Amount of energy deposited per kg of tissue	Rad	Gray (Gy) 1 Gy= 100 Rad
Relative effective dose	Amount of energy deposited per kg of tissue normalized for biological effectiveness	Roentgen equivalent man (rem)	Sievert (Sv) 1 Sv= 100 rem

Cardiac MRI

Answer: 58. A. Need for iodinated contrast agents

Answer: 59. C. Assess coronary anatomy precisely

Answer: 60. D. Subendocardial enhancement

Answer: 61. D. All

Answer: 62. A. Idiopathic Dilated Cardiomyopathy

Answer: 63. C. Cardiac MRI

Answer: 64. D. All of the above. Coronary stents, heart valves, artificial joints, and vertebral plates are not contraindications.

Answer: 65. D. All of the above.

Answer: 66. A. Shortens T1 and increases signal on T1-weighted images.

The seven unpaired electrons on gadolinium couple with excited water spins and hasten relaxation, thereby reducing T1.

Advantages of Cardiac MRI:

No ionizing radiation

Imaging less affected by body habitus

Disadvantages of MRI:

Availability and high cost

Claustrophobia

Long acquisition time

Contraindicated in patients with foreign metallic objects in eye or brain, Starr-Edwards mechanical valve, pacemakers and ICDs

Nephrogenic systemic fibrosis with gadolinium

Indications of MRI:

Coronary artery disease:

Stress perfusion to detect CAD and assessment of myocardial viability by late gadolinium enhancement (LGE).

Subendocardial or transmural enhancement is suggestive of ischemic cause

More than 50% transmural enhancement has a low likelihood of functional recovery after revascularization.

Cardiomyopathy:

Cardiac MRI provides accurate measurements of biventricular function, volume and tissue characterization for diagnosis.

Myocarditis:

LGE is typically subepicardial (focal or widespread)

Increased T2 intensity is suggestive of myocardial edema

Sarcoidosis: LGE in basal septal wall, subepicardial and medmyocardial areas.

Amyloidosis:

Global subendocardial left and right ventricular LGE because of distribution of amyloid protein.

HCM:

Increased wall thickness and accurate quantification of LV mass

Hemochromatosis:

T2* sequences used for quantification of iron and cardiac involvement in hemochromatosis.

T2* <20 ms is suggestive of hemochromatosis.

Non-compaction cardiomyopathy:

A diastolic ratio of non-compacted to compacted myocardium > 2.3 is suggestive.

Congenital heart diseases:

Assessment of cardiac anatomy, great vessels, collaterals, coronary anomalies, shunt calculation, post operative LV and RV volumes and ejection fractions

Cardiac tumors:

Visualization and characterization of cardiac masses with good contrast resolution

Pericardial diseases:

Assessment of pericardial masses and constrictive pericarditis

Cardiac MRI scan sequences:

Dark Blood Imaging

Flowing blood appears dark while slow moving structures such as myocardium is bright.

T2 weighted images are sensitive to water content and will be represented as high signal in areas of acute injury such as myocarditis and infarction.

Bright blood Imaging

Allows acquisition of cine images for assessment of cardiac function. Steady state free precession technique is commonly used for this purpose

Phase-contrast

Allows measurement of **velocity and quantification of blood flow**

Perfusion

Contrast agents such as gadolinium (Gd), which shortens T1 relaxation time, can be imaged as it transits through cardiac structures

MR angiography

Allows 3-dimensional examination of complex cardiac and vascular structures

Late gadolinium enhancement

Delayed hyperenhancement of Gd (~10 min after administration) is seen in areas of myocardial necrosis and fibrosis

Cardiac nuclear imaging:

Answer: 67. C. Aminophylline

Answer: 68. D. 73 hours

Answer: 69. B. Thallium – 201

Answer: 70. A. Fluorine-18

Answer: 71. B. Differential washout is minimal for Thallium-201 & Tc 99m teboroxime

Answer: 72. C. Fluorine -18

Answer: 73. C. Reduced perfusion and preserved glucose metabolism

Myocardial perfusion imaging:

MPI is performed in the context of stress testing to determine the presence and extent of myocardial ischemia.

Either treadmill exercise or a pharmacologic stressor can be used.

Pharmacologic stress agent: Adenosine, Ragadenoson, Dipyridamole, Dobutamine.

In presence of LBBB, pharmacologic stressor is preferred as in place of exercise.

Vasodilator stress agents:

Adenosine:

Non-selective agonist of A_1, A_{2A}, A_{2b}, A_3 and A_4 receptors.

Half-life = < 10 seconds.

Regadenoson:

Recently approved selective A_{2A} agonist.

Half-life of 30 minutes.

Similar side effects as adenosine but lower incidence due to increased selectivity.

Dipyridamole:

Produced coronary hyperemia by impairing cellular reuptake of adenosine.

Contraindications of vasodilator stress agents: Severe asthma, COPD, High degree AV block, sick sinus syndrome, SBP<90, HR<40, MI less than 2 days.

Inotropic stress agent:

Dobutamine: Beta 1 receptor agonist, used when exercise or vasodilator stressing is not feasible or contraindicated.

Radionuclides (Tracers) for nuclear imaging:

Radionuclides commonly used for SPECT myocardial perfusion imaging include technetium-99m (99mTc) and thallium-201 (201TI)

Positron emission tomography (PET) utilizes Rubidium (82Rb), oxygen (15O), nitrogen (13N), carbon (11C), and fluorine (18F)

Common tracers used:

SPECT	Production	Half life	
Technetium-99m (^{99m}Tc)-Sestamibi	On site generator	6 hours	Most commonly used for medical procedures
Thallium-201(^{201}Tl)	Cyclotron	73 hours	
PET			
Rubidium (^{82}Rb)	Cyclotron	76 seconds	Better spatial and temporal resolution compared with SPECT.

Radionuclide tracers used for MPI

SPECT tracers

Thallium-201:

Injection of tracer at peak exercise or with pharmacologic agent followed by immediate imaging and subsequent redistribution images 3-4 hours later.

Uptake of thallium is active whereas uptake of technetium tracer is passive.

Infarcted myocardium- Appears as fixed dense thallium defect on both initial and delayed images

Hibernating myocardium- Initial defect similar to infarcted myocardium, but shows uptake in delayed images (i.e. rest redistribution).

Technetium-99m: 2 agents are available

Sestamibi- Accumulates in mitochondria of cell with ATP requiring process, thus is an indicator of viability. There is minimal redistribution.

Tetrofosmin- Similar utility to sestamibi.

Protocol- Requires two injections of technetium 99m labelled tracer in order to obtain images at rest and stress.

Technetium-99m labelled tracers are less prone to soft tissue attenuation artefact as compared to thallium and LVEF can also be calculated with ECG gated imaging.

PET tracers

Perfusion tracers: Rubidium-82, 13-N ammonia, Oxygen-15, Fluorine-18.

Myocardial metabolism:

Glucose metabolism: F-18 (FDG) (glucose analogue, used to assess myocardial viability)

Fatty acid metabolism: C-11 palmitate

Oxidative metabolism: C-11 acetate

Important points:

Hibernating myocardium on PET: Reduced perfusion and preserved glucose metabolism.

Scarred myocardium: Reduced perfusion as well as reduced glucose metabolism.

Transient ischemic dilatation (TID):

Ratio of heart cavity size in stress to rest >1.20, is associated with abnormal perfusion.

Increased lung uptake is also associated with poor prognosis and is suggestive of significant ischemia.

3 Cardiac Pharmacology

Beta Blockers

1. Which beta-blocker from following is excreted through kidney?

A. Propranolol B. Atenolol
C. Carvedilol D. Metoprolol

2. In a patient with acute anterior MI, post primary PCI, and an EF of 30%, which of the following may reduce the risk of death in the ensuing 3 months?

A. Digoxin B. Amiodarone
C. Carvedilol D. Flecainide

3. Contraindications to Beta-blockers:

A. Severe depression
B. Raynaud phenomenon
C. Peripheral vascular disease
D. All of the above

4. Mortality benefit of beta blocker in congestive heart failure is seen with all of the following except:

A. Bucindolol B. Carvedilol
C. Bisoprolol D. Metoprolol

5. A 50 year old male was recently started on antihypertensive therapy with multiple drugs. He reported 3 months later with skin lesions diagnosed as psoriasis. Which drug is most likely responsible?

A. Atenolol B. Amlodipine
C. Olmesartan D. Spironolactone

6. All of the following are B blocker contraindicated in renal failure except?

A. Atenolol B. Carvedilol
C. Sotalol D. Nodalol

7. Beta blocker with least mortality benefit in patients with heart failure is?

A. Metoprolol succinate
B. Bisoprolol
C. Nevibolol
D. Carvedilol

ACE Inhibitors, ARBs and Aldosterone Antagonists

8. Which of the following drug is renin inhibitor?

A. Ivabradine B. Eplerenone
C. Aliskiren D. Satavaptan

9. Which of the following is true about ACE inhibitors in acute STEMI?

A. Prevents infarct expansion
B. Treatment should be initiated with long acting ACE inhibitors for sustained action
C. Started 3-5 days after acute MI
D. Combination of ARB and ACE inhibitors results in better outcomes

10. Which one of the following drug has long half life?

A. Losartan B. Irbesartan
C. Telmisartan D. Valsartan

11. A 56-year old male patient has Type-2 DM with micro-albuminuria, hypertension, and serum creatinine of 1.5 mg%. He was started on olmesartan at the recommended doses. After 2 months, the creatinine has increased to 1.9 mg%, the blood pressure is well controlled. The appropriate step in this patient will be:

A. Continue same treatment and monitor renal function
B. Switch olmesartan to amlodipine
C. Initiate dialysis
D. Decrease the dose of olmesartan to half and reassess renal function

12. A 36 Y/M presents with chest pain, associated with bilateral nipple tenderness and sensitivity. Which of the following medications in this patient's profile can mostly likely cause these symptoms?

A. Triamterene/hydrochlorothiazide
B. Spironolactone
C. Labetalol
D. Ranolazine

13. All of the following are true regarding ACE inhibitor induced angioedema except:

A. Overall incidence has been estimated between 0.1% and 0.7%
B. ARBs are prohibited in such patients with heart failure
C. Most commonly affects non-dependent areas
D. Not related to dose

14. PARADIGM-HF studied the effect of which drug?

A. Tolvaptan
B. Valsartan/sacubitril combination
C. Telmisartan/sacubitril combination
D. Levosimendan

15. Half life of digoxin is:

A. 1 hour B. 5 days
C. 36 hours D. 1 week

Drugs for AHF

16. All are true for furosemide except:

A. Urinary chloride excretion is increased
B. May be given as a continuous infusion in refractory heart failure
C. In non-congested patients it causes activation of RAS
D. In case of sulphonamide allergy, bumetanide should be given in place of furosemide

17. The diuretic which may be used in a patient with a confirmed Stevens–Johnson reaction to trimethoprim-sulfamethoxazole?

A. Furosemide
B. Hydrochlorothiazide
C. Metolazone
D. Ethacrynic acid

18. Which of the following is not true about nesiritide?

A. It is recombinant BNP
B. Studied in ASCEND-HF trial
C. Causes cAMP mediated vasodilation
D. Venous as well as arterial dilator

19. Which drug was studied in SURVIVE trial?

A. Milrinone B. Levosimendan
C. Nesiritide D. Ivabradine

20. Which of the following is cardiac myosin activator?

A. Omecamtiv mecarbil
B. Istaroxime
C. Serelaxin
D. Rolofylline

21. Which of the following is PDE-IIIa inhibitor?

A. Levosimendan
B. Conivaptan
C. Milrinone
D. Aliskiren

22. Which one of following is not true for Milrinone?
A. It is a phosphodiesterase inhibitor
B. It is beta receptor stimulant
C. It has inotropic effect
D. It has vasodilator effect

23. All of the following are true about levosimendan which is used in ADHF except?
A. Decreased 30 days mortality VS dobutamine
B. Hypotension with I/V loading dose
C. AF is a known side effect
D. BNP markedly decreased

24. Identify the wrong statement in the management of acute heart failure?
A. Nitroprusside can cause cyanide toxicity
B. Infusion of dobutamine for > 72 hours can develop tachyphylaxis
C. Milrinone is a more effective vasodilator than dobutamine
D. Levosimendan acts on B1 and B2 receptors

25. All of the following are true about levosimendan except:
A. ATP dependent K^+ channel opener
B. Reduced BNP
C. Inotropic and vasoconstrictor
D. May lead to atrial fibrillation

Anticoagulants

26. The genetic test which you could order as a send-out before initiating warfarin in a patient?
A. VKORC1 genotype
B. HLA-B*5701 allele
C. HLA-B*1502 allele
D. CYP2C19 genotype

27. All of the following are direct thrombin inhibitors except:
A. Bivalirudin B. Dabigatran
C. Argatroban D. Apixaban

28. Chronic use of heparin may cause all except:
A. Osteoporosis
B. Hyperkalemia
C. Bilateral adrenal hyperplasia
D. Cutaneous necrosis

29. The most appropriate step for a patient of acute coronary syndrome who developed heparin induced thrombocytopenia (HIT) on unfractionated heparin (UFH) should be?
A. Switch UFH to low molecular weight heparin (LMWH)
B. Reduced the dose of UFH to half
C. Switch to bivalirudin
D. Switch to warfarin

30. All are true regarding heparin induced thrombocytopenia (HIT) except:
A. Fondaparinux is safe in patients with normal renal function
B. Warfarin must be given for 3 months in patients with thrombosis
C. Presence of heparin-PF4 antibodies is diagnostic
D. Surgical patients are at higher risk of HIT compared to medical patients

31. Which one of following is not true for Bivalirudin?
A. It is direct thrombin inhibitor
B. It has half life of 3 hours
C. It does not cause thrombocytopenia
D. It is used in percutaneous coronary interventions

32. Which of the following should not be used as the sole anticoagulant during PCI?
A. Enoxaparin
B. Bivalirudin
C. Fondaparinux
D. None of the above

33. One among the following drug has 100% bioavailability:

A. Heparin B. Enoxaparin
C. Fondaparinux D. Rivaroxaban

34. All of the following are correct about fondaparinux except:
A. Indirect factor Xa inhibitor
B. Can be used in place of heparin as sole anticoagulant in PCI
C. Can be used for anticoagulation post-thrombolysis in acute STEMI
D. There is decreased risk of bleeding vs enoxaparin

35. A 30-year-old patient has undergone percutaneous transvenous mitral commissurotomy (PTMC). He developed cardiac tamponade during the procedure. A total of 5,000 units of unfractionated heparin (UFH) was given during the procedure. All of the following statements are true for administration of protamine sulphate to neutralize UFH except?
A. Each mg of protamine neutralizes 100 units of active heparin
B. It should be given as fast bolus for immediate action
C. It can cause pulmonary hypertension
D. Maximal dose which can be given is usually 50 mg

36. All of the following are true for HIT except?
A. Antibodies against PF4 form immune complexes
B. Prognosis of early HIT is poorer
C. Thrombocytopenia is accompanied by paradoxical thrombosis
D. It is treated with thrombin inhibitors

37. Which of the following is true about protamine sulphate?
A. 1 mg of protamine is required to neutralise 1000 U of heparin
B. Bolus doses are given for immediate action
C. Can be given in repeated doses for subcutaneous heparin
D. Causes pulmonary hypertension

38. A 40 year old man develops thrombocytopenia followings heparin administration for acute pulmonary embolism. For further management which statement is true?
A. Low molecular weight heparin can be safely substituted for intravenous unfractionated heparin
B. A direct thrombin inhibitor, such as lepirudin, could be safely substituted for heparin
C. Intravenous heparin should be continued because the low platelet count represents a laboratory artefact without clinical significance
D. This is a transient reaction to heparin and does not preclude future heparin treatment for this patient

39. Novel anticoagulant mostly excreted through the kidneys is:
A. Dabigatran B. Rivaroxaban
C. Apixaban D. Edoxaban

40. Which of the following novel anticoagulants is a direct thrombin inhibitor?
A. Rivaroxaban B. Apixaban
C. Dabigatran D. Edoxaban

41. Based on the RE-LY trial, which of the following statements is false?
A. Dabigatran 110 mg was noninferior to warfarin in preventing stroke or embolism
B. Dabigatran 150 mg was superior to warfarin in preventing stroke/embolism
C. Dabigatran was associated with more gastrointestinal bleeds
D. Dabigatran was associated with more intracranial bleeds

42. Which of the following test is used to assess dabigatran activity?
A. Prothrombin time
B. Partial thromboplastin time

C. Heptest
D. Prothrombinase induced clotting time

43. Which of the following drugs has been approved by the US Food and Drug Administration for use to reverse the effect of dabigatran?
A. Idarucizumab B. Andexanet alfa
C. Aripazine D. Protamine

44. Which of the following drugs is a anti-Xa inhibitor?
A. Idarucizumab
B. Andexanet alfa
C. Aripazine
D. Protamine

45. Which of the following drugs is being evaluated as a universal anticoagulant reversal agent?
A. Idarucizumab
B. Andexanet alfa
C. Aripazine
D. Protamine

Antiplatelets

46. Which of the following statements is incorrect regarding prasugrel use?
A. It reduces risk of stent thrombosis compared with clopidogrel
B. It has a higher risk of bleeding in those above 75 years of age or weigh <60 kg
C. It is safe in those with prior stroke or transient ischemic attack (TIA)
D. It is used 10 mg once a day.

47. One of the following drug has long platelet bound half life:
A. Abciximab B. Eptifibatide
C. Tirofiban D. All of the above

48. Dose adjustment is needed for all of the following antithrombotic agents in patients with chronic kidney disease (estimated creatinine clearance <60 mL/min):
A. Eptifibatide B. Tirofiban
C. Clopidogrel D. Bivalirudin

49. What is false regarding Ticagrelor?
A. 180 mg loading dose followed by 90 mg BD maintenence dose
B. Concurrent Aspirin dose is 150 mg OD
C. PLATO trial concluded that ticagrelor as compared with clopidogrel significantly reduced major adverse cardiovascular events without an increase in the rate of overall major bleeding.
D. ONSET OFFSET trial concluded that ticagrelor achieved more rapid and greater platelet inhibition than high-loading-dose clopidogrel.

50. Select the true statement?
A. Levels of abciximab may remain detectable upto 2 weeks after discontinuation
B. The correlation of Anti Xa/Anti IIa for low molecular weight heparin is a good predictor of potency
C. Dalteparin has the highest IIa:Xa ratio
D. Lepirudin is reversible inhibitor of thrombin

51. Which of the following is true regarding ADP receptor antagonists?
A. Thienopyridines predominantly act through P2Y 1 receptors
B. Prasugrel use is safe in elderly patients
C. Ticagrelor is directly-acting, oral thienopyridine agent
D. Cangrelor is a reversible platelet inhibitor

52. Which of the following is an intravenous P2Y12 receptor inhibitor?
A. Ticagrelor B. Clopidogrel
C. Prasugrel D. Cangrelor

53. The platelet bound half-life is longest for:
A. Eptifibatide B. Abciximab
C. Tirofiban D. Fondaparinux

54. Which of the following medications has an active metabolite with the longest half-life?

A. Aspirin B. Clopidogrel
C. Prasugrel D. Ticagrelor

55. The proposed rationale behind avoiding concomitant use of ticagrelor with aspirin doses above 100 mg per day is:
A. Concomitant use of ticagrelor and aspirin >100 mg daily may result in decreased efficacy of aspirin
B. Concomitant use of ticagrelor and aspirin >100 mg daily may result in decreased efficacy of ticagrelor
C. Concomitant use of ticagrelor and aspirin >100 mg daily may result in intolerable gastrointestinal adverse events that may lead to drug discontinuation
D. Concomitant use of ticagrelor and aspirin >100 mg daily may result in increased hypersensitivity to aspirin

56. 60/M patient presented with a new STEMI and underwent primary PCI to LAD. Past medical history includes HTN, diabetes mellitus type 2, hyperlipidemia, and history of transient ischemic attack. Which of the following P2Y12 receptor antagonists may not be used with aspirin 81 mg for dual antiplatelet therapy to prevent stent thrombosis?
A. Clopidogrel B. Prasugrel
C. Ticagrelor D. Cangrelor

57. A common adverse drug reaction to ticagrelor is:
A. Leukocytosis B. Hyperkalemia
C. Weight loss D. Dyspnea

58. All of the following are true about ticagrelor except:
A. Uricosuric
B. Increase serum creatinine
C. Contraindicated in AV block/sick sinus syndrome patients
D. Increases bleeding complications when used with ketaconazole

59. A two-step CYP enzyme dependent metabolism to become an active drug is required for?
A. Aspirin B. Clopidogrel
C. Prasugrel D. Ticagrelor

60. Which of the following is a reversible antiplatelet agent?
A. Aspirin B. Clopidogrel
C. Prasugrel D. Ticagrelor

61. In TRITON-TIMI 38 trial clopidogrel was compared with:
A. Cangrelor B. Prasugrel
C. Ticagrelor D. Vorapaxar

62. All of the following is true regarding anti-thrombotic therapy except:
A. Ticagrelor should be stopped 24 hours before urgent CABG
B. Aspirin should be stopped 24 hours before urgent CABG
C. Clopidogrel should be stopped 24 hours before urgent CABG
D. Tirofiban should be stopped 2-4 hours before urgent CABG

63. All of the following are true match except:
A. Prasugrel-ADP receptor inhibitor
B. Congrelor-I/v ADP inhibitor
C. Ticagrelor-Reversible ADP inhibitor
D. Cilostazol-Adenosine reuptake blocker

64. Which of the following is antiplatelet drug with shortest half-life?
A. Ticagrelor
B. Prasugrel
C. Clopidogrel
D. Cangrelor

65. Which of the follow glycoprotein IIb/IIIa inhibitors has longest observed platelet antagonism effects:
A. Abciximab
B. Eptifibatide
C. Tirofiban
D. Orbofiban

Anti-anginals

66. Which one of following is not true for Ranolazine?

A. It inhibits late inward sodium current.
B. It is used in angina
C. It prolongs QT interval
D. It decreases heart rate

67. All of the following drugs are diabetogenic except:

A. Ranolazine
B. Atenolol
C. Hydrochlorthiazide
D. Atorvastatin

68. All of the following drugs are diabetogenic except:

A. Atenolol
B. Hydrochlorothiazide
C. Atorvastatin
D. Ranolazine

69. All of the following are true about these drugs except:

A. Perhexiline inhibit FA oxidation
B. Ivabradine impair night vision
C. Ranolazine increases QT
D. Trimetazidine increases glucose levels

70. Ivabradine acts as

A. Inhibitor of late sodium current
B. If current inhibitor
C. Potassium channel opener
D. Calcium channel blacker

71. Which of the following drug acts on I_f channels?

A. Istaroxime B. Ivabradine
C. Sacubitril D. Nesiritide

72. Which of the following drug is known to improve morbidity or mortality?

A. Tazosentan for heart failure
B. Ivabradine for heart failure
C. Dalcetrapib for lipid modification
D. Glimeperide in macrovascular disease

73. Phosphenes (visual disturbance) may be seen with all except:

A. Ivabradine B. Nicorandil
C. Sildenafil D. Tadalafil

74. Which of the following is wrong about these antianginals?

A. Perhexiline: Fatty acid oxidation inhibitor
B. Trimetazidine: Fatty acid oxidation inhibitor and increases blood sugar levels in diabetics
C. Ranolazine: Prolongs QT interval
D. Ivabradine: Causes night vision problems

75. Verapamil does not increase blood level of following drug:

A. Digoxin B. Atorvastatin
C. Aspirin D. Ketoconazole

76. Which one of following is not true for Nicorandil?

A. It is potassium channel activator
B. It can produce ulcerations in gastrointestinal tract
C. It has negative chronotropic effect
D. It is venodilator & coronary dilator

Miscellaneous

77. Drug NOT metabolized by CYP2D6?

A. Propafenone B. Metoprolol
C. Codeine D. Clopidogrel

78. All of the following drugs are metabolized by CYP- 2D6 except:

A. Simvastatin B. Carvedilol
C. Codeine D. Metoprolol

79. All of the following are true about P- glycoprotein except:

A. It is involved in BBB (blood brain barrier) transport
B. Amiodarone inhibits P-glycoprotein

C. Ritonavir induces P-glycoprotein
D. It is coded by ABCB1 gene

80. All of the following are hepatotoxic drugs except:
A. Bosentan B. Dabigatran
C. Dronedarone D. Statin

81. Hypokalemia is caused by all except:
A. Ingestion of avocados
B. Insulin overdose
C. Licorice
D. Acute theophylline toxicity

82. NSAID which is least cardiotoxic?
A. Diclofenac B. Etoricoxib
C. Rofecoxib D. Naproxen

83. Increased diuretic resistance is seen with all except:
A. Decreased RA pressure
B. Decreased K^+
C. Associated ACE-I use
D. NSAIDs use

84. All of the following are true about diuretic resistance except:
A. Low mean RA pressure
B. Concomitant use of ARB
C. NSAIDs
D. Severe hypokalemia

85. All of the following may be responsible for diuretic resistance except:
A. Indomethacin B. Dehydration
C. Hypokalemia D. Enalapril

86. Which of the following is best agent for anaphylactic reactions in beta blocking?
A. Dopamine B. Vasopressin
C. Glucagon D. Salbutamol

ANSWERS

BETA BLOCKERS:

Answer: 1. B. Atenolol

Answer: 2. C. Carvedilol

Answer: 3. D. All

Answer: 4. A. Bucindolol

Answer: 5. A. Atenolol

Answer: 6. B. Carvedilol

Answer: 7. C. Nevibolol

B1 selective: Acebutolol, Atenolol, Bisoprolol, Esmolol, Metoprolol

Non-selective: Act on both B1 as well as B2. Nadolol, Pindolol, Propranolol.

Agents with intrinsic sympathomimetic activity: Have partial beta agonist activity and prevent resting bradycardia. Acebutolol, Pindolol.

Nebivolol: Selective beta1 antagonist which also reduces SVR by producing an endothelium-derived NO dependent vasodilation.

Low lipid solubility (Renal excretion): Acebutolol, Atenolol, Bisoprolol, Esmolol, Nadolol, Sotalol

High lipid solubility (Liver excretion): Propranolol, Carvedilol, Metoprolol, Timolol, Pindolol

Contraindications: Hypersensitivity to beta-blockers, asthma, heart block greater than first degree, overt heart failure, severe peripheral arterial disease.

Major clinical trials:

Three beta blockers have been shown to be effective in reducing the risk of death in patients with chronic HF: bisoprolol and sustained release metoprolol succinate both selectively block the β1 receptor, and carvedilol which competitively blocks the α1, β1, and β2 receptors.

MERIT-HF: Metoprolol improved survival in CHF.

CIBIS-I and II: Bisoprolol reduced mortality in CHF.

COPERNICUS: Carvedilol reduced mortality in CHF.

CAPRICORN: Carvedilol reduced total mortality in patients with LV dysfunction after MI.

COMET: Carvedilol improved survival and LVEF greater than immediate release metoprolol tartrate. There are no trials to ascertain benefits of carvedilol are greater than metoprolol succinate.

BEST: Bucindolol (which is nonselective beta 1 and beta 2 blocker with some alpha 1 blocking activity) showed non significant reduction in overall mortality in CHF.

SENIORS: Nebivolol (which is selective beta 1 receptor antagonist with vasodilatory properties mediated by nitric oxide) did not reduce total mortality but reduced cardiovascular hospitalizations.

Answer: 8. C. Aliskiren

Answer: 9. A. Prevents infarct expansion

Answer: 10. C. Telmisartan

Answer: 11. A. Continue same treatment and monitor renal function

Answer: 12. B. Spironolactone.

Gynecomastia and nipple tenderness are dose- and duration-dependent side effect of spironolactone. Gynecomastia may be reversible following discontinuation of therapy, but on rare occasions may persist.

Answer: 13. B. ARBs are prohibited in such patients with heart failure

ACE inhibitors are contraindicated after ACE inhibitor induced angioedema because this side effect is a class effect and one ACE inhibitor should not be substituted with another ACE inhibitor. Although ARBs can also cause angioedema, they can be precautiously considered in such patients.

ACE inhibitors:

Not a prodrug: Lisinopril

Side effects: Cough, acute renal failure, angioedema, hyperkalemia, proteinuria, hypotension, neutropenia/ agranulocytosis.

Contraindications: Pregnancy, bilateral renal artery stenosis, unilateral renal artery stenosis in patients with solitary kidney.

Major clinical trials:

SAVE: Captopril decreased mortality in asymptomatic LV dysfunction following MI.

GISSI-3: Lisinopril reduced mortality after MI.

TRACE: Trandolapril reduced mortality in diabetic patients after MI.

HEART: Early use of ramipril after acute MI decreased LV remodelling and resulted in swift LV recovery.

CONSENSUS: Enalapril reduced mortality in severe CHF.

V-HeFT II: Enalapril reduced mortality in CHF more than hydralazine-isosorbide combination.

ARBs:

Cough is not seen (because do not alter metabolism of bradykinin, rest side effects similar to ACE inhibitors. Angioedema may occur but is rare.

CHARM: Candesartan reduced mortality in heart failure in patients who were intolerant of ACE inhibitors.

Val-HeFT: Valsartan reduced mortality in CHF. When given in combination with ACE inhibitors it increased mortality.

RESOLVD: Candesartan and enalapril safe and effective in treatment of CHF.

Aldosterone receptor antagonists: Spironolactone, Eplerenone

Side effects: Hyperkalemia, gynecomastia (not seen with eplerenone), hypotension, sexual dysfunction.

RALES: Addition of spironolactone to standard therapy of CHF reduced mortality in NYHA III and IV.

EPHESUS: Eplerenone decreased mortality in patients with CHF post-MI.

EMPHASIS-HF: Eplerenone reduced mortality in NYHA II HF with EF < 35%.

Renin inhibitor:

Aliskiren: Orally active direct renin inhibitor which blocks conversion of angiotensinogen to angiotensin I.

ALOFT: Aliskiren decreased NT-proBNP in urinary aldosterone excretion.

ASTRONAUT and ATMOSPHERE trials: Aliskiren failed to improve outcomes in HFrEF patients. Hence, it is not presently recommended as an alternative to ACE inhibitors or ARB in heart failure.

Angiotensin Receptor Neprilysin Inhibitors (ARNI):

Answer: 14. B. Valsartan/sacubitril combination

ARNI

Combination of valsartan (ARB) with sacubitril (a neprilysin inhibitor) in a 1:1 mixture.

Combination of an angiotensin receptor and neprilysin inhibitor (ARNI) slows the degradation of natriuretic peptides, bradykinin, and adrenomedullin, thereby enhancing diuresis, natriuresis, and myocardial relaxation

PARADIGM-HF: Fixed-dose sacubitril/valsartan combination resulted in reductions in all-cause mortality, CV mortality, and HF hospitalizations compared with an ACEI (enalapril) alone in patients with mild to moderate HF (NYHA Class II to IV; LVEF 35%).

In patients with HFrEF NYHA Class II or III who are tolerating an ACEI or ARB, ARNIs are recommended as a replacement for ACEI/ARB to further reduce morbidity and mortality.

Side Effects of ARNIs hypotension, hyperkalemia, cough, and extremely low incidence of angioedema.

Oral neprilysin inhibitors, used in combination with ACEIs, leads to increased incidence of angioedema; thus the concomitant use of ACEIs and ARNIs is contraindicated (class III recommendation).

For patients who are switching from ACEIs to sacubitril/valsartan, the ACEI should be withheld for at least 36 hours before initiating sacubitril/valsartan, to minimize the risk of angioedema caused by overlapping ACE and neprilysin inhibition.

Digoxin:

Answer: 15. C. 36 hours

Used as adjunctive treatment for heart failure and to slow ventricular rate in patients with atrial fibrillation

Digoxin inhibits the **sodium-potassium ATPase pump** on the cell membrane, blocking sodium transport out of the cell, thus increasing intracellular sodium concentrations. This results in an increase in cardiac contractility.

Digoxin enhances parasympathetic tone, leading to an increase in AV nodal refractory period, as observed by increases in the P-R interval.

Side effects: Nausea vomiting, blurred vision, visual colour distortion, atrial and ventricular arrhythmias.

Half-life of digoxin is **36 hours.**

Therapeutic levels: Between 0.5 to 1.0 ng/ml. Toxicity: More than 2.0 ng/ml.

Toxicity of digoxin increased by hypokalemia, hypomagnesemia or hypercalcemia.

Antidigoxin Fab- Used to reverse potentially life threatening digoxin toxicity.

Concomitant use of quinidine, verapamil, spironolactone, flecainide, propafenone, and amiodarone increase the serum digoxin levels.

DIG trial: Digoxin had a neutral effect on the primary endpoint of mortality, but reduced hospitalizations for HF.

DRUGS FOR ACUTE DECOMPENSATED HEART FAILURE:

Answer: 16. D. In case of sulphonamide allergy, bumetanide should be given in place of furosemide

Answer: 17. D. Ethacrynic acid

Answer: 18. C. Causes cAMP mediated vasodilation

Answer: 19. B. Levosimendan

Answer: 20. A. Omecamtiv mecarbil

Answer: 21. C. Milrinone

Answer: 22. B. It is beta receptor stimulant

Answer: 23. A. Decreased 30 days mortality VS dobutamine

Answer: 24. D. Levosimendan acts on B1 and B2 receptors

Answer: 25. C. Inotropic and vasoconstrictor

Diuretics:

Loop diuretics are preferred decongestive agents in ADHF.

DOSE trial: No significant difference between intermittent bolus dosing or continuous iv infusion of furosemide in ADHF patients.

In presence of diuretic resistance, thiazide like diuretic (chlorothiazide or metolazone) and potassium sparing diuretic (spironolactone, eplerenone) may be added to loop diuretic.

Common drugs avoided in sulfa allergy:

Antibacterial agents: Sulfadiazine, Sulfamethoxazole, Sulfisoxazole, Sulfapyridine (in sulfasalazine)

COX-2 inhibitors: Celecoxib, Etoricoxib

Carbonic anhydrase inhibitors: Acetazolamide

Diuretics: Bumetanide, Chlorthalidone, Furosemide, Hydrochlorothiazide, Indapamide, Metolazone, Torsemide

Sulfonylureas: Chlorpropamide, Glibenclamide, Glimepiride, Glipizide, Glyburide, Tolbutamide, Tolazamide

Others: Ibutilide, Sotalol, Topiramate, Zonisamide

Vasodilators:

In the absence, vasodilators can be used in combination of diuretics for rapid relief of symptoms.

ALARM-HF: Patients treated combination of diuretics and vasodilators had better survival than patients treated with diuretics alone or those treated with inotropes.

Venous dilators- Reduce preload

Arterial dilators- Decrease afterload

Balanced dilators- Act on both venous as well as arterial system.

Nitrates, Sodium nitroprusside and Nesiritide- All these drugs act by activating soluble guanosine monophosphate (cGMP) and lead to vascular relaxation.

Nitrates:

Potent venodilator but at higher doses also act as arterial dilators reducing afterload.

Headache is most common adverse effect. Hypotension is also common which is exacerbated with recent use of sildenafil or tadalafil.

Sodium nitroprusside:

Reduces both preload as well as afterload and is particularly effective in setting of hypertensive AHF and moderate -severe mitral regurgitation.

Very short acting, requires continuous iv infusion.

Not recommended for patients with active myocardial ischemia because of myocardial steal phenomenon.

It can rarely cause cyanide toxicity.

Nesiritide:

It is recombinant human BNP and causes potent cGMP mediated vasodilation in the venous and arterial system which helps in ADHF.

VMAC trial: Nesiritide produced more fall in PCWP compared to nitroglycerin in ADHF patients.

ASCEND-HF: Nesiritide did not reduce death or rehospitalization for HF as compared to placebo in ADHF.

ROSE-HF: Nesiritide had no beneficial effect on urine output or cystatin C or clinical outcomes but increased the rates of symptomatic hypotension.

Inotropes and Inodilators:

Dobutamine:

Dobutamine or dopamine are preferred inotrope in hypotension and renal dysfunction, given renal excretion of milrinone.

Concomitant use of beta blocker therapy will result in competitive antagonism of effects of dobutamine.

Dopamine:

Agonist of both adrenergic and dopaminergic receptors.

Low dose dopamine (d"2 mcg/kg/min)- Specific dilation of renal, splanchnic, and cerebral arteries, causes natriuresis by increasing renal blood flow.

Intermediate dose dopamine (2 to 10 mcg/kg/min)- Enhances NE release, causes positive inotropic effect.

High dose dopamine (10 to 20 mcg/kg/min)- Causes peripheral and pulmonary artery vasoconstriction, mediated by agonist of alpha 1 receptors.

Epinephrine:

Full beta receptor agonist and potent inotropic agent with balanced vasodilator and vasoconstrictor effects.

Milrinone:

Inhibits phosphodiesterase IIIa and increases cAMP concentration. Inotropic effect as well as causes peripheral and pulmonary vasodilation.

OPTIME-CHF: Milrinone increased the sustained hypotension and new atrial arrhythmias without primary end points.

Levosimendan:

Increases myocardial contractility (by cardiac myofilament calcium sensitization) and produces peripheral vasodilation (by activation of smooth muscle potassium channels).

Potent vasodilator effect can cause significant hypotension.

REVIVE-II: Levosimendan showed significant improvement in **clinical status and BNP level** compared to standard care, but it was associated with more episodes of **hypotension, AF and ventricular ectopy as well as non-significant increase in early mortality**.

SURVIVE: Levosimendan was associated with lower incidence of worsening HF and **greater incidence of AF** compared to dobutamine.

Vasopressors:

Norepinephrine: Potent agonist of beta 1 and alpha 1 receptors resulting in marked vasoconstriction. It is a preferred vasopressor for cardiogenic shock.

Phenylephrine: Selective alpha 1 receptor agonist with potent arterial vasoconstrictor effects. May be used in hypotension related to systemic vasodilation.

Vaptans:

They are AVP antagonists and used for hyponatremia associated with heart failure.

Tolvaptan: Oral, selective V_2 receptor antagonist

Conivaptan: V_{1a}/V_2 receptor antagonist for iv use.

Both of these improve hyponatremia but don't improve long term outcomes in HF.

EVEREST: Tolvaptan improved signs and symptoms during hospitalization but survival and re-admission rates were not affected.

Novel therapies:

Serelaxin

Recombinant human relaxin-2, has beneficial effects on cardiac preconditioning, inflammation and fibrosis.

RELAX-AHF-2: Serelaxin did not improve CV mortality at 180 days compared to placebo in acute heart failure patients.

Natriuretic peptides

Urodilatin (a modified pro-ANP) and Ularitide (a synthetically produced urodilatin.

TRUE-AHF: Ularitide did not improve CV mortality and had no beneficial effects on secondary end points.

Omecamtiv mecarbil

Cardiac myosin activator, increases myocardial contractility. It increases systolic ejection time, stroke volume and EF without increasing intracellular cAMP or calcium.

Istaroxime

Mechanism: Positive inotropic effect by acting on two pathways, 1. By stimulation of Na-K ATPase and 2. Increasing the activity of SERCA2a.

HORIZON-HF: Istaroxime lowered PCWP and heart rate and increased SBP without any effect of renal function and troponin levels.

ANTICOAGULANTS:

Answer: 26. A. VKORC1 genotype

Answer: 27. D. Apixaban

Answer: 28. C. Bilateral adrenal hyperplasia

Answer: 29. C. Switch to bivalirudin

Answer: 30. C. Presence of heparin-PF4 antibodies is diagnostic

Answer: 31. B. It has half life of 3 hours

Answer: 32. A. Fondaparinux.

This is because of risk of catheter thrombosis.

Answer: 33. C. Fondaparinux

Answer: 34. B. Can be used in place of heparin as sole anticoagulant in PCI

Answer: 35. B. It should be given as fast bolus for immediate action

Answer: 36. B. Prognosis of early HIT is poorer

Type I HIT is also called as early HIT which has good prognosis.

Answer: 37. D. Causes pulmonary hypertension

Answer: 38. B. A direct thrombin inhibitor, such as lepirudin, could be safely substituted for heparin

Answer: 39. A. Dabigatran.

Among the drugs listed in the question, dabigatran is cleared through the kidneys (80%), while rivaroxaban (66%), apixaban (25%) and edoxaban (50%) have lower rates of renal clearance.

Answer: 40. C. Dabigatran.

Dabigatran is a direct thrombin inhibitor, while all the other agents are factor Xa inhibitors.

Answer: 41. D. Dabigatran was associated with more intracranial bleeds.

Answer: 42. B. Partial thromboplastin time (aPTT)

Heptest is used for LMWH monitoring.

Warfarin:

Oral coumarin derivative, vitamin K antagonist initially developed as a rodenticide.

Interferes with the synthesis of vitamin K–dependent clotting proteins, which include prothrombin (factor II) and factors VII, IX, and X.

Also impairs synthesis of the vitamin K–dependent anticoagulant proteins C and S.

It inhibits vitamin K–dependent gamma-carboxylation of these factors by inhibiting vitamin K epoxide reductase enzyme.

Plasma half life: 36 hours

Metabolized by CYP2C9 and VKORC1 enzymes.

Monitoring: Prothrombin time

Side effects: Bleeding, Skin necrosis, Fetal abnormalities.

Unfractionated heparin (UFH):

Side effects: Bleeding, thrombocytopenia (benign type I and more severe type II, which may cause thrombosis), elevation in AST/ALT, osteoporosis, cutaneous necrosis and hyperkalemia

Monitoring: aPTT or anti factor Xa level

Heparin induced thrombocytopenia (HIT):

HIT is associated with thrombocytopenia but is not marked by bleeding; instead, venous thromboembolism is the most common complication. Less often arterial thrombosis may occur.

Pathophysiology: HIT is a prothrombotic disorder caused by antibodies to complexes of platelet factor 4 (PF4) and heparin.

Antibodies to PF4 are also present in many patients (especially patients undergoing cardiac procedures) who have been exposed to heparin but who do not have clinical manifestations of HIT. Hence, presence of these antibodies is not diagnostic of HIT.

Heparin-induced platelet aggregation assay (HIPA) and the serotonin release assay (SRA) are more specific test for diagnosis of HIT.

Type I: Non-antibody-mediated reaction, occurs within 1st two days, platelet count normalizes with continued heparin use

Type II: Antibody-mediated reaction-typically IgG, occurs within 5-14 days after exposure to heparin, associated with life threatening thrombotic complications

Thromboembolic complications (e.g., deep vein thrombosis [DVT], MI, stroke) are associated with type II HIT and can be life threatening.

The incidence of thrombocytopenia is 10% to 15%, but the incidence of developing type II HIT is less than 1%.

HIT is more common with Heparin than LMWH.

More common in surgical patients than medical patients.

Females are more prone for HIT complications than males.

Thrombosis may precede thrombocytopenia in up to 25% of patients with HIT.

Management of HIT

Stop all heparin.

Give an alternative anticoagulant, such as lepirudin, argatroban, bivalirudin, fondaparinux, or rivaroxaban.

Do not give platelet transfusions.

Do not give warfarin until the platelet count returns to baseline levels; if warfarin was administered, give vitamin K to restore the INR to normal.

Warfarin should be started with other anticoagulant which can be discontinued when warfarin has been therapeutic for at least 2 days.

Evaluate for thrombosis, particularly deep vein thrombosis.

Antidote for Heparin: Protamine sulphate

Can be used for heparin and LMWH overdose.

1mg of Protamine reverses 100 units of heparin.

Common side effect is hypotension, allergic reactions and hence rapid infusions or bolus doses are not given.

It can also cause pulmonary hypertension.

Low-Molecular-Weight Heparin

Dalteparin, Enoxaparin, Tinzaparin

Risk of HIT and osteoporosis lesser as compared to UFH.

Monitoring: Anti factor Xa level; therapeutic 0.5 to 1.2 units/ml; prophylactic 0.2 to 0.5 units/ml.

SYNERGY: Enoxaparin non-inferior to UFH in NSTEMI with slight increased bleeding risk.

Direct thrombin inhibitors:

Bivalirudin, Lepirudin (Irreversible), Argatroban, Dabigatran

Bivalirudin, lepirudin, and argatroban are given intravenously, and dabigatran is available orally

Trials:

HERO-2: Bivalirudin decreased infarction rates as compared to heparin in acute MI with slight increase in risk of bleed.

RE-LY: Dabigatran 150 mg BD better than warfarin in atrial fibrillation with similar rates of bleeding. Dabigatran 110 mg BD non-inferior to warfarin with lesser risk of bleeding.

ACUITY: Bivalirudin found to have significantly reduced rates of major bleeding and was noninferior compared to heparin plus GP IIb/IIIa inhibitor for ischemic events.

HORIZONS-AMI: Rates of major adverse cardiac events less with Bivalirudin in STEMI patients undergoing PCI as compared to heparin plus IIb/IIIa inhibitor.

Factor Xa inhibitors:

Parenteral: Fondaparinux; Oral: Rivaroxaban, Apixaban, Edoxaban.

Fondaparinux: Intravenous. Associated with significant guiding **catheter related thrombosis** during primary PCI after MI when used alone.

Rivaroxaban: Oral

Rivaroxaban may be started for DVT treatment and does not require overlap therapy with a parenteral agent.

Warfarin, dabigatran, and edoxaban must be started concomitantly with at least 5 days of a parenteral agent, such as enoxaparin or heparin.

Monitoring of newer anticoagulants:

Qualitative assessment of anticoagulant activity: the prothrombin time for factor Xa inhibitors and partial thromboplastin time (APTT) for dabigatran.

To measure plasma level of factor Xa inhibitors: Chromogenic anti–factor Xa assays

To measure plasma level of direct thrombin inhibitors: Diluted thrombin clotting time or ecarin clotting or chromogenic assays

OASIS 6: Fondaparinux decreased more mortality in MI patients than UFH. Was associated with more catheter thrombotic events.

RE-LY trial:

Patients with non-valvular AF.

High dose dabigatran vs low dose dabigatran vs warfarin.

High-dose dabigatran was associated with reduced incidence of stroke 1.11% versus 1.69% without any major bleeding when compared with warfarin.

ROCKET AF: Rivaroxaban was non-inferior to warfarin in nonvalvular AF. Major GI bleed less than heparin. Overall bleeding similar.

ENGAGE AF: Edoxaban was non-inferior to warfarin in preventing strokes or embolism in nonvalvular AF.

ARISTOTLE: Apixaban was superior to warfarin in preventing stroke

Antidotes for newer anticoagulants:

Answer: 43. A. Idarucizumab.

Answer: 44. B. Andexanet alfa

Answer: 45. C. Aripazine.

Idarucizumab:

Idarucizumab is a humanized, monoclonal, antibody fragment that specifically binds with high affinity to dabigatran.

It acts by competitively displacing dabigatran from thrombin to reverse anticoagulation and restore fibrin formation.

Dabigatran has an affinity for idarucizumab that is 350 times greater than its affinity for thrombin.

Andexanet alfa:

It is a modified recombinant FXa molecule intended for I/V administration, has been developed as an antidote to reverse anticoagulant activity of oral direct (e.g., apixaban, edoxaban, and rivaroxaban) and injectable indirect (e.g., enoxaparin and fondaparinux) FXa inhibitors.

Studied in ANNEXA-R trial, normalization of coagulation parameters was achieved within 2 min of completing the IV bolus infusion; the effect lasted 1–2 h with the IV bolus dose.

Aripazine (Ciraparantag):

It is a small, synthetic molecule designed with broad reversal activity and administered as a single IV bolus dose.

It binds to oral FXa inhibitors and direct thrombin inhibitors, as well as to injectable unfractionated heparin and LMWH via noncovalent bonding and charge–charge interactions to neutralize anticoagulation and bleeding.

ANTIPLATELETS:

Answer: 46. C. It is safe in those with prior stroke or transient ischemic attack (TIA)

Answer: 47. A. Abciximab

Answer: 48. C. Clopidogrel

Answer: 49. B. Concurrent Aspirin dose is 150 mg OD

Answer: 50. A. Levels of abciximab may remain detectable upto 2 weeks after discontinuation

Answer: 51. D. Cangrelor is a reversible platelet inhibitor

Answer: 52. D. Cangrelor

Answer: 53. B. Abciximab

Answer: 54. D. Ticagrelor.

àTicagrelor has an active metabolite with the longest half-life of approximately 9 h.

Answer: 55. B. Concomitant use of ticagrelor and aspirin >100 mg daily may result in decreased efficacy of ticagrelor.

Answer: 56. B. Prasugrel.

Answer: 57. D. Dyspnea.

Answer: 58. C. Contraindicated in AV block/sick sinus syndrome patients

Answer: 59. B. Clopidogrel.

Answer: 60. D. Ticagrelor.

Answer: 61. B. Prasugrel

Irreversible antiplatelets: Aspirin, Clopidogrel, Ticlopidine, Prasugrel

Reversible antiplatelets: Ticagrelor, Cangrelor

Aspirin: Irreversible inhibitor of platelet cyclo-oxygenase.

Aspirin irreversibly inhibits the platelet cyclo-oxygenase (COX-1 and COX-2) enzymes

Clopidogrel: Irreversibly inhibits P2Y12 component of ADP receptor.

Clopidogrel is metabolized extensively via two oxidative steps that are dependent predominantly on CYP2C19 to an active drug.

CYP2C19 inhibitors, such as proton pump inhibitors, may lead to reduced serum concentrations of clopidogrel's active metabolite.

Prasugrel: Prodrug, when activated irreversibly inhibits P2Y12 portion of ADP receptor.

It is contraindicated in patients with **history of TIA/stroke**. Use in **patients >75 years** of age is not recommended due to increased risk of fatal and intracranial bleeding. For patients of low weight (<60 kg), it should be avoided or a lower maintenance dose should be considered.

Ticagrelor: Reversibly binds to the ADP P2Y12 receptor.

Dyspnea is common side effect which is seen in 15% of patients, triggered by adenosine because it inhibits the clearance of adenosine. Discontinuation due to dyspnea in 4.3% patients. More likely to occur in initial 7 days.

Efficacy may be reduced if used with aspirin doses higher than 100 mg daily. Therefore, dose of aspirin should be <100 mg when used with ticagrelor.

Cilostazole:

It acts as a phosphodiesterase III inhibitor, suppressing breakdown of cAMP and thus leading to vasodilation and platelet inhibition.

Improves intermittent claudication. Contraindicated in CHF.

Major trials:

ISIS-2: Aspirin and streptokinase independently reduced mortality in patients with AMI. Combination better than 2 drugs because of synergistic effects.

CURE: Combination of clopidogrel with aspirin reduced cardiac events in NSTEMI when compared to aspirin alone.

CREDO: After PCI, long term clopidogrel therapy (1 year) reduced ischemic events.

CLARITY-TIMI 28: Early clopidogrel loading after fibrinolysis in patients who subsequently proceeded to PCI was associated with lower risk of ischemic events.

TRITON-TIMI 38: Prasugrel compared to clopidogrel in ACS patients scheduled for PCI, reduced rates of ischemic events and stent thrombosis, with significant increase in major bleeding.

PLATO: Ticagrelor compared to clopidogrel in ACS patients, decreased mortality and ischemic events without increasing overall bleeding.

Intravenous Antiplatelet Therapy/ Glycoprotein IIb/IIIa Inhibitors

Abciximab: Murine-derived monoclonal antibody Fab fragment

Abciximab may sometimes cause sudden profound thrombocytopenia.

Eptifibatide: Heptapeptide antagonist that reversibly inhibits GP IIb/IIIa receptor

Tirofiban: Nonpeptide antagonist that reversibly inhibits GP IIb/IIIa receptor

Eptifibatide and tirofiban are renally cleared and require dose adjustment in renal impairment.

Abciximab is metabolized via proteolytic cleavage and its clearance is not dependent on renal function, but its antiplatelet effects can last up to **7–14 days.**

Cangrelor is a **reversible** and intravenous antiplatelet; it is not dependent on renal or hepatic function and its antiplatelet effect wears off after **1 hour.**

Answer: 62. B. Aspirin should be stopped 24 hours before urgent CABG

→Aspirin should not be stopped before emergency CABG.

Answer: 63. D. Cilostazol-Adenosine reuptake blocker

→Cilostazole is PDE- 3 inhibitor and causes arterial vasodilation and prevents platelet aggregation. It does not affect adenosine metabolism.

Answer: 64. D. Cangrelor

→Half-lives: Ticagrelor- 7 hours, Prasugrel- 7 hours, Clopidogrel- 6 hours, Cangrelor- 3 to 5 minutes

Answer: 65. A. Abciximab.

→Dissociation of abciximab from the glycoprotein IIb/IIIa receptor occurs through proteolytic cleavage, resulting in slow elimination and consequently profound platelet antagonism that can last up to 12 h post-infusion. Platelet function may remain abnormal up to 7–14 weeks after infusion.

Antianginals:

Answer: 66. D. It decreases heart rate

Answer: 67. A. Ranolazine

Answer: 68. D. Ranolazine

Answer: 69. D. Trimetazidine increases glucose levels

Answer: 70. B. If current inhibitor

Answer: 71. B. Ivabradine

Answer: 72. B. Ivabradine for heart failure

Answer: 73. B. Nicorandil

Common drugs causing phosphenes:

Alcohol, LSD, Ivabradine, PDE5 inhibitors (Sildenafil, Tadalafil).

Answer: 74. B. Trimetazidine: Fatty acid oxidation inhibitor and increases blood sugar levels in diabetics

Answer: 75. D. Ketoconazole

Answer: 76. C. It has negative chronotropic effect

Antianginals:

The various drugs used to relieve angina include: Beta blockers, Nitrates, Calcium channel blockers, Ranolazine, Nicorandil, Trimetazidine, Ivabradine

Mechanism of action of Nicorandil- Dual-action **potassium channel opener** that relaxes vascular smooth muscle through membrane hyperpolarization via increased transmembrane potassium conductance and increased intracellular concentration of cyclic GMP

Mechanism of action of Trimetazidine- Trimetazidine is an anti-anginal metabolic agent, improves myocardial glucose utilization through inhibition of fatty acid metabolism, also known as fatty acid oxidation inhibitor.

In diabetic patients with CAD trimetazidine decreases blood glucose, increases glucose uptake, and improves endothelial function. It may worsen Parkinson's disease.

Ranolazine:

Causes inhibition of the late phase of the inward sodium channel (I_{Na}) in ischemic cardiac myocytes.

Does not have cardioinhibitory action, does not decrease BP and heart rate.

Used for chronic stable angina.

Prolongation of QT interval is seen.

Contraindicated in significant hepatic impairment.

Ranolazine **decreases** HbA1c and blood sugar level.

Ranolazine also acts as anti-arrhythmic agent and reduces AF.

Studies of Ranolazine: CARISA, MARISA, ERICA, RIVER-PCI, MERLIN-TIMI-36.

Ivabradine:

Ivabradine reduces heart rate by selectively inhibiting the **pacemaker funny (I_f) current** in SA node in a dose-dependent manner.

I_f channel controls the spontaneous depolarization of the sinoatrial node.

Initially developed as antianginal agent, also shown to improve outcomes in LV dysfunction.

Used in symptomatic management of stable angina and heart failure not fully managed by beta blockers; also, being used off-label in the treatment of inappropriate sinus tachycardia.

Heart failure: When used LVEF lower than 35 percent inadequately controlled by beta blockers alone and whose heart rate exceeds **70 beats per minute**, decreases the risk of hospitalization for heart failure.

Side effects: Bradycardia, Headache, Luminous phenomenon **(Phosphenes).**

Around 14.5% of patients taking ivabradine experience luminous phenomena (by patients described as sensations of enhanced brightness in a fully maintained visual field).

Studies of Ivabradine:

BEAUTIFUL study: Stable CAD and left ventricle dysfunction (ejection fraction < 40%).

In patients with a heart rate of more than 70 bpm, ivabradine significantly reduced the secondary endpoints including coronary events, fatal and nonfatal myocardial infarction, coronary revascularization.

SIGNIFY trial: Coronary artery disease and a heart rate greater than 70, but without clinical heart failure to ivabradine or placebo in addition to standard therapy. Ivabradine did not improve outcomes in this patient group.

SHIFT study:

Ivabradine significantly reduced the risk of the primary composite endpoint of hospitalization for worsening heart failure and cardiovascular death significantly compared with placebo on top of optimal therapy.

Miscellaneous:

Answer: 77. D. Clopidogrel

Answer: 78. Simvastatin

Protein	**Substrates**
CYP3A4, CYP3A5	Erythromycin, Clarithromycin, quinidine, Mexiletine, Cyclosporine, Tacrolimus HMG CoA reductase inhibitors (**Except pravastatin)**
CYP2D6	**Beta blockers:** Propranolol, Timolol, Metoprolol, Carvedilol Propafenone, TCA (Desipramine), Amitriptyline, Codeine
CYP2C9	**Warfarin,** Phenytoin, Tolbutamide, Losartan, **Clopidogrel**
CYP2C19	**Omeprazole, Clopidogrel**
P-glycoprotein	**Digoxin**
N-acetyl transferase	Procainamide, Hydralazine, Isoniazid
Thiopurine methyltransferase	6-Mercaptopurine, Azathioprine
SLCO1B1	**Simvastatin** and other statins, Methotrexate, Bosentan

Answer: 79. C. Ritonavir induces P-glycoprotein

P-glycoproteins:

It is an **ATP-dependent efflux pump** which pumps many foreign substances out of cells.

P-gp is extensively distributed in the intestinal epithelium, bile ducts, proximal tubule of the kidney, in the capillary endothelial cells composing the **blood–brain barrier** and blood-testis barrier.

P-gp is a glycoprotein that in humans is encoded by the **ABCB1 gene**.

P-gp transports **digoxin** inside the cells.

Common pharmacological inhibitors of P-glycoprotein include: **amiodarone**, clarithromycin, **erythromycin**, ciclosporin, colchicine, **CCBs** (diltiazem, verapamil, nifedipine, felodipine), lansoprazole, **omeprazole**, paroxetine, sertraline and quinidine.

Common inducers: Phenytoin, Rifampicin, Tenofovir, Carbamazepine, Phenobarbitone, St. Johns wort.

Substrates: Digoxin, Dabigatran, Colchicine, Cyclosporine, Morphine

Answer: 80. B. Dabigatran

Answer: 81. A. Ingestion of avocados

Avocados is a fruit which is rich in potassium.

Answer: 82. D. Naproxen

Answer: 83. C. Associated ACE-I use

Answer: 84. B. Concomitant use of ARB

Answer: 85. D. Enalapril

Answer: 86. C. Glucagon

4 Coronary Artery Disease

Acute Coronary Syndrome

1. **The third universal definition of MI defines MI associated with PCI as elevation of cardiac Troponin values of:**
   A. >3 × 99thpercentile URL in patients with normal baseline values
   B. >5 × 99thpercentile URL in patients with normal baseline values
   C. >10 × 99thpercentile URL in patients with normal baseline values
   D. >20 × 99thpercentile URL in patients with normal baseline values

2. **Myocardial infarction associated with coronary artery bypass grafting:**
   A. Type 2 MI B. Type 3 MI
   C. Type 4 MI D. Type 5 MI

3. **Troponin level does not increase in following condition:**
   A. STEMI
   B. Myocarditis
   C. Renal disease
   D. Liver disease

4. **Which of the following is cardiac biomarker with longest duration of presence after acute MI?**
   A. CK-MB
   B. Troponin I
   C. Troponin T
   D. Heart type fatty acid binding protein (H-FABP)

5. **Following criteria favours myocardial infarction in presence of LBBB except:**
   A. ST segment elevation greater than 1 mm & concordant with QRS complex
   B. ST segment depression greater than 1 mm in v1 , v2 , v3
   C. ST segment depression greater than 1 mm in II , III , AVF
   D. ST segment elevation greater than 5 mm & discordant with QRS complex

6. **Time to reperfusion therapy is the most important determinator of outcomes in acute MI. In this context, which of the following is a recommended treatment goal?**
   A. First medical contact (FMC) to ECG & diagnosis 60 minutes
   B. First medical contact to fibrinolysis (FMC to needle time) 60 minutes
   C. First medical contact to primary PCI (FMC to balloon time) 90 minutes
   D. None of the above

7. **Absolute contraindication for fibrinolytic therapy:**
   A. Aortic dissection
   B. Recent internal bleeding
   C. Active peptic ulcer
   D. Prolonged CPR

8. **Absolute contraindications to fibrinolytic therapy include all except:**

A. Previous intracranial haemorrhage or stroke of unknown origin at any time
B. Pregnancy or within 1 week postpartum
C. Ischaemic stroke in the preceding 6 months
D. Aortic dissection

9. Absolute contraindication to thrombolytic therapy for acute myocardial infarction include (s):
a. Prolonged CPR for more than 10 minutes
b. Ischemic stroke of 1-hour duration
c. Intracranial haemorrhage 3 months back
d. All of the above

10. Which of the following is correct regarding acute STEMI qualifying for reperfusion therapy?
A. Desired door to needle is ≤30 min and door to balloon time is ≤90 min
B. Desired door to needle and door to balloon times are ≤90 min
C. There is no indication for thrombolysis
D. Delayed thrombolysis is associated with better outcomes

11. Perioperative MI in non-cardiac surgery:
A. Intraoperative B. 4 hrs
C. 24-48 hrs D. 1 week

12. All of the following statements are true regarding acute myocardial infarction except:
A. Following thrombolysis, all high risk patients should be electively transferred to a PCI capable centre
B. Prehospital fibrinolysis does not significantly reduce mortality as compared to hospital based management
C. Recent trials suggest that non-culprit artery PCI may be done in patients undergoing primary PCI
D. Therapeutic hypothermia should be started as early as possible in comatose patients with STEMI and out of hospital cardiac arrest

13. Killips class-III is:
A. Shock
B. S3 gallop
C. Elevated JVP
D. Frank pulmonary edema

14. Which of the following is not a feature of right ventricular infarction?
A. Square root sign
B. Kussmaul sign
C. Acute pulmonary edema
D. Pulsus paradoxus

15. Which one of following is not true for right ventricular infarction?
A. Hypotension
B. Kussmaul sign
C. Elevated JVP
D. Basal crepitations in lungs

16. A 48-year-old man with acute inferior MI has a heart rate of 74 bpm, BP of 90/60 mmHg. JVP is elevated and there are no murmurs and crepitations. What would the appropriate treatment for low BP include?
A. Intravenous bolus of normal saline
B. Normal saline and dobutamine infusion if BP is still low
C. Intravenous Lasix
D. Infusion of norepinephrine

17. Hemodynamic findings suggestive of right ventricular myocardial infarction:
A. Wide pulmonary artery pulse pressure
B. Systemic hypertension
C. Decrease in right atrial pressure with amplitude
D. Right ventricular pressure curve shows dip and plateau

18. All of the following may be first line agent in the treatment of Inferior wall MI, all except:
A. AV sequential pacing
B. Intravenous nitroglycerine

C. Primary angioplasty
D. Aggressive hydration

19. All are features of RV MI except:
A. ST segment elevation in V4R
B. Increased LV filling pressure
C. Increased RA pressure
D. Steep Y descent in JVP

20. Which of the following is not true about heart blocks associated with IWMI?
A. Generally, first degree or Mobitz type I, but sometimes worse
B. Generally intranodal problem due to ischemia or increased vagal tone
C. May respond to atropine
D. Always permanent pacemaker

21. All of the following are true about heart blocks associated with AWMI, except:
A. Generally, Mobitz type II or complete heart block
B. Generally due to increased parasympathetic activity
C. In Mobitz type II AV block, atropine can make it worse by dropping the ventricular rate by increasing atrial rate
D. Generally needs permanent pacemaker

22. One of the following is a mechanical complication after acute MI:
A. Ventricular fibrillation
B. Ventricular septal rupture
C. Ventricular aneurysm
D. Pericardial effusion

23. Which of the following characteristics is not true for free wall rupture following acute MI?
A. More frequent in elderly
B. Associated with large infarctions
C. Most common between 1st & 4th day of MI
D. More common in normotensives than hypertensives

24. Which one of following is not true for pseudoaneurysm of LV after infarction?
A. It lacks any elements of myocardial wall
B. It is made up of organized thrombus & pericardium
C. It communicates with LV cavity through a narrow neck
D. It communicates with LV cavity through a wide neck

25. Which of the following statements is true regarding acute mitral regurgitation following acute myocardial infarction (MI)?
A. Occurs more commonly due to anterolateral papillary muscle
B. Can occur with both large or focal area of MI
C. Occurs more commonly with anterior wall MI than inferior wall MI
D. Usually occurs within 24 hours of MI

26. The statement regarding ventricular free wall rupture complicating myocardial infarction (MI) include all of the following except:
A. It is more likely to occur in patients with a history of prior MI
B. It typically occurs within the first 4 days after infarction
C. It is more common in elderly patients and in women
D. A history of hypertension is a risk factor for free wall rupture

27. In what is left ventricle free wall rupture in the presence of acute MI more common?
A. Elderly
B. Women
C. Those without prior infarcts
D. Large infarcts
E. All of the above

28. Which of the following are true about left ventricle free wall rupture?

A. It tends to occur at the junction of infarct and normal muscle
B. Generally occurs after 1–4 days of infarct, but can occur as late as 3 weeks
C. Usually occurs in left ventricle, but may involve right ventricle or atria
D. All of the above

29. A 54/M patient with inferior STEMI, post primary PCI, became suddenly short of breath, rapidly evolving into pulmonary edema needing endotracheal intubation. On examination, his heart rate was 130 bpm, BP 80/50 mmHg, bilateral rales, and high jugular venous pressure and there was no murmur. The ECG showed sinus tachycardia with normal ST segments. What is the most likely diagnosis?
A. Coronary stent thrombosis
B. Acute pulmonary embolism
C. Papillary muscle rupture
D. Large RV infarct

30. Which of the following statements are true regarding papillary muscle rupture?
A. It can occur with small subendocardial infarcts affecting tip of papillary muscle
B. More commonly involves posteromedial papillary muscle
C. Anterolateral papillary muscle may derive dual blood supply from LAD and circumflex arteries and is less prone to rupture
D. All of the above

31. All are the causes of new systolic murmur after MI except:
A. Dynamic LV outflow obstruction
B. MR
C. VSD
D. Dynamic RV outflow obstruction

32. Dressler syndrome occurs after:
A. Acute myocardial infarction
B. Acute rheumatic fever
C. Infective endocarditis
D. Congestive heart failure

33. A 60-year-old patient presents 3 weeks after an acute MI with fever and pleuritic chest pain. There was no cough, and chest X-ray showed blunting of costophrenic angles. ECG showed inferior Q waves with no ST elevation. ESR was 100 mm, WBC 20 000 with neutrophilia. What would the best treatment be?
A. Azithromycin
B. Aspirin 650 mg q 6 h
C. NSAIDs
D. Prednisone 40 mg/day
E. Immediate PCI

34. Which of the following is true about immediate Post MI acute pericarditis?
A. Corticosteroids are the treatment of choice
B. Aspirin is given for symptomatic relief
C. Due to subendocardial ischemia
D. Heparin dose needs to be modified

35. What minimum level of damage to left ventricular myocardium is required in patients with STEMI for cardiogenic shock?
A. 50%
B. 60%
C. 70%
D. 40%

36. Which of the following patients with STEMI will have worst prognosis?
a. 40-year male diabetic with inferior wall MI, clear chest, no LVS3
b. 70-year old patient with inferior wall MI and basal crepts and LVS3
c. 60-year male with anterior wall MI and clear chest, no LVS3
d. 7 5-year male with old anterior wall MI, acute IWMI, LVEF 45%, clear chest

37. Presence of ST elevation & Q waves in the ECG are markers of transmural infarction & necrosis. Select the false statement amongst the following?

A. LBBB conduction abnormality may have Q wave not secondary to myocardial infarction.
B. Generally, an amplitude of Q wave more than 25% of R wave represents a necrosis Q wave.
C. Brugada Syndrome & hypothermia may cause ST segment elevation in absence of ischemic heart disease.
D. In cases of inferior wall MI, ST segment elevation in lead III more than lead II is suggestive of occlusion of proximal left circumflex artery

38. Following is true for atrial infarction incidence in patients with STEMI:
A. 10% B. 5%
C. 15% D. 25%

39. All are true for atrial infarction except:
A. LA is more commonly involved than RA
B. Usually associated with ventricular infarction
C. Associated with increased incidence of thromboembolism
D. P-Ta depression is diagnostic (part between P and Q wave)

40. Plaque fissuring / disruption is less common in?
A. Lipid burden in atheroma 70%
B. Thin cap atheroma
C. Thick cap atheroma
D. Luminal area of stenotic area 4.0 mm square

41. In a patient with non-ST elevation ACS, early coronary angiography is not appropriate in which of the following situations?
A. TIMI score of 5
B. Continuing chest pain
C. EF <40%
D. Normal cardiac biomarkers

Chronic Stable Angina

42. How many patients of stable CAD may have normal resting ECG?
A. About 10% B. About 50%
C. About 75% D. 100%

43. How many patients of stable CAD may develop new ECG changes during episode of angina?
A. 100% B. 50%
C. 75% D. 25%

44. Which of the following is most common finding in the ECG in stable CAD patients during an episode of angina?
A. ST segment depression
B. ST segment elevation
C. Normalization of previous ST abnormalities (pseudonormalization)
D. None of the above

45. In a patient with chest pain and moderate probability of CAD and a normal resting ECG, what is the best test to order to evaluate for ischemia?
A. Exercise stress ECG
B. Exercise echo
C. Dobutamine stress echo
D. Stress nuclear

46. A stress nuclear test is helpful in which of the following situations?
A. Abnormal resting ECG changes
B. LBBB
C. LV hypertrophy
D. All of the above

47. Which of the following is a true statement?
A. Stress test in females is associated with low rate of false-positive results compared with males
B. Stress test in females is associated with higher false-positive results compared with males

C. Stress test in females is associated with higher rates of false negative results compared with males
D. Stress test in females is associated with low rates of false-negative results compared with males

48. In a diabetic patient with symptomatic CAD, with three-vessel CAD on coronary angiography and an EF of 40%, what would the best approach be?
A. Multivessel PCI with DES
B. Multivessel PCI with bare metal stents
C. Coronary artery bypass grafting (CABG) including left internal mammary artery (LIMA) to LAD artery
D. Medical therapy only

49. According to the SYNTAX trial, what was a low SYNTAX score?
A. 23–32 B. ≥33
C. ≤22 D. 50

Miscellaneous

50. Regarding use of nitrates in patients with STEMI, following is not an indication:
A. Post MI angina
B. Hypertension
C. LV failure
D. 48 hours after anterior wall MI with no angina

51. All of the following are true about linked angina except?
A. Precipitated by GERD acid reflux
B. Increases by bending forward
C. Normal coronaries
D. Increases after fatty food

52. All of the following are true about linked angina except:
A. Precipitated by food
B. Increases on forward bending
C. Coronary arteries are normal on angiography
D. Mimicked by esophageal acid stimulation

53. Earliest change in coronary artery occlusion:
A. Regional dyskinesia
B. Increased LVEDP
C. Angina
D. ECG changes

54. Periprocedural MI most commonly occurs during non cardiac surgery:
A. Intraoperative
B. Within 4 hours of surgery
C. 24-48 hours of surgery
D. 7 days of surgery

55. Ischemic mitral involvement with systolic anterior motion, all can be used except:
A. B blockers
B. ACE inhibitors
C. I/V fluids
D. Alpha agonist

56. A 60 years old male underwent PCI to proximal LAD for symptoms of angina. His echocardiogram showed ejection fraction of 35%. He is on aspirin, clopidogrel, metoprolol and atorvastatin. Prior to discharge, what other medication is indicated?
A. Angiotensin-converting inhibitor
B. Hydrochlorothiazide
C. Diltiazem
D. Ivabradine

57. A 62-year-old man underwent PCI to LAD in view of acute anterior wall STEMI within 4 hours of chest pain. Echo showed EF of 30%. He is on DAPT, beta blocker, ACE inhibitor and high dose statin. What else is likely to improve his outcome, if done before discharge?
A. Implantation of an implantable cardioverter-defibrillator

B. Amiodarone 200 mg daily to reduce risk for VT/Vfib
C. Eplerenone 25 mg daily
D. Warfarin to get an INR to 2-3 to prevent LV thrombus

58. Which one of following has no survival benefit in coronary artery disease?

A. Aspirin B. Beta blockers
C. Ace inhibitors D. Antioxidants

ANSWERS

Acute coronary syndrome

Answer: 1. B. >5 × 99thpercentile URL in patients with normal baseline values

Answer: 2. D. Type 5 MI

Diagnosis of STEMI

STEMI (ST-elevation myocardial infarction): New ST elevations in 2 contiguous leads 0.2 mV in men or 0.15 mV in women in leads V2–V3 and/or 0.1 mV in other leads; new LBBB (left bundle branch block) is suggestive.

Posterior MI (myocardial infarction): ST depression V1 and V2 (particularly if horizontal ST depression with upright T wave and tall R wave) and/or ST elevation V7–V9

Approximately 4 % of acute MI patients have isolated posterior ST elevations; detecting the presence is important since it qualifies for acute reperfusion therapy.

RV (right ventricular) MI: ST elevation 1 mm in V1, and/or V4R

Clinical Classification of Different Types of Myocardial Infarction

Type 1

Spontaneous myocardial infarction related to ischemia due to a primary coronary event such as plaque erosion and/or rupture, fissuring or dissection

Type 2

Myocardial infarction secondary to ischemia due to either increased oxygen demand or decreased supply, eg, coronary artery spasm, anemia, arrhythmias, hypertension, or hypotension

Type 3

Sudden unexpected cardiac death, including cardiac arrest with features suggestive of MI.

Type 4a

Myocardial infarction associated with PCI; Troponin should be more than 5 time the URL in patients with normal baseline values.

Type 4b

Myocardial infarction associated with stent thrombosis as documented by angiography or at autopsy

Type 5

Myocardial infarction associated with CABG; Troponin should be more than 10 time the URL in patients with normal baseline values.

Cardiac biomarkers:

Answer: 3 D. Liver disease

Answer: 4. C. Troponin T

Cardiac biomarkers:

Cardiac biomarkers are helpful for diagnosis as well as prognostication.

Troponins:

The cTn complex comprises 3 subunits: 1) cTnC binds calcium, 2) cTnI inhibits actin-myosin interaction, and 3) cTnT binds tropomycin.

Most cTn elevations by 2 to 3 hours after the onset of MI and nearly 100% by 6 hours.

cTn values typically peak at 24 hours and can remain elevated for 1 to 2 weeks. cTnT stays elevated slightly longer than cTnI.

cTn levels are highly specific for myocardial damage, as opposed to CK-MB

Non MI causes of Tn elevation:

Demand ischemia: Sepsis, Hypotension, Hypovolemia

Myocardial ischemia: Coronary vasospasm

Direct myocardial damage: Cardiac contusion, DC cardioversion, Myocarditis, Pericarditis

Myocardial strain: CHF, Pulmonary embolism, PAH

CKD

Creatine Kinase

Isoenzymes are 1) CK-MB (predominantly in myocardium, but 1%–7% is in skeletal muscle, and traces are in the small intestine, tongue, diaphragm, uterus, and prostate); 2) CK-BB (in brain and kidney); and 3) CK-MM (in skeletal muscle).

Much like cTn, CK may be elevated within 3 to 6 hours after onset of symptoms and peak at 24 hours.

However, unlike cTn, CK typically decreases to the baseline value by 36 to 48 hours.

Advantage of CK-MB: To diagnose reinfarction and infarct extension more effectively

Cardiac Biomarkers of Myocardial Injury

Biomarker	Time to Elevation (h)	Mean Time to Peak Elevation	Return to Normal Range
CK-MB	3	24 h	48–72 h
cTnI	3	24 h	5–10 d
cTnT	3	12 h to 2 d	5–14 d
Myoglobin	1	6–7 h	24 h

Diagnosis of AMI

99th percentile of a normal reference population as the appropriate metric for defining an elevation in cTn

cTn elevations 5 times normal should be considered abnormal and suggestive of a postoperative MI.

NB: In renal dysfunction, cTnT is high in 82%, and cTnI is high in 6%.

Answer: 5. C. ST segment depression greater than 1 mm in II , III , AVF

Answer: 6. C. First medical contact to primary PCI (FMC to balloon time) 90 minutes

Answer: 7. A. aortic dissection

Answer: 8. B. Pregnancy or within 1 week postpartum

Answer: 9. c. Intracranial haemorrhage 3 months back

Answer: 10. A. Desired door to needle is d"30 min and door to balloon time is d"90 min

Answer: 11. C. 24-48 hrs

Answer: 12. B. Prehospital fibrinolysis does not significantly reduce mortality as compared to hospital based management

Prehospital fibrinolysis significantly reduce time to reperfusion and is associated with reduction in mortality.

Answer: 13. D. frank pulmonary edema

ECG criteria for MI in presence of LBBB (Sgarbossa criteria):

ST elevation ≥1 mm, concordant with QRS

ST depression ≥1 mm, in lead V1, V2, or V3

ST elevation ≥5 mm, discordant with QRS

Killip class:

Class	Finding
I	No S 3 or rales
II	Rales in less than half of lung field
III	Rales in more than half of lung field
IV	Cardiogenic shock

PRIMARY PCI FOR STEMI:

Door to balloon time at PCI capable centre should be **less than 90 minutes.**

First contact to balloon time should be **less than 120 minutes** if patients presents at non PCI enabled centre and patient is transferred to PCI enabled centre, including transfer time of 30 minutes.

FIBRINOLYTIC THERAPY

If primary PCI is not available or appropriate, then the **door-to-needle time should be <30 min**.

Survival benefit is greatest when fibrinolytics are administered within the first 3 h of symptom-onset but patients presenting within the first 12 h are eligible.

Absolute contraindications: history of intracranial hemorrhage, closed head or facial trauma within the past 3 months, recent bleeding or bleeding diathesis, suspected aortic dissection, known structural cerebrovascular lesion, known malignant intracranial neoplasm, and ischemic stroke within the past 3 months.

Relative contraindications: uncontrolled hypertension (>180/110 mmHg), ischemic stroke more than 3 months previously, dementia, any known intracranial disease that is not an absolute contraindication, traumatic or prolonged (>10 min) CPR (cardiopulmonary resuscitation), major surgery within the preceding 3 weeks, internal bleeding within the preceding 2–4 weeks or an active peptic ulcer, noncompressible vascular punctures, pregnancy, current warfarin therapy, prior exposure or allergic reaction (for streptokinase or anistreplase).

NB: Routine, or transfer for, coronary angiography 3–24 h after fibrinolysis is reasonable even in hemodynamically stable STEMI patients with evidence of successful reperfusion.

RV infarction:

Answer: 14. C. Acute pulmonary edema

Answer: 15. D. Basal crepitations in lungs

Answer: 16. B. Normal saline and dobutamine infusion if BP is still low.

The patient has classical RV infarct with raised jugular venous pressure, Kussmaul's sign, and clear lungs in the setting of inferior MI. Other signs may include ST elevation in right chest leads. Intravenous fluids help improve RV output, and dobutamine will recruit noninfarcted RV myocardium to increase its performance. BP may fall with diuretics and NTG.

Answer: 17. D. Right ventricular pressure curve shows dip and plateau

Answer: 18. B. Intravenous nitroglycerine

Answer: 19. B. Increased LV filling pressure

RV infarction:

Isolated RV MI is rare, but an estimated 30% of patients with acute inferior MI have clinical or echocardiographic evidence of RV dysfunction or infarction

Most RV infarctions usually result from occlusion of the proximal RCA; mid and distal RCA occlusion usually spares enough RV branches of the RCA that RV infarction does not occur

Other causes of RV infarction: Dominant LCx or Type 3 LAD occlusion

Clinical presentation:

Classic triad of hypotension, increased jugular venous pressure, and clear lung fields

Other features: Kussmaul sign, pulsus paradoxus, and a positive hepatojugular reflux

Treatment:

Early reperfusion of the culprit artery (with thrombolysis or percutaneous coronary intervention),

Maintenance of RV preload- administration of isotonic saline

Inotropic support of the ventricular septum (which has a dual blood supply from the RCA and the left anterior descending coronary artery) and the dysfunctional RV,

Reduction of RV afterload, and maintenance of atrioventricular synchrony.

Specific Therapy to Avoid: Nitrates and diuretics may decrease the preload and can cause profound hypotension.

Complete heart block in MI:

Answer: 20. D. Always permanent pacemaker

Answer: 21. B. Generally due to increased parasympathetic activity

Complete heart block may occur with either an anterior or an inferior MI.

With inferior infarcts, the conduction defect is likely to be in the AVN, with escape rhythms exceeding 40 beats per minute and exhibiting a narrow QRS complex.

With an anterior MI, the conduction defect is infranodal and the escape rhythm (if present) is usually less than 40 beats per minute with a wide QRS complex.

Permanent pacing is almost always required for high grade block with anterior MI; the prognosis is poor because of the large amount of myocardium involved.

Complete heart block with inferior MI is usually transient and rarely requires permanent pacing; usually resolves spontaneously.

Mechanism:

Anterior infarction: extensive necrosis of infra-His conduction system due to severe ischemia

Multiple mechanisms in inferior MI: Increased parasympathetic tone or Ischemic "stunning" of AV node

Blood supply of cardiac conduction system:

SA node: RCA

LCX or dual blood supply

AV node: RCA 80%

LCX or dual blood supply 20%

Bundle of His: LAD 80%

AV bundle: RCA or dual blood supply 20%

Right bundle branch: LAD

Left bundle (Anterior fascicle): LAD

Left bundle (Posterior fascicle): LAD and RCA

Blood supply of papillary muscles:

The anterolateral papillary muscle: Dual arterial blood supply from the left anterior descending coronary artery and either its diagonal branch or a marginal branch of the left circumflex coronary artery.

The posteromedial papillary muscle: Single arterial blood supply from either the left circumflex or right coronary artery, depending on coronary dominance, which makes it particularly susceptible to ischemic injury.

MECHANICAL COMPLICATIONS OF MI:

Answer: 22. B. Ventricular septal rupture

Answer: 23. D. More common in normotensives than hypertensives

Answer: 24. D. It communicates with LV cavity through a wide neck

Answer: 25. b. Can occur with both large or focal area of MI

Answer: 26. a. It is more likely to occur in patients with a history of prior MI

Answer: 27. E. All of the above.

Answer: 28. D. All of the above.

Answer: 29. C. Papillary muscle rupture.

In view of flash pulmonary edema and hypotension. Hypotension combined with high left atrial pressure and large regurgitant orifice may not result in an MR murmur because of low driving pressure and lack of turbulence in the MR jet. Acute stent thrombosis is less likely in view of lack of ST elevation. Acute pulmonary embolism and RV infarct won't cause pulmonary edema.

Answer: 30. D. All of the above.

Posteromedial papillary muscle has blood supply from right coronary artery only and is more likely to rupture.

Answer: 31. D. Dynamic RV outflow obstruction

True and False Ventricular Aneurysms

True LV aneurysm is a discrete, thinned segment of the left ventricle that protrudes during both systole and diastole and has a broad neck. Rarely ruptures.

False LV aneurysm has a narrow neck, a result of a prior LV free wall rupture, and is contained solely by the adherent pericardium. Rupture is quite common.

The presence of hypertension and the use of corticosteroids and NSAIDs may promote aneurysm formation

Rupture of ventricular free wall:

Significant predisposing factors for early ventricular rupture are **old age and female sex**. Other commonly identified risk factors for cardiac rupture include hypertension, absence of ventricular hypertrophy, **absence of previous infarction**, poor collateral flow, and lateral wall MI.

Rupture typically occurs at the junction of normal and infarcted myocardium

Thrombolysis does not increase the overall risk of cardiac rupture but may accelerate the process of cell necrosis and **lead to earlier ventricular wall rupture**, usually within 24 hours of administration. PCI is associated with decreased free wall rupture.

Rupture of the Ventricular Septum

Frequently a serpiginous tract

Presents abruptly with hypotension

Acute RV failure, and a new pansystolic murmur

Inferior infarctions cause septal rupture in the basal inferior septum, whereas anterior infarctions cause rupture in the apical septum

Septal rupture from inferior wall MI has a worse prognosis than that associated with anterior wall infarction

Acute Mitral Regurgitation

Acute mitral regurgitation after MI can be due ischemia of the papillary muscle, papillary muscle rupture (either partial or complete), or mitral annular dilatation associated with LV failure

The blood supply to the **posteromedial papillary muscle** (derived only from PDA) is **more tenuous** than that to the anterolateral papillary muscle (derived from both the LAD and the LCX). Consequently, **90%** of papillary muscle ruptures involve the posteromedial papillary muscle

Infarctions associated with papillary muscle rupture are **usually small**, and frequently there is only single-vessel coronary disease

The classic systolic murmur of mitral regurgitation **may be absent** in acute severe mitral regurgitation

PERICARDIAL EFFUSION AND PERICARDITIS

Answer: 32. A. acute myocardial infarction

Answer: 33. B. Aspirin 650 mg q 6 h.

→ This is classic Dressler's syndrome, which is thought to be autoimmune. NSAIDs and steroids are best avoided as they may impair the left ventricle healing process and may promote rupture.

Answer: 34. B. Aspirin is given for symptomatic relief

Early pericarditis and pericardial effusion occur in about 20% of patients that do not receive reperfusion therapy for acute MI.

In contrast only 5% of patients who receive reperfusion therapy will develop this complication

Treatment is with **aspirin**, 650 mg every 4 to 6 hours.

Corticosteroids are generally **contraindicated** association with myocardial aneurysm formation and myocardial rupture

Postinfarction Syndrome (Dressler Syndrome)

Results from injury to mesothelial pericardial cells that release cardiac antigens and subsequently generate an inflammatory response in the pericardium, pleura, and lungs.

It typically occurs several weeks after infarction (mean duration is 1 to 8 weeks) and may be recurrent

Treatment is with aspirin, 650 mg every 4 to 6 hours, or NSAIDs

Cardiogenic shock in MI:

Answer: 35. D. 40%

Answer: 36. b. 70-year old patient with inferior wall MI and basal crepts and LVS3

→ Patient has features of cardiogenic shock

Most common cause of death in patients hospitalized with acute myocardial infarction is cardiogenic shock.

Defined as systolic blood pressure <90 mm Hg along with signs of inadequate tissue perfusion.

Cardiac index is typically **<2.2 L/min/m2** and pulmonary capillary wedge pressure (PCWP) is elevated, typically >18 mm Hg.

On examination, crepitations in chest, LVS3, cold peripheries, decreased urine output, altered mentation.

Develops after loss of **40%** of LV myocardium.

SHOCK trial: LV failure was most common cause of cardiogenic shock. In hospital mortality **59%.**

Answer: 37. D. In cases of inferior wall MI, ST segment elevation in lead III more than lead II is suggestive of occlusion of proximal left circumflex artery

→ ST elevation in II > III is suggestive of LCx involvement whereas III > II is s/o RCA occlusion.

Atrial infarctions:

Answer: 38. A. 10%

Answer: 39. A. LA is more commonly involved than RA

Atrial infarctions:

Seen in **10%** of STEMI patients and is usually associated with ventricular infarction.

More common in **RA** than LA.

Diagnosed by abnormalities of PTa segment, P wave morphology and development supraventricular arrhythmias.

Frequently complicated by **atrial arrhythmias** and has higher incidence of thromboembolism.

Associated with **reduced** secretion of atrial natriuretic peptide.

Answer: 40. C. Thick cap atheroma

High risk (vulnerable) plaques:

Associated with high risk of rupture and myocardial infarctions.

Features:

Thin fibrous cap, High lipid burden, Large necrotic core, intraplaque haemorrhage.

Whereas, thick fibrous cap, large amount of smooth muscles in plaque shoulder and low lipid burden are associated with low risk of rupture.

Answer: 41. D. Normal cardiac biomarkers

Indications of early angiography (Early invasive strategy) in USA/NSTEMI:

Angina in the presence of heart failure symptoms (pulmonary edema, an S3 gallop, or new mitral regurgitation)

Known left ventricular dysfunction

Hemodynamic instability

Positive non-invasive stress test (large area of ischemia)

Sustained ventricular tachycardia

Prior revascularization (prior coronary artery bypass grafting [CABG], or PCI within the last 6 months)

High risk scores (TIMI ≥3, GRACE score >140)

Newer guidelines recommend early PCI in rest angina despite intensive anti-ischemic therapy or with new ST depressions or elevated cardiac biomarkers also.

TIMI risk score for UA/NSTEMI

- Risk factor (each worth 1 point)
- Age ≥65 years
- ≥ 3 CAD risk factors
- Known CAD (stenosis ≥ 50 %)
- ASA use in past 7 days
- ≥ 2 anginal episodes within past 24 h
- ST segment deviation ≥ 0.5 mm
- Elevated cardiac biomarkers

→ High risk score is **≥3**.

GRACE score: Variables included in the score include age, history of CHF, history of MI, heart rate and blood pressure, presence of ST-segment depression, serum creatinine and elevated cardiac biomarkers, and no percutaneous coronary intervention (PCI) performed during hospitalization.

A score of **>140** is considered high.

Chronic stable angina

Answer: 42. B. About 50%.

Answer: 43. B. 50%.

Answer: 44. A. ST segment depression.

The most common finding on a resting ECG during an episode of angina is ST depression.

ECG in CSA:

Approximately half of the patients with chronic stable angina have a normal resting ECG.

The most common ECG findings in chronic CAD include nonspecific ST-T wave changes

During an anginal episode, the ECG becomes abnormal in about 50% of the patients with a normal baseline ECG

Noninvasive Stress Testing:

Diagnostic stress testing is valuable when the pretest probability of CAD is intermediate (10%–90%)

Exercise ECG

Mean sensitivity is 68% and specificity is 77%

Stress myocardial imaging

For patients who have abnormal resting ECGs (eg, from repolarization abnormalities, left ventricular hypertrophy, electronically paced ventricular rhythm, preexcitation syndromes, left bundle branch block, or digitalis effect), exercise perfusion imaging is superior to exercise ECG alone in localizing diseased vessels, identifying multivessel disease, and detecting areas of ischemia or infarction

Answer: 45. A. Exercise stress ECG.

Exercise stress ECG is probably the best test to order in this situation. The stress ECG will be very useful to evaluate for ischemia especially when the resting ECG is normal and the patient is able to exercise and achieve a good workload.

Note:

In the presence of anti-anginal therapy, the sensitivity of stress ECG is reduced and a negative stress test cannot be used to rule out significant CAD. Long-acting nitrates and beta blockers need to be stopped 2–3 days prior to the test.

Answer: 46. D. All of the above.

See chapter cardiac investigations.

Answer: 47. B. Stress test in females is associated with higher false-positive results compared with males.

→ Exercise stress ECG is associated with a higher rate of false-positive rates.

Answer: 48. C. Coronary artery bypass grafting (CABG) including left internal mammary artery (LIMA) to LAD artery.

→ CABG has received a class 1 recommendation in patients with diabetes mellitus and multivessel CAD (three vessel or complex two vessel including proximal LAD artery provided a LIMA graft can be anastomosed to the LAD artery).

Answer: 49. C. $\leq$22.

→ A low SYNTAX score is defined as $\leq$22. This score is based on location, severity, and extent of stenosis, with a low score indicating less complicated anatomy. A score of 23 to 32 is defined as intermediate, and a score $\geq$33 is defined as a high-risk score.

Miscellaneous:

Linked angina:

Answer: 50. D. 48 hours after anterior wall MI with no angina

Answer: 51. C. Normal coronaries

Answer: 52. C. Coronary arteries are normal on angiography

Linked angina:

The term "Linked angina" was coined by Smith et al which implies that gastrointestinal factors (GERD) bring on attacks of genuine angina in patients with **established CAD**.

Studies have suggested acid infusion in esophagus results in reduced coronary blood flow and brings out ischemic ECG changes in CAD patients.

Reflex coronary vasoconstriction is initiated by vagal irritation in the gastrointestinal tract

Also called as **cardio-esophageal reflex** is absent in Post cardiac transplant patients suggesting the neural mechanism of this phenomenon.

Patients have **significant coronary obstruction** which is further worsened with reflex vasoconstriction causing symptoms and ECG changes.

Answer: 53. A. Regional dyskinesia

Answer: 54. C. 24-48 hours of surgery

Periprocedural MI is common within 48 hours of surgery.

Answer: 55. B. ACE inhibitors

Behaves as dynamic LVOT obstruction due to systolic anterior motion of mitral leaflet

Answer: 56. A. Angiotensin-converting inhibitor.

Since his LV EF is <40%, he should be started on angiotensin converting enzyme inhibitor.

Answer: 57. C. Eplerenone 25 mg daily.

As the EF is <35%. There is no indication for an implantable cardioverter-defibrillator unless EF after 40 days remains <35%.

Answer: 58. Antioxidants

5 Risk Factors for Coronary Artery Diseases

Dyslipidemia and Atherosclerosis

1. **One of the following lipoprotein is not secreted from liver:**
   A. VLDL B. HDL
   C. Chylomicrons D. Lipoprotein (a)

2. **Enzyme stimulated after intracellular uptake of cholesterol:**
   A. LDL receptor
   B. ACAT (Acyl Co-A acyl transferase)
   C. HMG CoA reductase
   D. HMG CoA synthase

3. **Coconut oil contains:**
   A. Saturated fatty acids
   B. Monounsaturated fatty acids
   C. Polyunsaturated fatty acids
   D. Trans fatty acids

4. **Effects of exercise on lipid profile demonstrates greatest effect on?**
   A. LDL
   B. HDL
   C. Triglycerides
   D. Small dense LDL

5. **Metabolic syndrome is typically associated with all of the following except?**
   A. Increased waist circumference
   B. Elevated LDL-Cholesterol
   C. Impaired fasting glucose
   D. Low HDL-Cholesterol

6. **Following are features of vulnerable plaque except:**
   A. Increased macrophages
   B. Increased smooth muscle cells
   C. Increased T cells
   D. Neovascularization

7. **All of the following are true about Lipoprotein (a) except:**
   A. Statin and bile acid sequestrants do not decrease their level
   B. Diet and lifestyle modification decrease their level
   C. Positive family history increases risk of CAD
   D. Screened only in selected patients of established CAD

8. **Tangier disease is:**
   A. Familial hypercholesterolemia
   B. Familial HDL deficiency
   C. Lipoprotein lipase deficiency
   D. Abetalipoproteinemia

9. **"Plucked chicken" appearance of the skin in the axillae and skinfolds of a young person is characteristic of:**
   A. Type III hyperlipoproteinemia
   B. Type II hyperlipoproteinemia
   C. Pseudoxanthoma elasticum
   D. Abetalipoproteinemia

10. All of the following are true about pseudoxanthoma elasticum except?
A. Can cause CAD
B. Angioid streaks
C. Massive GI bleed is usually seen
D. ABCC6 gene

11. All of the following are true about pseudo-xanthoma elasticum except:
A. Calcium mitigates disease progression
B. Arteriosclerosis of coronary arteries
C. Angioid streaks on retina
D. It can cause massive GI haemorrhage

12. Palmer xanthomas are seen in which hyperlipoproteinemia?
A. Type I B. Type II
C. Type III D. Type IV

13. Intestinal microorganisms produce TMAO (Trimethylamine N-oxide) which is associated with increased risk of?
A. Atherosclerosis
B. Rheumatic heart disease
C. Neural tube defects and congenital heart disease
D. Dilated cardiomyopathy

14. Regarding fibrates all are true except:
A. Good efficacy in lowering fasting as well as post-prandial triglyceride levels
B. HDL-C-raising effects are modest
C. Antagonists of peroxisome proliferator-activated receptor- alpha (PPAR- alpha)
D. Reported to raise both serum creatinine and homocysteine in both short-term and long-term studies

15. Which of the following therapy has conclusively shown to increase HDL and decrease cardiovascular mortality?
A. Anacetrapib
B. Niacin
C. Fibrates
D. None of the above

16. Which of the following is associated with microalbumnuria?
A. Atorvastatin
B. Metoprolol
C. Amlodipine
D. Lisinopril

17. Which of the following is not a cause of hypertriglyceridemia?
A. Oral estrogens
B. Excessive alcohol intake
C. Amiodarone
D. Diabetes mellitus

18. Which of the following may result in elevation of LDL-C?
A. Diuretics
B. Cyclosporine
C. Amiodarone
D. Biliary obstruction
E. All of the above

19. Atorvastatin blocks formation of which of the following substrate by 3-hydroxy 3–methylglutaryl CoA inhibition:
A. Squalene
B. Isopentenyl 5 pyrophosphate
C. Mevalonic acid
D. Acetoacetyl CoA

20. All of the following are true about pitavastatin all except:
A. Increases HDL also
B. Metabolised by CYP 3A4
C. Less drug interaction
D. Less myositis

21. Which of the following is not primary prevention trial for lipids?
A. WHO
B. WOSCOPS
C. AFCAPS
D. 4S

Hypertension

22. All are true about management of hypertension in black patients except:
A. Multiple drug combinations are often required
B. ACE inhibitors are less effective
C. Thiazide diuretics have high BP lowering efficacy
D. Significantly low incidence of angioedema with ACE inhibitors

23. Which of the following food/nutrients has convincing effect on lowering hypertension?
A. Dark Chocolate
B. High calcium intake
C. Vitamin D
D. Soy foods

24. Drug of choice for malignant hypertension with renal ischemia?
A. Fenoldopam B. Nitroprusside
C. Nicardipine D. Enalaprilat

25. A 25-year-old female patient has history of chronic kidney disease (CKD) stage 2. She denies any cardiac symptoms. Her vitals are heart rate 76 bpm, BP 170/98 mmHg. Her physical exam is otherwise normal. She is on furosemide 40 mg daily. What would your add-on drug of choice in this patient be?
A. Amlodipine B. Clonidine
C. Lisinopril D. Hydralazine

26. What is the BP goal for a 62-year-old patient according to the JNC 8 guidelines?
A. <140/90 mmHg
B. <150/90 mmHg
C. <160/100 mmHg
D. <160/90 mmHg

27. What is the BP goal for a 42 year old patient with diabetes mellitus according to the JNC 8 guidelines?
A. <140/90 mmHg
B. <150/90 mmHg
C. <160/100 mmHg
D. <160/90 mmHg

28. Which is the most preferred drug to treat hypertension in pregnancy according to the JNC 8 guidelines?
A. Labetalol B. Nifedipine
C. Methyldopa D. ACEI

29. An elderly patient presents with BP of 170/90 mmHg. All of the following are the first line antihypertensive drugs except:
A. B blocker B. Amlodipine
C. Chlorthalidone D. ACE inhibitor

30. Which antihypertensive agent may reduce uric acid levels?
A. Diuretic B. CCB
C. Losartan D. Candesartan

31. Which antihypertensive agent may reduce migraine attacks?
A. Diuretic B. CCB
C. Losartan D. Candesartan

32. Which antihypertensive agent may result in gynecomastia?
A. Spironolactone B. CCB
C. Losartan D. Candesartan

33. What is the recommended daily Na restriction in hypertension?
A. <2400 mg B. <1200 mg
C. <500 mg D. None of the above

34. What systolic BP (SBP) goal does the Systolic Blood Pressure Intervention Trial (SPRINT) support?
A. <120 mmHg B. <130 mmHg
C. <140 mmHg D. <150 mmHg

35. Clinical characteristics of Hypertensive crisis:
A. Diastolic BP >120 mm of Hg
B. Congestive heart failure

C. Microangiopathic hemolysis
D. All of the above

Diabetes Mellitus

36. In diabetes all of the following are true for PCI as compared to CABG except?
A. PCI increases mortality
B. PCI increases MI
C. CABG decreased incidence of stroke
D. CABG decreases rate of revascularization

37. Which of the following antidiabetic drug doesn't cause weight gain?
A. Insulin
B. Sulfonylurea
C. Pioglitazone
D. Canagliflozin

38. Which of the following statements is not true?
A. The FREEDOM trial showed that coronary artery bypass grafting (CABG) surgery is superior to percutaneous coronary intervention (PCI)
B. The benefit of CABG was due to lower rates of myocardial infarction and death from any cause
C. CABG was associated with lesser number of stroke rates as compared to PCI
D. All-cause mortality was higher with PCI

Miscellaneous

39. Red wine exerts cardiovascular benefits by:
A. Resveratrol
B. Selenium
C. Berberine
D. Arginine

40. Which of the following NSAIDs does not cause hypertension?
A. Indomethacin
B. Aspirin
C. Piroxicam
D. Colecoxib

41. Prehypertension in children is defined as:
A. B/W 90-95th percentile N for age and sex
B. B/W 85-90th perrcentile N for age and sex
C. B/W 80-85 percentile N for age and sex
D. B/W 95-99 perrcentile N for a e and sex

42. Framingham risk score includes all except:
A. Family history B. Smoking
C. Age D. Diabetes

ANSWERS

Dyslipidemia

Answer: 1. C. Chylomicrons

Chylomicrons are synthesized in enterocytes.

Answer: 2. B. ACAT (Acyl Co-A acyl transferase)

Metabolism of lipids:

Lipids are transported in the body in the form of lipoprotein (combination of lipids and lipoprotein), in which protein part is known as apolipoprotein.

IDL is the most atherogenic lipoprotein, but LDL (which carries 70% of plasma cholesterol) is the principle lipoprotein responsible for atherosclerosis.

TG rich lipoproteins: Chylomicrons, VLDL.

1. Chylomicrons are synthesized by enterocytes from the lipids absorbed in the gut. VLDL are synthesized in the liver. Both chylomicrons and VLDL transfer energy rich triacylglycerol to cells in the body. TAG is removed from chylomicrons and VLDL by lipoprotein lipase found on endothelial cells.
2. After removal of TAG from VLDL, VLDL particles become condensed and they are remodelled in liver into LDL. The function of LDL is to transfer cholesterol to cells for synthesis of membrane or hormones. LDL binds to LDL receptor and is internalized in an endocytic vesicle.
3. Excess cholesterol is removed from the body by two pathways. Liver removes LDL from circulation by receptor mediated endocytosis. Additionally, excess cholesterol from cells is brought back to liver by HDL by reverse cholesterol transport.

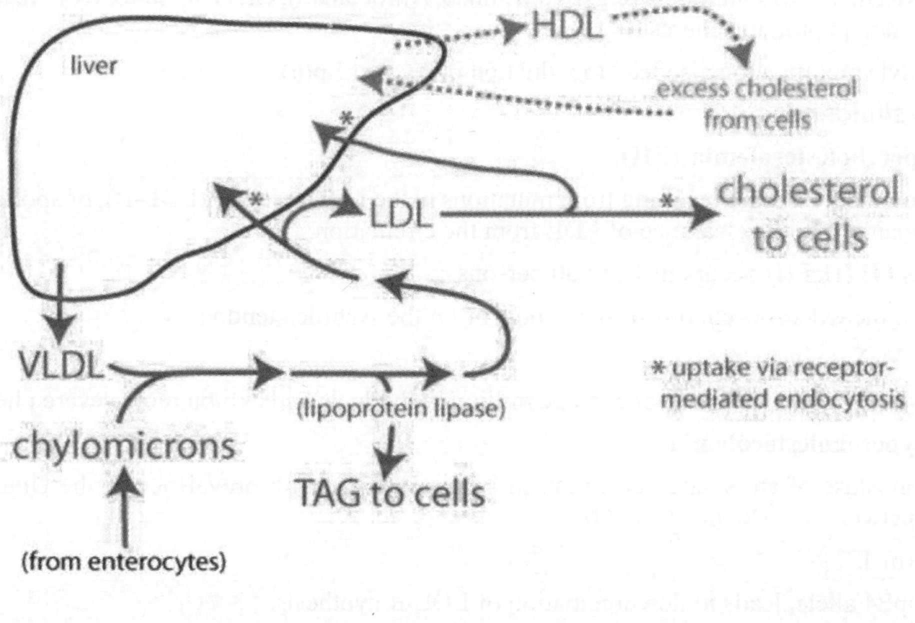

Answer: 3. A. Saturated fatty acids

Answer: 4. C. Triglycerides

Answer: 5. B. Elevated LDL-Cholesterol

Answer: 6. B. Increased smooth muscle cells

Increased smooth muscle cells are seen in stable non-vulnerable plaque.

Answer: 7. B. Diet and lifestyle modification decrease their level

Answer: 8. B. Familial HDL deficiency

Answer: 9. C. Pseudoxanthoma elasticum

Answer: 10. C. Massive GI bleed

Answer: 11. A. Calcium mitigates disease progression

Answer: 12. C. Type III

Lipoprotein (a):

Lipoprotein (a), or Lp(a), is an LDL-like particle but unlike LDL, apoB 100 on the surface of Lp(a) is bound to a protein called apolipoprotein (a), or apo(a), which has strong homologies to plasminogen. Promotes prothrombotic state and increases risk of CAD.

Statins don't decrease their level.

Reduced by Niacin, PCSK9 inhibitors (e.g. Evolocumab, Alirocumab), CETP inhibitors (eg Anacetrapib), Mipomersen and lipoprotein apheresis.

Diet and lifestyle modification also lead to reduction in level of Lp(a)

Primary Dyslipidemias

Familial hypercholesterolemia (FH)

Autosomal dominant disorder resulting from mutations in the LDL receptor (LDL-R), or apoB receptor, leading to impaired hepatic clearance of LDL from the circulation.

Heterozygous FH (HeFH) occurs in 1 in 500 persons

Xanthomas on the extensor tendons of the hands, or on the Achilles tendons

High risk of CAD at young age.

Homozygous FH (HoFH) occurs in one in one million individuals and exhibit more severe phenotype.

Polygenic hypercholesterolemia:

Most common cause of an isolated elevation in TC or LDL-C, with prevalence in the United States estimated at between 1 in 20 and 1 in 100.

TG levels normal.

Presence of apE4 allele, leads to downregulation of LDL-R synthesis.

Xanthomas are absent.

Familial combined hyperlipidemia:

One of the commonest dyslipidemia, population prevalence of 1% to 3%.

Two to fivefold increased risk of CHD.

High total cholesterol, TG, LDL and low HDL.

Arcus cornea and xanthelasmas are commonly seen, but tendon xanthomas are unusual

Hyperapobetalipotroteinemia:

Very high levels of TG

Arcus xanthoma, xanthelasma present but no tendon xanthomas.

Familial Dysbetalipoproteinemia (Type III hyperlipidemia):

Defective apoE, usually AR, high CAD risk

Planar xanthomas of palmer creases

Tuberous xanthomas of knees and elbows not attached to tendons

Familial mixed hypertriglyceridemia:

High TG level

No xanthomas, CAD risk not elevated.

Familial chylomicronemia:

LPL or apoC-II mutations leads to accumulation of chylomicrons

AR, very high TG levels

Eruptive xanthomas on extensor limb surfaces, hepatosplenomegaly, pancreatitis

Unclear association with CAD.

Secondary dyslipidemia:

Elevated TC and LCL-C:

Diet rich in saturated fat, drugs (oral contraceptives or OCPs, HRT, HAART, Thiazide diuretics, cyclosporine, amiodarone), hypothyroidism, nephrotic syndrome, chronic liver disease, and chronic biliary tract disease (classically, primary biliary cirrhosis).

Elevated TG: Diet rich in carbohydrates, drugs (blockers, thiazide diuretics, isotretinoin, glucocorticoids, HAART, OCP HRT), excessive alcohol consumption, obesity, DM, hypothyroidism, CRI, chronic pancreatitis, and pregnancy.

Metabolic Syndrome

1. Waist circumference over 40 in. (men) or 35 in. (women)
2. Blood pressure over 130/85 mmHg
3. Fasting triglyceride (TG) level over 150 mg/dl
4. Fasting HDL cholesterol less than 40 (men) or 50 (women) mg/dl
5. Fasting blood sugar over 100 mg/dl

Tangier's disease:

Familial alpha-lipoprotein deficiency (defective ABCA1 transporter) causing severe **reduction in HDL**. **Yellow/orange discolouration of tonsils** by deposition of various esters.

Risk factor for CAD

Pseudoxanthoma elasticum:

AR mutation in ABCC6 gene on chromosome 16 affecting skin and eyes.

Features:

Plucked chicken appearance

Angioid streaks in retina and retinal hemorrhages

GI haemorrhage, rarely can be massive.

Premature atherosclerosis and CAD, aortic regurgitation.

Xanthomas:

Palmer crease xanthoma: Type III hyperlipoproteinemia

Tendon xanthoma: Type II hyperlipoproteinemia

Eruptive xanthoma: Type I and V hyperlipoproteinemia; Not associated with coronary artery disease.

Answer: 13. A. Atherosclerosis

Some type of human gut flora converts dietary carnitine to TMAO.

In the presence of TMAO, there is increased deposition and decreased removal of cholesterol from the peripheral cells increasing risk of atherosclerosis.

Lipid lowering drugs:

Answer: 14. C. Antagonists of peroxisome proliferator-activated receptor- alpha (PPAR- alpha)

Answer: 15. D. None of the above

Drugs which can increase HDL levels: Niacin, Fibrates, Anacetrapib.

HDL lowering with any drug has not been associated with reduction in cardiovascular mortality.

Answer: 16. A. Atorvastatin.

Answer: 17. C. Amiodarone.

Answer: 18. E. All of the above.

Answer: 19. C. Mevalonic acid

Answer: 20. B. Metabolised by CYP 3A4

Answer: 21. D. 4S

Statins:

Inhibit HMG-CoA reductase (the rate limiting enzyme in cholesterol synthesis) and prevent the formation of mevalonic acid which upregulates LDL-R and increases hepatic LDL clearance.

$$\text{HMG CoA} \xrightarrow{\text{HMG CoA reductase}} \text{Mevalonic acid}$$

Decrease TC, LDL, TG and increase HDL.

Adverse effects: Myopathy, rhabdomyolysis, increased hepatic transaminases, microalbuminuria

Resins:

Cholestyramine, Colestipol, Colesevelam

Bind intestinal bile acids, interrupt enterohepatic recycling and increase stool elimination of bile acids.

Decrease TC, LDL and increase HDL and TG.

Side effects: Constipation, diarrhoea, flatulence, **hypertriglyceridemia**

Fibrates: Agonist of PPAR-alpha, increase catabolism of triglyceride and increases HDL-C.

Increase HDL, decrease TG, TC and LDL.

Nicotinic acid:

Increase HDL, decrease LDL, TG and Lp (a).

Side effects: Hepatotoxicity, gout, flushing, hyperuricemia, hyperglycemia.

Ezetimibe:

Cholesterol absorption inhibitors.

Decrease cholesterol transport across intestinal brush border.

Decrease TC, LDL and TG

IMPROVE IT trial: Combination of ezetimibe with a statin showed modest benefit in reducing heart disease.

Omega-3 fatty acids: Fish oil.

Decrease TG and increase HDL and LDL.

Proprotein convertase subtilisin/kexin type 9 (PCSK9) inhibitors:

PCSK9 is a protein which binds to LDL receptors and targets them for breakdown. Hence, PCSK9 inhibitors prevent degradation of LDL receptors and increase clearance of LDL from the body. E.g.: Alirocumab, Evolocumab

Lipids trials:

Primary prevention trials: WHO, HHS, WOSCOPS, AFCAPS, ASCOT-LLA

Secondary prevention trials: 4S, CARE, LIPID, HPS

Current ATP-III guidelines:

Risk Category	LDL-C Goal	Initiate TLC	Consider Drug Therapy[a]
High risk: CHD[b] ro CHD risk equivalents[c] (10-y risk >20%)	<100 mg/dL (optional goal: <70 mg/dL)[d]	≥100 mg/dL[e]	≥100 mg/dL[f](<100 mg/dL: consider drug options)[a]
Moderately high risk: 2+ risk factors (10-y risk >20%)[g]	<130 mg/dL (optional goal: <100 mg/dL)	≥130 mg/dL[e]	≥130 mg/dL (<100–129 mg/dL: consider drug options)[a]
Moderate risk: 2+ risk factor (10-y risk <10%)[g]	<130 mg/dL	≥130 mg/dL	≥160 mg/dL
Lower risk: 0–1 risk factor[i]	<160 mg/dL	≥160 mg/dL	≥190 mg/dL (<160–189 mg/dL: LDL-lowering drug options)[a]

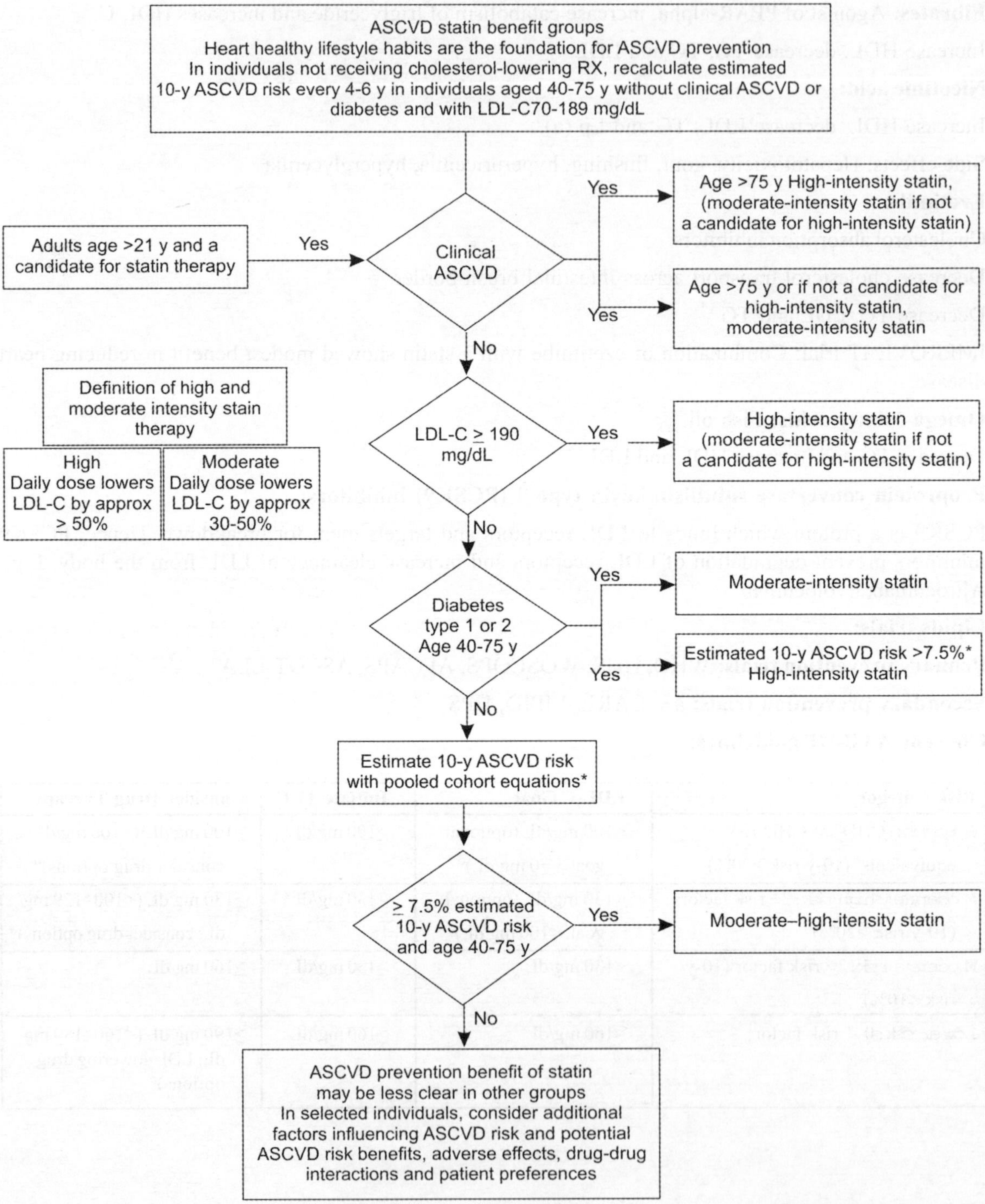

ASCVD statin benefit groups
Heart healthy lifestyle habits are the foundation for ASCVD prevention
In individuals not receiving cholesterol-lowering RX, recalculate estimated 10-y ASCVD risk every 4-6 y in individuals aged 40-75 y without clinical ASCVD or diabetes and with LDL-C70-189 mg/dL
Adults age >21 y and a candidate for statin therapy
Yes
Clinical ASCVD
Yes
Age >75 y High-intensity statin, (moderate-intensity statin if not a candidate for high-intensity statin)
Yes
Age >75 y or if not a candidate for high-intensity statin, moderate-intensity statin
No
Definition of high and moderate intensity stain therapy
High
Daily dose lowers LDL-C by approx ≥ 50%
Moderate
Daily dose lowers LDL-C by approx 30-50%
LDL-C ≥ 190 mg/dL
Yes
High-intensity statin (moderate-intensity statin if not a candidate for high-intensity statin)
No
Diabetes type 1 or 2 Age 40-75 y
Yes
Moderate-intensity statin
Yes
Estimated 10-y ASCVD risk >7.5%* High-intensity statin
No
Estimate 10-y ASCVD risk with pooled cohort equations*
≥ 7.5% estimated 10-y ASCVD risk and age 40-75 y
Yes
Moderate–high-itensity statin
No
ASCVD prevention benefit of statin may be less clear in other groups
In selected individuals, consider additional factors influencing ASCVD risk and potential ASCVD risk benefits, adverse effects, drug-drug interactions and patient preferences

Hypertension

Answer: 22. D. Significantly low incidence of angioedema with ACE inhibitors

Answer: 23. A. Dark Chocolate

Answer: 24. A. Fenoldopam

Labetalol as per newer guidelines.

Answer: 25. C. Lisinopril.

Answer: 26. B. <150/90 mmHg.

Answer: 27. A. <140/90 mmHg.

Answer: 28. A. Labetalol.

Nifedipine and methyldopa are acceptable. An ACEI is contraindicated.

Answer: 29. A. B blocker

Answer: 30. C. Losartan.

Answer: 31. D. Candesartan.

Answer: 32. A. Spironolactone.

Answer: 33. A. <2400 mg.

Answer: 34. A. <120 mmHg.

Answer: 35. D. All of the above

Hypertension is the single greatest modifiable risk factor for CV disease, causing more disability and premature death than smoking, dyslipidemia, obesity, diabetes and the other classical risk factors for heart disease.

Hypertension in black patients:

1. Incidence and prevalence of cardiovascular and renal complications of hypertension are greater in blacks.
2. Relative risk of stroke is twice than whites.
3. Greater risk of treatment resistant hypertension and often multiple drugs are required.
4. ACE inhibitors are less effective and cause high incidence of angioedema in blacks.
5. Thiazides and CCBs maintain high BP lowering efficacy.

BP Measurement

Seated comfortably for 5 minutes with back fully supported

Brachial artery maintained at heart level

Use a cuff with a bladder that encompasses at least 80% of the upper arm

Individuals must not talk during BP measurement; talking increases BP by up to 20 mm Hg

Ambulatory blood pressure monitoring (ABPM)

Average blood pressure does not exceed in a sustained fashion 135/85 mm Hg in the awake state or 125/75 mm Hg while asleep

JNC 8 Recommendations

Recommendation 1: Aged ≥60 years, initiate pharmacologic treatment to lower BP at SBP ≥150 mmHg or DBP ≥90 mmHg and treat to an SBP goal of <150 mmHg and a DBP goal of <90 mmHg. (Strong recommendation – grade A).

Recommendation 2: Aged <60 years, initiate pharmacologic treatment to lower BP at SBP ≥140 or DBP ≥90 mmHg and treat to an SBP goal of <140 and DBP goal of <90 mmHg. (For ages 30–59 years).

Recommendation 3: Aged ≥18 years with CKD, initiate pharmacologic treatment to lower BP at SBP ≥140 mmHg or DBP ≥90 mmHg and treat to an SBP goal of <140 mmHg and a DBP goal of <90 mmHg.

Recommendation 4: Aged ≥18 years with diabetes, initiate pharmacologic treatment to lower BP at SBP ≥140 mmHg or DBP ≥90 mmHg and treat to an SBP goal of <140 mmHg and a DBP goal of <90 mmHg.

Recommendation 5: General nonblack population, including those with diabetes, initial antihypertensive treatment should include a thiazide-type diuretic, CCB, ACEI, or ARB. Note that beta blocker is not a first-line drug.

Recommendation 6: General black population, including those with diabetes, initial antihypertensive treatment should include a thiazide-type diuretic or CCB.

Recommendation 7: Aged ≥18 years with **CKD**, initial (or add-on) antihypertensive treatment should include an **ACEI or ARB** to improve kidney outcomes. This applies to all CKD patients with hypertension regardless of race or diabetes status.

Resistant Hypertension

Defined as blood pressure not controlled with use of three drugs including one diuretic in recommended doses.

All patients with resistant hypertension should be evaluated for secondary hypertension.

Hypertensive crisis (Malignant hypertension)

Severely elevated blood pressure (SBP > 180 or DBP > 120) is referred as hypertensive crisis.

2 types:

1. Hypertensive emergency

Diagnosed when there is evidence of direct damage to one or more organs due to severely elevated blood pressure

May include hypertensive encephalopathy, retinal papilledema or exudates, Chest pain, Pulmonary edema due to CHF, AKI, Microangiopathic hemolytic anemia

2. Hypertensive urgency

Severely elevated blood pressure when there is no evidence of target organ damage.

Trials:

SPRINT trial: Patients with hypertension and SBP >130 mmHg and at high cardiovascular risk (renal disease, heart disease, stroke), but not diabetes, were randomized to intensive BP control (SBP <120 mmHg) versus traditional control (SBP <140 mmHg).

Both the cumulative events and deaths were about 25% lower the in intensive treatment group.

ACCORD trial: Type 2 diabetes patients aged 40–79 years at high risk for cardiovascular disease (CVD) events. Participants were randomly assigned to hemoglobin A1c goals of <6.0% (<42 mmol/mol; intensive glycemia) or 7.0–7.9% (53–63 mmol/mol; standard glycemia) and then randomized a second time to either (1) SBP goals of <120 mmHg (intensive BP) or <140 mmHg (standard BP) or (2) simvastatin plus fenofibrate (intensive lipid) or simvastatin plus placebo (standard lipid).

Compared with combined standard treatment, intensive BP or intensive glycemia treatment alone improved major CVD outcomes, without additional benefit from combining the two.

Diabetes mellitus

Answer: 36. C. CABG decreased incidence of stroke

Answer: 37. D. Canagliflozin

Answer: 38. C. CABG was associated with lesser number of stroke rates as compared to PCI

Diagnosis of Diabetes mellitus:

A. Hemoglobin (Hb) A1C >6.5%

B. Fasting glucose >126 mg/dL

C. 2 h glucose >200 mg/dL

Indication of bariatric surgery in obese patients:

BMI >40 kg/m2 with no comorbidities or BMI >35 kg/m2 with an obesity-related comorbidity with no response to behavioral or pharmacological treatment

Drugs producing weight gain:

A. Thiazolidinediones

B. Insulin

C. Glinides

D. Sulfonylureas

Dipeptidyl peptidase inhibitors are weight neutral

Drugs producing weight loss:

A. Metformin

B. Pramlintide

C. Exenatide

D. Liraglutide

E. Sodium-glucose cotransporter-2 inhibitors

Thiazolidinediones:

Both rosiglitazone and pioglitazone are associated with weight gain and fluid retention, and should be used with caution in CHF.

Rosiglitazone is associated with excess risk for nonfatal MI

Sodium-Glucose cotransporter 2 (SGLT2) inhibitors:

Examples- Empagliflozin, Canagliflozin, Dapagliflozin, Ertugliflozin.

Mechanism of action- Block SGLT2 receptor in the proximal tubule of the kidney, increase urinary excretion of glucose as well as sodium.

Hence reduce sugars, blood pressure and body weight.

EMPA-REG OUTCOME TRIAL- Empagliflozin showed significant 14% reduction in CV death, MI and stroke as compared to placebo in high risk diabetic patients on optimal medical therapy. All reduced all cause mortality, hospitalizations for heart failure.

CANVAS Trial- Canagliflozin reduced MACE rates in high risk diabetic patients as compared to the placebo but did not reach clinical significance.

Two additional hazards were seen, which were doubling risk of **lower limb amputations** and smaller increase in **risk of fracture**.

DM and CAD trials:

ACCORD: Intensive therapy in CAD patients resulting in HbA1c of 6.4 % is associated with increased mortality.

BARI 2D:

No clear benefit from early elective revascularization with PCI or CABG as compared with optimal medical therapy.

In patients with DM2, mortality was lower with CABG than multi-vessel PCI

SYNTAX:

Patients with DM2 and 3VD or LM disease have better outcome with CABG than PCI.

FREEDOM:

Showed superiority of CABG over PCI in diabetic patients with advanced CAD in terms of MI and all-cause mortality.

However, strokes were more frequent in the CABG group.

Primary prevention of CAD in DM

For primary prevention, AHA recommends aspirin (75 to 162 mg) per day for patients with diabetes, age 50 years or older with one or more additional CVD risk factors.

Therapeutic lifestyle counselling (TLC) interventions- Regular physical activity, nutritional counselling for weight management and healthy food choices, and counseling for smoking abstinence

Medical nutrition therapy should be targeted at caloric restriction for weight management, increased dietary fiber intake, and limited fat intake (<30% of daily energy; <7% from saturated fats)

Intake of total cholesterol <200mg/day and trans-fatty acids should be <1% of daily fat intake.

Leisure time physical activity targets are at least 150 minutes weekly of modest-intensity exercise, or at least 90 minutes weekly of vigorous exercise.

Miscellaneous

Answer: 39. A. Resveratrol

Answer: 40. B. Aspirin

Answer: 41. A. B/W 90-95th percentile N for age and sex

Answer: 42. A. Family history

Framingham risk score:

Gender specific score used to predict 10-year cardiovascular risk of an individual.

Modified in 2008, includes the following points:

1. Age
2. Total cholesterol
3. Smoking
4. HDL cholesterol
5. Systolic blood pressure

Prior version of Framingham risk score published in 2002, included Age, Sex, LDL, HDL, Blood pressure, Diabetes and smoking. Updated version in 2008 excluded diabetes, type 2 diabetes is now considered as CHD risk equivalent, having same 10-year risk as patient with prior CHD.

6 Heart Failure, Cardiomyopathies and Pericardial Diseases

Physiology of Heart Failuret Failure

1. **Which of the following pathways contribute to cardiac dysfunction in Heart failure:**
   A. Necrosis
   B. Apoptosis
   C. Autophagy
   D. All of the above

2. **Which of the following is a marker of Oxidative stress in Heart failure?**
   A. Myeloperoxidase
   B. Tumor necrosis factor
   C. Brain natriuretic peptide
   D. Matrix metalloproteinases

3. **One of the following does not belong to Natriuretic peptide family:**
   A. ANP B. BNP
   C. Urodilantin D. Urotensin

4. **Brain natriuretic peptide levels are increased in all of the following, except:**
   A. Constrictive pericarditis
   B. Restrictive cardiomyopathy
   C. Non-ischemic cardiomyopathy
   D. Severe aortic stenosis with left ventricular dysfunction

5. **Decreased BNP concentrations may be found in?**
   A. Older individuals
   B. Females
   C. Obesity
   D. Cirrhosis

6. **What is the increase in myocardial contractile force with increase in preload called?**
   A. Frank–Starling phenomenon
   B. Anrep phenomenon
   C. Bowditch phenomenon
   D. None of the above.

7. **What is the increase in myocardial contractile force with acute increase in afterload called?**
   A. Frank–Starling phenomenon
   B. Anrep phenomenon
   C. Bowditch phenomenon
   D. None of the above.

8. **What is the increase in myocardial contractile force with increase in heart rate called?**
   A. Frank–Starling phenomenon
   B. Anrep phenomenon
   C. Bowditch phenomenon
   D. None of the above.

9. **What is true about Bowditch effect is?**
   A. Also called as treppe phenomenon or Force frequency relationship
   B. This phenomenon is muted in heart failure
   C. This phenomenon occurs only upto an optimal heart rate (usually upto 150-180/min)
   D. All the above

10. Maximum systolic tension develops at sarcomere length of:

A. 2.4 mm B. 2.2 mm
C. 2.8 mm D. 1.2 mm

11. Compared with atrial myocyte, ventricular myocyte is which of the following?

A. Longer
B. Broader
C. Has more T tubules
D. All of the above

12. T tubules are absent in?

A. Ventricular myocyte
B. Atrial myocyte
C. Purkinje cells
D. None of the above

13. Which of the following has most abundant gap junctions?

A. Ventricular myocyte
B. Atrial myocyte
C. Purkinje cells
D. None of the above

HFrEF

14. Major criteria for the diagnosis of Heart failure with normal Ejection fraction (EF):

A. Ankle edema
B. Hepatojugular reflex
C. Hepatomegaly
D. Nocturnal cough

15. Not a major criterion in Framingham's criteria for heart failure is:

A. PND
B. Rales
C. Hepatomegaly
D. Hepatojuglar reflux

16. Which of the following is not a major Framingham Criteria for diagnosis of heart failure?

A. Paroxysmal nocturnal dyspnea
B. Hepatojugular reflux
C. Hepatomegaly
D. Response to diuretics

17. The major Framingham criteria for HF include:

A. S3
B. Paroxysmal nocturnal dyspnea
C. Basal rales
D. All of the above

18. The minor Framingham criteria for HF include which of the following:

A. Shortness of breath
B. Edema
C. Nocturnal cough
D. All of the above

19. Which of the following agents has not shown improvement in survival in heart failure with reduced ejection fraction (HFrEF)?

A. Carvedilol and metoprolol succinate
B. Digoxin
C. Angiotensin-converting-enzyme inhibitor (ACEI)
D. Spironolactone

20. In a patient with systolic heart failure on optimal doses of carvedilol and spironolactone, which drug is likely to produce maximum mortality and HF admission benefit?

A. ACEI
B. Angiotensin receptor blocker
C. Neprilysin inhibitor
D. Diuretic

HFpEF

21. Which of the following agents has shown improvement in survival in heart failure with preserved ejection fraction?

A. Carvedilol and metoprolol succinate
B. ACEI

C. Spironolactone
D. None of the above

22. In diastolic HF, findings in echo all except:
A. Normal LV size
B. Increased LA size
C. Near normal LVEF
D. Eccentric LVH

Heart Transplant

23. Which of the following is level 3 in INTERMACS criteria heart failure?
A. Critical cardiogenic shock
B. Stable but inotrope dependent
C. Recurrent advanced heart failure
D. NYHA III sypmtoms

24. Which of the following drugs may retard cardiac allograft vasculopathy?
A. Sirolimus
B. Everolimus
C. Statins
D. Mycophenolate mofetil
E. All of the above.

25. Which of the following are potential side effects of tacrolimus?
A. Diabetes mellitus
B. Tremor
C. Anemia
D. All of the above

26. Potential side effects of cyclosporine include which of the following?
A. Hypertension
B. Hypercholesterolemia
C. Increase in creatinine
D. All of the above

27. Which statin has least interaction with immune suppressants?
A. Simvastatin B. Pravastatin
C. Atorvastatin D. Rosuvastatin

28. Which immunosuppressant may increase serum creatinine level?
A. Sirolimus
B. Cyclosporine
C. Mycophenolate mofetil
D. Corticosteroid

Myocarditis

29. Dallas criteria is used for diagnosis of:
A. Post partum cardiomyopathy
B. Myocarditis
C. Acute rheumatic fever
D. Marfan's syndrome

Cardiomyopathies

30. What is the most common mode of inheritance in DCMP?
A. Autosomal dominant
B. Autosomal recessive
C. X-linked
D. Mitochondrial

31. A 19-year-old patient has DCM with EF of 10%, complete heart block, junctional escape rhythm with left bundle branch block (LBBB), and muscle weakness. What is the likely mutation in?
A. Lamin A/C gene
B. Troponin T gene
C. Desmin gene
D. Titin gene

32. Which of the following is not a standard indication for starting anticoagulation in a patient with dilated cardiomyopathy?
A. Male, 30 years, DCM, EF of 10%
B. Male, 30 years, DCM, EF of 25%, apical thrombus
C. Male, 30 years, DCM, EF is 20%, multiple TIAs
D. Male, 30 years, DCM, EF 35%, left ven-

tricle is hypertrabeculated with non-compacted to compacted ratio of 2.5

33. Arrhythmogenic right ventricular dysplasia (ARVD) was coined for the first time in 1978 for "total or partial replacement of right ventricular muscle by adipose and fibrous tissue associated with arrhythmias." True regarding ARVD is:

A. No familial predilection of ARVD/C has been recognized
B. The sites of involvement are found in the so-called "triangle of dysplasia", namely, the right ventricular inflow, tricuspid valve and moderator band.
C. The ECG in patients with ARVD/C usually shows sinus rhythm and a terminal deflection within or at the end of the QRS complex (called epsilon wave) in leads V5 & V6
D. The tachyarryhythmias occurring in ARVD are characteristically monomorphic and LBBB morphology, usually with inferior QRS axis

34. Arrhythmogenic right ventricular cardiomyopathy is a disease of:

A. Tropomyosin
B. Intercalated disc
C. Myosin light chain
D. Mitochondrial DNA

35. Epsilon waves are seen in:

A. Ebstein anomaly
B. Endomyocardial fibrosis
C. Arrhythmogenic Right ventricular dysplasia
D. Hypertrophic cardiomyopathy

36. Takotsubo cardiomyopathy is related to?

A. Peripartum
B. Stress
C. Inflammation
D. Tachycardia

37. Which one of following is not true for Takotsubo cardiomyopathy?

A. It is irreversible
B. It is known as apical ballooning syndrome also.
C. ECG may mimic acute myocardial infarction
D. Most common in postmenopausal woman

38. All of the following are true about Takotsubo cardiomyopathy except?

A. Coronary angiography is normal/shows insignificant coronary artery stenosis
B. Most commonly seen in young males
C. Catecholamine induced cardiotoxicity
D. Reversible LV dysfunction

39. Takotsubo cardiomyopathy all except:

A. LGE on CMR generally absent
B. Precordial ST elevation essential to diagnose
C. Blood catecholamine level is not uniformly elevated
D. RWMA typically extends beyond a single epicardial coronary artery distribution

40. Following a post-premature beat the left ventricular outflow gradient is increased with a reduction in the pulse pressure of the aortic contour. In this regard, identify the false statement:

A. This maneuver is called as Brockenbrough maneuver.
B. A premature ventricular beat may also accentuate the spike-and-dome configuration of the aortic pressure waveform.
C. This is classically associated with restrictive cardiomyopathy.
D. The paradoxical haemodynamic response to post extrasystolic potentiation is explained by dynamic narrowing of the LVOT.

41. In patients with HOCM, echo screening of their son/daughter should be started at age of:

A. 5 years B. 9 years
C. 12 years D. 23 years

42. Which of the following statements is not accurate regarding screening of first degree relative of newly diagnosed hypertrophic cardiomyopathy patient?

A. It is appropriate to screen first-degree relatives with an echocardiogram
B. It is strongly recommended to screen first-degree relatives for high risk genotypes
C. It is appropriate to perform a physical examination and an electrocardiogram (ECG) in first-degree relatives
D. It is appropriate to screen adult first-degree relatives every 5 years and children every 12–18 months.

43. A 20 years old gentleman has been detected to have same MHC gene mutation as his father who is a known case of HCM. The son has normal physical examination, ECG, and an echocardiogram. How frequently would you repeat an echocardiogram on this son?

A. No need to repeat
B. Every 12–18 months
C. Every 5 years
D. Only if symptoms occur or ECG becomes abnormal

44. Which of the following is not a non-sarcomeric protein mutation causing hypertrophic cardiomyopathy?

A. Danon (LAMP2) disease
B. Fabry's disease
C. PRKAG2 cardiac syndrome
D. Beta myosin heavy chain gene mutation

45. Which of the following mutation is not associated with hypertrophic cardiomyopathy (HCM)?

A. Myosin heavy chain
B. Myosin light chain
C. Troponin T
D. Desmin

46. All are established risk factors for sudden cardiac death in patients with hypertrophic cardiomyopathy except?

A. Severe cardiac hypertrophy
B. Left ventricular outflow tract gradient
C. Causal mutations
D. Modifier genes

47. Prevalence of hypertrophic cardiomyopathy in humans is approximately

A. One in 50 B. One in 500
C. One in 1000 D. One in 1500

48. The prevalence of HOCM in general population:

A. 1: 2000 B. 1: 500
C. 1: 5000 D. 1: 10,000

49. Which of the following is true about "Brockenbrough Braunwald phenomenon" on aortic pulse pressure?

A. Decrease in pulse pressure
B. Increase in pulse pressure
C. Wide pulse pressure
D. None of the above

50. The following features contribute to left ventricular outflow tract obstruction in hypertrophic cardiomyopathy, except:

A. Apical displacement of papillary muscles
B. Systolic anterior motion of mitral valve
C. Asymmetric septal hypertrophy
D. Apical hypertrophy

51. Which of the following therapies is class I indication in asymptomatic HCM patients with no outflow obstruction?

A. Beta blocker to reduce atrial fibrillation risk
B. Calcium channel blocker as positive lusiotropic agents to improve cardiac performance

C. Amiodarone to reduce risk of sudden death
D. None of the above

52. In a hypotensive patient with HOCM with high outflow gradient, in addition to intravenous fluids, which intravenous drug would be most useful?
A. Phenylephrine
B. Norepinephrine
C. Dopamine
D. Verapamil

53. Which of the following markers may not be associated with elevated SCD risk in HCM patients?
A. Family history of HCM
B. Syncope
C. Non-sustained VT
D. LV wall thickness >30 mm

54. All of the following risks are higher with alcohol septal ablation as compared to surgical myectomy in HOCM except:
A. Right bundle branch block
B. LBBB
C. Complete heart block
D. Sustained VT

55. What is the risk of needing a permanent pacemaker implantation with alcohol septal ablation in HOCM?
A. 2% B. 5%
C. 15% D. 60%

56. Which of the following is correct regarding residual outflow obstruction after surgical myectomy versus septal ablation?
A. Similar
B. More with surgical myectomy
C. More with alcohol septal ablation
D. None of the above

57. All of the following are risk factors for sudden cardiac death in HCM except:
A. Family history of SCD
B. Syncope on exertion
C. Frequent ventricular ectopics seen on Holter
D. LV thickness > 30 mm

58. Alcohol septal ablation is contraindicated in:
A. LBBB B. LVOT> 80
C. Syncope D. SAM with MR

59. All of the following statements are true for cardiac amyloidosis except:
A. Atrial septal thickening on echocardiography is a specific finding
B. Diltiazem is useful for improving diastolic dysfunction
C. Hypertension is an unusual finding
D. Low-voltage complexes are seen in the limb leads of ECG

60. Which of the following is true about cardiac amyloidosis?
A. Atrial septal thickening on echo is specific
B. CCB are treatment of choice for diastolic dysfunction
C. Hypertension is common
D. Cardiac silhouette is enlarged due to LV dilatation

61. All of the following are true about cardiac amyloidosis except:
A. Cardiac transplantation may be curative in transthyretin deposits
B. Beta blockers and ACE-I are poorly tolerated in CHF of cardiac amyloidosis
C. Cardiac MRI is not specific in picking up amyloid deposits before it is seen in echocardiography
D. ICD may not be useful in secondary prevention of arrhythmias

62. Select the true statement for Sarcoidosis:
A. There is predilection for granulomatous infiltration to upper septal area
B. Conduction disturbance is more common than pump dysfunction

C. Both of the above
D. None of the above

63. The following statements are true of sarcoid heart disease, except:
A. Results in left ventricular dysfunction
B. Complete heart block is a dominant feature
C. Pleomorphic ventricular tachycardia is frequent
D. Characteristic absence of delayed enhancement on MRI

64. Senile cardiac amyloidosis results from deposition of:
A. Transthyretin
B. Calcitonin
C. Atrial natriuretic peptide derived amyloid
D. Serum prealbumin

Pericardium

65. Normal amount of pericardial fluid is:
A. 0 ml
B. 20–50 ml
C. 50–100 ml
D. 100–200 ml

66. Correct statement about pericardial sinuses?
A. The transverse sinus is between ascending aorta and pulmonary trunk anteriorly and superior vena cava posteriorly
B. The oblique sinus is posterior to the left atrium and lies between left and right pulmonary veins
C. Both A and B are correct
D. Neither A nor B are correct

67. Normal intrapericardial pressure is:
A. 0 ± 3 mmHg
B. 5 ± 3 mmHg
C. 10 ± 3 mmHg
D. 15 ± 3 mmHg

Pericarditis

68. Pericarditis is seen with:
A. Lithium B. Procainamide
C. Methysergide D. Indomethacin

69. Which of these drugs can cause pericarditis?
A. Hydralazine
B. Methyldopa
C. Penicillin
D. Sodium cromoglycate
E. All of the above

70. Some of the characteristics of pericardial rub include which of the following?
A. Scratchy or grating superficial sound that is heard close to the ears; best heard with diaphragm with pressure
B. Best heard sitting up, leaning forward, in expiration
C. May vary with position and heartbeats
D. All of the above

71. Most common etiology of acute pericarditis is:
A. Idiopathic B. Viral
C. Bacterial D. Autoimmune

72. ECG changes during acute pericarditis include:
A. Concave-up ST elevation with upright T in most of the leads; ST depression in aVR
B. PR segment depression in most of the leads
C. PR segment elevation in aVR
D. All of the above

73. Acute pericarditis can be differentiated from early repolarization by:
A. Progressive changes over days
B. PR segment depression
C. ST segment/T wave height ratio of >0.25
D. All of the above

Pericardial Effusion

74. Beck triad is seen in:
A. Pericardial effusion
B. Acute pericarditis
C. Cardiac tamponade
D. Constrictive pericarditis

75. Most common cause of malignant pericardial effusion with tamponade:
A. Lung cancer B. Breast cancer
C. Lymphoma D. Renal cancer

76. A 70-year-old female patient is a case of breast cancer. She is receiving active chemotherapy. She has presented to the emergency with cold extremities. The blood pressure is 100/70, heart rate 100 beats/minute, Sa02 98%. JVP raised with blunted Y descent. The likely diagnosis is:
A. Constrictive pericarditis
B. Cardiac tamponade
C. Left ventricular systolic dysfunction
D. Acute pulmonary embolism

77. All of the following are true regarding the hemodynamics of cardiac tamponade, except:
A. Paradoxical pulse may be absent in patients with concomitant left ventricular dysfunction
B. The normal decline of systemic venous pressures on inspiration is preserved.
C. The left and right heart pressures are 180 degrees out of phase.
D. Right atrial pressure and jugular venous pressure are usually discordant in tamponade

Constrictive Pericarditis

78. Enhanced expiratory flow reversal in hepatic veins is a feature of:
A. Constrictive pericarditis
B. Restrictive Cardiomyopathy
C. Both
D. None

79. Normal pericardial thickness is:
A. <3 mm on echo
B. <2 mm on computed tomography (CT)
C. <4 mm on MRI
D. All of the above

80. Pericardial calcification is best detected by:
A. Fluoroscopy B. CT scan
C. MRI D. Echocardiography

81. The ECG finding in acute pericarditis is?
A. ST depression
B. PR segment elevation
C. PR segment depression
D. Bundle branch block

82. Risk of constrictive pericarditis is highest with:
A. Idiopathic pericarditis
B. Tubercular pericarditis
C. Uremic pericarditis
D. Malignant pericarditis

83. Dip and plateau in diastolic pressure wave is seen in all except:
A. Constrictive pericarditis
B. RCM
C. Cardiogenic shock
D. RVMI

84. Most common cause of chronic constrictive pericarditis is:
A. Viral
B. Cryogenic
C. Tubercular
D. Recurrent idiopathic pericarditis

Miscellaneous

85. Which of the following is true about Batista procedure?
A. Endoventricular patch plasty (using Dacron)

B. Latissimus dorsi cardiomyoplasty
C. Percutaneous repair of mitral valve
D. Left ventricular reduction surgery

86. Reversible LV dysfunction is caused by all except:
A. Selenium deficiency
B. Hypercalcemia
C. Hypophosphatemia
D. Thiamine deficiency

87. LBBB is a marker of one of the 4 underlying conditions, associated with increased risk of cardiovascular mortality and morbidity. Among the options given below, which one is not true?
A. CAD with LV dysfunction
B. Hypertensive heart disease
C. Aortic valve disease
D. Arrhythmogenic right ventricular dysplasia

88. Inotrope of choice for treatment of hyperdynamic shock with associated tachyarrhythmia?
A. Phenylephrine B. Dobutamine
C. Epinephrine D. Milrinone

89. Which one of following is true for development of alcoholic cardiomyopathy?
A. Consumption of more than 80 gm of ethanol per day for at least 10 years
B. Consumption of more than 80 gm of ethanol per day for at least 5 years
C. Consumption of more than 40 gm of ethanol per day for at least 5 years
D. Consumption of more than 40 gm of ethanol per day for at least 10 years

ANSWERS

Physiology of heart failure

Answer: 1. D. All of the above
Answer: 2. A. Myeloperoxidase
Answer: 3. D. Urotensin
Answer: 4. A. Constrictive pericarditis.
Answer: 5. C. Obesity
Answer: 6. A. Frank–Starling phenomenon.
Answer: 7. B. Anrep phenomenon.
Answer: 8. C. Bowditch phenomenon.
Answer: 9. D. All
Answer: 10. B. 2.2 mm
Answer: 11. D. All of the above.
Answer: 12. C. Purkinje cells.
Answer: 13. C. Purkinje cells.

Adaptive responses to heart failure

Short term adaptations: Activation of the Frank-Starling mechanism and activation of the sympathetic nervous system (SNS).

Long-term adaptations: Increased activity of the renin-angiotensin-aldosterone system (RAS) and alterations in the size and the shape of the heart (the so-called left ventricular [LV] remodelling).

Autonomic dysfunction:

SNS is activated

Elevated plasma NE levels are observed

The failing heart tissue is relatively depleted of NE, thus rendering the heart less responsive to sympathetic stimulation

Renin angiotensin aldosterone system

RAAS is over-active in the circulation and in the tissue in heart failure

Angiotensin II has a vast array of biologic activities:

- Vasoconstriction
- Vascular and cardiac myocyte growth, hypertrophy
- Activation of fibroblasts with increased collagen production
- Stimulation of aldosterone release
- Volume expansion
- Proinûammatory activity
- Direct toxicity to the myocardium

Inflammation and oxidative stress

Inflammatory markers are increased, C-reactive protein (CRP) and proinûammatory cytokines (TNF-a, IL- 1, IL-6, and IL-18).

Oxidative stress marker: myeloperoxidase (MPO)

Left ventricular remodelling

- Increased myocardial mass (hypertrophy)
- Increased myocyte size (elongation and increased width)
- Cellular necrosis, apoptosis and autophagy (cell dropout)
- Collagen deposition (reactive and replacement)

Abnormal cellular mechanisms

- Decreased beta receptor density in the heart
- Increased G_1 coupling protein in the heart
- Alpha to beta myosin heavy-chain transition (decreased myosin ATPase enzyme velocity) in the myocytes
- Defect in sarcolemma calcium uptake
- Defect in calcium-ATPase (SERCA) and phospholamban (Ca exchange)

Counter-regulatory systems (Natriuretic peptides)

BNP is a modest vasodilator also has antigrowth activity and reduces collagen synthesis

Both atrial natriuretic peptide (ANP) and BNP are produced from the ventricles in response to increased volume and pressure load.

Role of Brain Natriuretic Peptide in Heart Failure

1. BNP >400 pg/mL or N-terminal prohormone of BNP (NT-proBNP) >2000 pg/mL supports diagnosis of HF.
2. If BNP <100 pg/mL or NT-proBNP <400 pg/mL in a patient with dyspnea, consider alternate diagnosis.
3. Persistently elevated levels predict poor prognosis and recurrent hospital admissions for HF.
4. May **be** false negative **in obesity because of being metabolized by adipocytes.**

Frank-Starling law:

States that the stroke volume of the heart increases in response to an increase in the volume of blood in the ventricles. Occurs as result of length tension relationship.

In the human heart, maximal force is generated with an initial **sarcomere length of 2.2 micrometers**

Anrep effect:

Autoregulation method in which myocardial contractility increases with afterload.

Bowditch effect (Treppe phenomenon):

Autoregulation method by which myocardial tension increases with an increase in heart rate.

Also known as the **Treppe phenomenon or staircase effect.**

Otherwise known as the force–frequency relationship. Contractile force is maximal at a rate of about 150 bpm.

Cardiac myocytes:

Ventricular myocytes are **longer, broader, and have more T tubules, mitochondria and sarcomeres** as compared to atrial myocytes. Ventricular myocytes are about 60–140 μm in length, compared with 20 μm for atrial myocytes. The diameter of a ventricular myocyte is about 20 μm, compared with 5 μm for an atrial myocyte.

Purkinje cells: These have no T tubules as they do not contract and their function is mainly electrical conduction. To facilitate rapid electrical conduction, they have lot of gap junctions.

Heart failure with reduced ejection fraction

Answer: 14. B. Hepatojugular reflex

Answer: 15. C. Hepatomegaly

Answer: 16. C. Hepatomegaly

Answer: 17. D. All of the above.

Answer: 18. D. All of the above

Answer: 19. B. Digoxin.

Answer: 20. C. Neprilysin inhibitor.

Framingham Criteria for Diagnosis of Congestive Heart Failure

Validated CHF if 2 major or 1 major and 2 minor are present concurrently

Major criteria:

- PND
- Orthopnea
- Elevated JVP
- Rales
- S3
- CXR cardiomegaly
- CXR pulmonary edema

Minor criteria:

- Peripheral edema
- Night cough
- DOE
- Hepatomegaly
- Pleural effusion
- HR >120/min
- Weight loss ≥4.5 kg in 5 days with diuretic

Heart Failure Stages

Stage A: Risk factors for heart disease such as hypertension, diabetes, or CAD, but no functional or structural changes.

Stage B: Structural or functional changes such as LV hypertrophy, low EF, abnormal LV diastolic function, or abnormal valve function, but no clinical HF.

Stage C: Ambulatory clinical HF.

Stage D: HF with symptoms at rest.

Treatment of Heart Failure with Reduced Ejection Fraction

1. General measures: Na restriction to <1–2 g/day, water restriction to <1 L/day in those with hyponatremia, treatment of underlying cause (e.g., alcohol or drug use, relief of ischemia), treatment of iron deficiency anemia.
2. IV diuretics: Treatment of acute decompensation with IV diuresis.
3. Beta blockers: Important disease-modifying agents by blocking toxic effects of catecholamines on myocardium and upregulating beta receptors; carvedilol, bisoprolol and metoprolol succinate have shown mortality benefit.
4. ACEIs or angiotensin receptor blockers (ARBs) reduce mortality. Neprilysin inhibitor, LCZ696, was superior to enalapril in PARADIGM-HF trial.

5. Ivabradine decreased heart rate without decreasing cardiac contractility. Used when LVEF <35% and heart rate >70 bpm, in spite of maximum tolerable beta blocker use.
6. Spironolactone or eplerenone improve survival.
7. Digoxin as an inotrope has neutral effect on mortality but may increase mortality in those with renal dysfunction, the aged, and women.
8. Combination of hydralazine and isorbide dinitrate (Isolazine) improves survival incremental to above drugs in black patients.
9. Inotropes increase mortality; they are used for palliative care and as bridge to heart transplant.
10. An implantable cardioverter-defibrillator (ICD) for primary prevention of death is recommended in those with EF <35%.
11. Cardiac resynchronization therapy (CRT) with biventricular pacer or ICD is recommended for those with EF <35% and QRS duration >150 ms with left bundle branch block morphology.
12. Cardiac transplant improves outcome in end-stage HF patients who are candidates for heart transplant.
13. LVADs improve survival in selected patients with end-stage HF who are not transplant candidates.

Heart failure with preserved ejection fraction

Answer: 21. D. None of the above.

Answer: 22. D. Eccentric LVH

HFpEF:

Of the total HF population, approximately half of patients with HF have HFpEF

Patients with HFrEF are more often male and more frequently have a history of coronary disease or antecedent myocardial infarction and ventricular conduction abnormalities.

In contrast, the dominant risk factors for HFpEF are older age, female sex, and history of hypertension, obesity and/or diabetes mellitus.

Earlier studies suggested that outcomes were better in HFpEF compared with HFrEF, but several recent studies have shown that morbidity and mortality are similar in both forms of HF

Pathophysiology: Diastolic dysfunction

Treatment:

No established treatment which reduces mortality in HFpEF.

PEP-CHF study: ACEIs in HFpEF patients, comparing perindopril 4 mg daily to placebo

No reduction in the primary end point of all-cause mortality or HF hospitalization at 3 years of follow-up.

CHARM-Preserved trial: HF and EF>40% to candesartan or placebo

Nonsignificant reduction in the composite end point in mortality and cardiovascular hospitalizations

I-PRESERVE trial: HF and an EF>45% to irbesartan or placebo

No difference in death or cardiovascular hospitalizations

DIG trial:

No benefit to digoxin in HFpEF

OPTIMIZE-HF: Use of β-blockers and ACEIs were not associated with any reduction in 1-year mortality or hospitalization rates of HFpEF patients, though each significantly improved both end points in HFrEF patients.

Heart transplant

Answer: 23. B. Stable but inotrope dependent

Answer: 24. E. All of the above.

Answer: 25. D. Gingival hyperplasia

Answer: 26. D. All of the above.

Answer: 27. B. Pravastatin.

Answer: 28. B. Cyclosporine.

Mechanical Ventricular Assist Devices

Bridge to transplant (BTT)

Destination therapy (DT)

Bridge to destination (BTD)

Bridge to recovery (BR)

REMATCH trial demonstrated that LVAD therapy was superior to medical therapy in advanced heart failure patients in terms of survival.

Continuous flow will likely have increased longevity compared to the older generation pulsatile flow pumps.

INTERMACS criteria for advanced heart failure

Level 1: critical cardiogenic shock

Level 2: progressive decline and heart failure despite inotropic therapy

Level 3: stable but inotropic-dependent patients

Level 4: recurrent, advanced heart failure

Level 5: exertion intolerance

Level 6: exertion-limited CHF

Level 7: advanced NYHA class III symptomatology

Selection criteria for heart transplant listing

1. Cardiogenic shock requiring either continuous inotropic support or mechanical support (IABP or ventricular assist device)
2. Persistent symptoms (NYA III-IV) refractory to maximal medical therapy (including resynchronization); LVEF < 20% and a maximal functional metabolic stress test showing a peak $VO_2 \leq 12$ ml/kg/min

3. Intractable or severe anginal symptoms with no revascularization options
4. Intractable life-threatening arrhythmias unresponsive to medical therapy, catheter-based intervention, or implantable cardioverter/defibrillator.

Absolute contraindications for cardiac transplant:

1. Any systemic illness with a life expectancy < 2 years
2. Active malignancy
3. AIDS
4. Amyloidosis with multisystem involvement
5. Irreversible renal or liver failure
6. Significant obstructive pulmonary disease
7. Fixed pulmonary artery hypertension

   PASP > 60 mmHg

   Mean TPG > 15 mmHg

   Pulmonary vascular resistance > 6 woods

Coronary allograft vasculopathy:

Most common cause of chronic rejection.

Both immune as well as non-immune mechanisms are involved in damage of endothelium.

Occurs months to years after transplantation and CMV infection increases the risk of CAV.

Incidence of CAV: 8% at 1 year, 20% at 3 years, 30% at 5 years, and >50% at 10 years.

Around 50% patients will have angiographically detected vasculopathy in 5 years.

CAV is more diffuse than native vessel atherosclerosis and also involves coronary veins.

Patient is not able to feel angina because of surgical denervation.

Coronary angiograms are routinely performed annually after 5 to 10 years of cardiac transplant, however angiograms are rather insensitive for detection of CAV, as they underestimate the presence and severity of CAV.

Intravascular ultrasonogram (IVUS) is more sensitive for detection and follow up of CAV.

Drugs used for prevention and treatment of CAV include statins, calcium channel blockers and immunosuppressive agents (sirolimus, everolimus, mycophenolate mofetil).

Drug Therapy in Cardiac Transplantation

Drugs	Side-effects
Cyclosporine	Nephrotoxcity Hypertension Hypomagnesemia Hypertrichosis Gout Gingival hyperplasia Hyperlipidemia

Tacrolimus	Nephrotoxicity Neurotoxicity (Tremors) HTN (< cyclosporine) Hyperlipidemia (< cyclosporine) Glucose intolerance Alopecia Diarrhea
Mycophenolate-mofetil	Anemia Diarrhea
Sirolimus Everolimus	Hyperlipidemia Thrombocytopenia Anemia Neutropenia Diarrhea
Azathioprine	Myelosuppression Leukopenia Keep WBC >3,000/mL

Myocarditis

Answer: 29. B. Myocarditis

Lake Louise Criteria: Criteria for diagnosis of myocarditis on MRI

Dallas Criteria for the Diagnosis of Lymphocytic Myocarditis

First biopsy

Active myocarditis (with or without fibrosis)

Borderline myocarditis (not diagnostic and requiring further biopsy)

No evidence of myocarditis

Subsequent biopsies

Ongoing (persistent) myocarditis

Resolving (healing) myocarditis

Resolved (healed) myocarditis

Treatment of Myocarditis

Myocarditis Treatment Trial

Trial of prednisolone plus cyclosporine or azathioprine for the treatment of biopsy-proven lymphocytic myocarditis

No benefit of immunosuppression over placebo in survival or improvement of LV function

IMAC trial

IVIG in patients with acute DCM who had an LV ejection fraction of less than 40% and heart failure symptoms for less than 6 months

Average increase in LV function of 14% **regardless** of treatment

Showed that immune modulation in most cases of acute DCM **does not** provide additional benefit beyond usual care

Giant Cell Myocarditis

Prone for arrhythmias (VT).

GCM is also associated with a worse prognosis than lymphocytic myocarditis; the median survival from the onset of symptoms is only 5.5 months, and the rate of death or transplant is 89%

Because of poor prognosis: consideration of immunosuppression and early evaluation for cardiac transplant

Cardiac Sarcoidosis

Clinical cardiac sarcoidosis in 5% of patients however, cardiac sarcoidosis in 25% patients.

Can present with ventricular tachycardia, heart block, or congestive heart failure.

Biopsy shows characteristic noncaseating granulomas.

Lyme Myocarditis

Infection by the spirochete Borrelia burgdorferi

High-grade AV block, history of travel to regions where Lyme disease is endemic or a history of a tick bite

Chagas Cardiomyopathy

Trypanosoma cruzi infection

Approximately 30% of patients with Chagas cardiomyopathy present with symptomatic heart block or ventricular arrhythmias

Cardiomyopathies

Dilated Cardiomyopathy

Answer: 30. A. Autosomal dominant

Answer: 31. A. Lamin A/C gene.

Answer: 32. A. Male, 30 years, DCM, EF of 10%.

DCM is the **one of the commonest** type of cardiomyopathy with an estimated prevalence in the general population of **1:2500**

More than 40 disease genes have been identified, and the most common mode of inheritance is **autosomal dominant** transmission

Mutations in genes encoding for cytoskeletal proteins (lamin A/C, phospholamban, dystrophin) as well as sarcomeric proteins (myosin heavy chain, cardiac troponin T, actin)

Analysis of asymptomatic relatives of patients with dilated cardiomyopathy indicates that familial disease accounts for one-third to one-half of cases

Dilated cardiomyopathy may develop in up to 50% of patients with acute myocarditis

Metabolic cardiomyopathies: deficiencies such as selenium, camitine, phosphate, calcium, and vitamin B deficiencies can all result in dilated cardiomyopathy

Treatment: Diuretics, beta blocker, ACE inhibitor, Aldosterone antagonist. Anticoagulation is **not** recommended even with severe LV dysfunction without any other associated risk factor.

Laminopathy: Mutations in the gene coding for **lamin A/C (LMNA gene),** associated with severe form of DCM, also involves other muscles, frequently associated with heart blocks.

Arrhythmogenic right ventricular dysplasia:

Answer: 33. D. The tachyarrhythmias occurring in ARVD are characteristically monomorphic and LBBB morphology, usually with inferior QRS axis

Answer: 34. B. Intercalated disc

Answer: 35. C. Arrhythmogenic Right ventricular dysplasia

Autosomal dominant disease predominantly aûecting the right ventricle by massive or partial replacement of myocardium by fatty or fibro-fatty tissue causing ventricular arrhythmias, and sudden death at a relatively young age.

Distributed in the so-called **"triangle of dysplasia",** i.e., right ventricular outflow tract, apex, and infundibulum.

Mutations in the genes of **intercalated discs;** plakoglobin and desmoplakin genes (recessive form of ARVC known as Naxos disease)

The **ECG** in patients with ARVD/C usually shows sinus rhythm and a terminal deflection within or at the end of the QRS complex (called **epsilon wave**) in anterior chest **leads V1 to V3.** RBBB may also be seen at baseline.

The **tachyarrhythmias (VT)** occurring in ARVD are characteristically monomorphic and LBBB morphology, usually with inferior QRS axis

Naxos disease: 1. Diffuse palmoplantar keratoderma, 2. Woolly hair and 3. Arrhythmogenic right ventricular cardiomyopathy. It has autosomal recessive inheritance.

Carvajal syndrome: A rare variant of Naxos disease characterized by woolly hair, striate palmoplantar keratoderma and left sided ventricular cardiomyopathy. Patient develop dilated cardiomyopathy at earlier age. It is inherited as autosomal recessive disorder and is due to mutation in desmoplakin gene.

Stress-induced ("tako-tsubo") cardiomyopathy

Answer: 36. B. Stress

Answer: 37. A. It is irreversible

Answer: 38. B. Most commonly seen in young males

Answer: 39. B. Precordial ST elevation essential to diagnose

First described in Japan, characterized by acute but rapidly **reversible** left ventricular systolic dysfunction in the **absence** of atherosclerotic coronary artery disease.

Typically brought on by profound **psychological stress**, predominantly affecting **postmenopausal women**, and preferentially involves the **apical portion of the left ventricle** (apical ballooning).

Also known as Broken heart syndrome.

ECG may show ST elevation in anterior leads, T wave inversion, non specific ST-T changes or QR prolongation.

Possible mechanisms:

Catecholamine induced myocyte injury

Transient vasospasm

Microvascular dysfunction

Hypertrophic cardiomyopathy:

Answer: 40. C. This is classically associated with restrictive cardiomyopathy.

Answer: 41. C. 12 years

Answer: 42. B. It is strongly recommended to screen first-degree relatives for high risk genotypes.

In the absence of genotyping the index case, it is inappropriate to screen relatives for possible mutations. Genetic testing is not indicated in relatives when the index patient does not have a definitive pathogenic mutation.

Answer: 43. C. Every 5 years.

In adults every 5 years, and 12–18 months in children. As the genotype is positive, periodic screening for phenotype is indicated even in the absence of symptoms or physical signs as an echocardiogram is a lot more sensitive.

Answer: 44. D. Beta myosin heavy chain gene mutation

Answer: 45. D. Desmin.

Answer: 46. B. Left ventricular outflow tract gradient

Answer: 47. B. One in 500

Answer: 48. B. l: 500

Answer: 49. A. Decreases in pulse pressure

Answer: 50. D. Apical hypertrophy

Answer: 51. D. None of the above

Answer: 52. A. Phenylephrine.

Answer: 53. A. Family history of HCM

Family history of HCM increases the chance of HCM in relatives but it does not increase the risk of SCD. Whereas, family history of sudden cardiac death is associated with increased risk of sudden cardiac death in patient.

Answer: 54. B. LBBB.

Risk of LBBB is higher with surgical myectomy whereas RBB is higher with alcohol septal ablation.

Answer: 55. C. 15%.

This is a lot higher than for surgical myectomy, where the risk is about 1–2%.

Answer: 56. C. More with alcohol septal ablation.

Answer: 57. C. Frequent ventricular ectopics seen on Holter

Answer: 58. A. LBBB

There is high risk of RBBB after alcohol septal ablation and patient with pre-existing LBBB will develop CHB.

Hypertrophic cardiomyopathy:

Most cases are familial disease with **autosomal dominant** inheritance

Premature sudden death occurs in approximately **1%** of HCM patients annually

HCM is present in approximately **1 in 500 persons**

Most of mutations involve the proteins of the cardiac **sarcomere**: **β-myosin heavy chain (M/C),** myosin-binding protein C, cardiac troponin T, cardiac troponin I, α-tropomyosin, essential myosin light chain, regulatory myosin light chain, cardiac α-actin, and titin.

The histologic hallmark of HCM is **myocardial disarray**: Short runs of severely hypertrophied fibers are interrupted by connective tissue

Adult family members of HCM patients undergo surveillance echocardiography every 5 years and that adolescents undergo screening every 12 to 18 months

LVOT obstruction is present under resting conditions or with physiologic provocation in up to **70% of patients**

Outflow obstruction is exacerbated in the presence of a decreased ventricular preload, decreased ventricular afterload, or increased ventricular contractility.

HCM vs Athlete's heart:

HCM: left ventricular septal wall thickness is typically unusual or asymmetric and more than 15 mm, the left atrium is dilated (>4 cm), and the left ventricular end-diastolic diameter is less than 45 mm.

Athletic heart: the distribution of hypertrophy is more commonly concentric, the left ventricular septal wall thickness is less than 15 mm, the left atrium is less than 4 cm, and, importantly, the left ventricular cavity is often dilated (left ventricular end-diastolic diameter >45 mm). In athletic heart, the left ventricular hypertrophy regresses after training stops, usually within 3 months. Diastolic function is normal in athletic heart but abnormal in HCM.

Examination: Bisferiens apical impulse or double apical impulse, triple ripple at apex, Spike and dome carotid contour

The murmur of HCM is increased by maneuvers that decrease left ventricular end-diastolic volume (decreased venous return, decreased afterload, increased contractility, pure vasodilators, inotropes, dehydration, and the Valsalva maneuver). The murmur decreases with squatting, passive leg raising, negative inotropes (e.g., β-blockers, verapamil, disopyramide), and any maneuver that increases left ventricular end-diastolic volume

NB: The **Brockenbrough** sign is a classic hemodynamic function in HCM

There is a decrease in pulse pressure and increase in left ventricular outflow tract gradient after the ventricular ectopic beat in **HOCM patients**. This phenomenon is known as Brockenbrough-Braunwald-Morrow phenomenon or sign. Occurs because of dynamic narrowing of LVOT.

Management of Obstructive HCM

All first-degree relatives of patients with HCM should undergo screening with either genetic testing or cardiac imaging

Surveillance echocardiography should be repeated every 5 years for adults; children and family members participating in competitive athletics should undergo screening every 12 to 18 months

HCM patients should avoid participating in competitive athletics or other strenuous activity

Avoid dehydration, pure vasodilators, high-dose diuretics, and positive inotrope

For patients who have obstructive cardiomyopathy and symptoms, β-Blockade is often the first-line therapy

If β-blockade does not adequately decrease the intraventricular gradient and control symptoms, a calcium channel blocker—either verapamil or diltiazem—may be administered (Avoid in severe outflow obstruction and advanced heart failure with CHF features.)

Dihydropyridine calcium channel blockers are contraindicated in obstructive HCM since they are pure vasodilators.

Disopyramide, a class I antiarrhythmic agent with strong negative inotropic properties, may also be used to treat HCM in conjunction with either a β-blocker or a calcium channel blocker

Phenylephrine is preferred as vasopressor agent (pure alpha stimulant) in hypotension.

Drugs to be avoided in HOCM:

Beta agonists, Nitrates, Diuretics, Digoxin, Nifedipine type calcium channel blockers, Positive inotropic agents.

Surgery (Morrow's procedure):

Patients with obstructive HCM and who continue to have severe symptoms despite appropriate medication, surgical septal myectomy through aortic route **(Morrow's procedure)** is usually the primary treatment. Complications <5% and mortality <1%. **LBBB** after surgery is very common. CHB requiring permanent pacemaker in <5% patients.

Indications: 1. Resting or provocable gradients greater than 50 mmHg; 2. Significant functional limitation (i.e. NYHA class III-IV) despite maximal medical therapy.

Alcohol Septal Ablation

When septal myectomy is high risk in view of comorbidities

Pure ethanol (1 to 3 ml) is injected into the septal perforator coronary artery that supplies the hypertrophied myocardium causing controlled infarct.

A relatively high rate of complete heart block necessitates permanent pacing (10%–20%) with mortality rates of <2%. **RBBB** is more common (may be seen in upto 80% patients).

Residual gradient is more with alcohol septal ablation and also relief of obstruction takes several weeks.

Risk Assessment for SCD in HCM

The annual rate of sudden cardiac death is approximately 1%.

HCM is the most common cause of sudden death in competitive and school-aged athletes.

Indications of ICD or high risk features in HCM

Prior cardiac arrest

H/o sustained VT or VF

F/H of SCD in first degree relative

Recent unexplained syncope

NSVT on Holter

IVS thickness more than 30 mm

LGE > 15% myocardium on MRI

Restrictive cardiomyopathy (RCM)

Answer: 59. B. Diltiazem is useful for improving diastolic dysfunction

Answer: 60. A. Atrial septal thickening on echo is specific

Answer: 61. A. Cardiac transplantation may be curative in transthyretin deposits

Answer: 62. C. Both of the above

Answer: 63. D. Characteristic absence of delayed enhancement on MRI

Answer: 64. A. Transthyretin

Primary RCM: Endomyocardial fibrosis, Loeffler's cardiomyopathy, Idiopathic RCM

Secondary RCM:

1. Infiltrative disease- Amyloidosis, Sarcoidosis, Post-irradiation therapy
2. Storage disease- Hemochromatosis, Glycogen storage disease, Fabry disease

Endomyocardial fibrosis: Endemic to tropical Africa, occurs in left and right ventricular apices with obliteration and involvement of subvalvular apparatus. Thromboemolism is frequently seen.

Loffler endocarditis: Endocardial thickening, obliteration of LV apex is seen and is associated with hypereosinophilia.

Amyloidosis:

Primary type (AL type): most common, and is associated with multiple myeloma. Fibrils are composed of immunoglobulin light chains

Secondary amyloidosis: rare, fibrils consisting of protein A.

Familial amyloidosis occurs because of production of **transthyretin (TTR).**

ECG: Low-voltage QRS complexes, Pseudoinfarct pattern (Q waves)

Echo: Biatrial enlargement, Increased interatrial septal thickness, granular myocardial texture, reduced E'.

MRI: Late gadolinium enhancement, diffuse throughout both ventricles, particularly **subendocarium.**

Catheterization: Dip and plateau (square root sign) in ventricular pressure, M or W waveform in atrial pressure tracing due to prominent Y and X descent.

Sarcoidosis:

Multisystem disease, formation of granulomas in many tissues.

Non caseating granulomas involving myocardium seen in 25% patients on autopsy. Clinical cardiac involvement is seen in 5% patients.

Associated with conduction abnormalities and arrhythmias (VT and AV blocks)

Pericardial diseases

Answer: 66. B. 20–50 ml.

Answer: 66. C. Both A and B are correct.

Answer: 67. A. 0 ± 3 mmHg.

Answer: 68. C. Methysergide

Answer: 69. E. All of the above.

Answer: 70. D. All of the above.

Answer: 71. A. Idiopathic.

Answer: 72. D. All of the above.

Changes in aVR are reciprocal to changes in all other leads. The ECG changes are progressive and progress to ST segment normalization with T wave flattening (stage 2), T wave inversion (stage 3, and normalization of ECG (stage 4).

Answer: 73. D. All of the above.

Answer: 74. C. Cardiac tamponade

Answer: 75. A. Lung cancer.

Answer: 76. B. Cardiac tamponade

Answer: 77. D. Right atrial pressure and jugular venous pressure are usually discordant in tamponade

Answer: 78. A. Constrictive pericarditis

Answer: 79. D. All of the above.

Answer: 80. B. CT scan.

Answer: 81. C. PR segment depression

Answer: 82. B. Tubercular pericarditis.

Answer: 83. C. Cardiogenic shock

Answer: 84. C. Tubercular

Anatomy and Function of the Pericardium

Two distinct layers:

1. Outer inelastic fibrous layer (fibrous pericardium)
2. Inner serous double layer (serous pericardium) is divided into the visceral pericardium (epicardium) and the parietal pericardium

Serous pericardium secretes a small amount of clear serous fluid **(normally about 25–50 mL)**

The normal thickness of the pericardium is **<2 mm**

Congenital Absence of the Pericardium

Complete absence of the pericardium is very rare and is usually asymptomatic.

Most common is the absence of a small portion of the pericardium, **usually on the left side.**

Diagnosed incidentally on chest radiography and displays a marked levoposition (left-sided shift) of the heart without tracheal deviation, also described as "Snoopy" dog cardiac silhouette.

Rarely, herniation of cardiac chambers through a partial defect of the pericardium may cause sudden death

Acute Pericarditis

Acute pericarditis usually is self-limited

Pain occurs because of inflammation of parietal pericardium (Visceral pericardium is devoid of pain fibers).

The pain is sharp, stabbing, and pleuritic and radiates to the scapula and back

Physical examination: A **Triphasic** pericardial friction rub, which is characterized by scratchy high-pitched sounds with 3 distinct components (coincidental with rapid ventricular filling, ventricular contraction, and atrial contraction).

Heard best at the left sternal border, with the patient leaning forward during held expiration.

ECG: ST-segment elevation is more **diffuse**, involving both limb and precordial leads, and it is **concave upward** and associated with upright T waves (In MI, ST elevation is convex upwards).

Depression of the PR segment because of atrial involvement

Cardiac tamponade:

If the rate of accumulation is rapid, even a small amount (50–100 mL) of fluid or blood in the pericardium can cause cardiac tamponade.

Classic findings of the Beck triad consist of 1) a decrease in systolic pressure, 2) an increase in systemic venous pressure, and 3) a quiet heart. Seen in only 10% to 40% of patients.

Swinging motion of heart inside pericardial sac on echo which translates on ECG in form of electrical alternans.

Other Echo features of tamponade:

1. Inspiratory decrease in the E-F slope of the mitral valve
2. Early diastolic collapse of the right ventricle
3. Late diastolic collapse of the right atrial free wall
4. Plethora of the inferior vena cava with a blunted respiratory change

Pulsus Paradoxus

Decrease (>10 mm Hg) in systolic blood pressure during inspiration

It may also occur in other conditions in which there is a significant decrease in forward stroke volume with inspiration, such as acute cor pulmonale (pulmonary embolism), chronic obstructive lung disease, right ventricular infarction, and asthma.

Cardiac tamponade vs constrictive pericarditis

Feature	Cardiac Tamponade	Constrictive Pericarditis
Pulsus paradoxus	Present	Present
Kussmaul sign	Absent	May be present
Pericardial knock	Absent	May be present
Systolic x descent	Large	Normal
Diastolic y descent	Small or absent	Large

Constrictive Pericarditis

Most common cause in developing countries and overall: **Tuberculosis**

Most common cause in developed countries: **Previous cardiac surgery**

Clinical features: Dyspnea, peripheral edema, marked systemic venous congestion with hepatomegaly, and ascites

Venous pressure increases with inspiration **(Kussmaul sign)** because of the inability of the right side of the heart to accept the increased cardiac input with inspiration.

Unlike patients with cardiac tamponade with x descent, patients with constrictive pericarditis have **rapid y descent**, which reflects the early diastolic decrease in right ventricular pressure

With high atrial pressure, rapid filling of the ventricle is accelerated, and this generates the **third heart sound (pericardial knock)**

Echo: abnormal ventricular septal motion (Septal bounce), increased pericardial thickness or calcification, dilated inferior vena cava with no significant changes on inspiration

Mitral inflow and pulmonary venous diastolic flow velocities decrease immediately after the onset of inspiration and increase with expiration. Reciprocal changes occur in tricuspid inflow and hepatic venous flow velocity.

Pericardial thickness

CT or MRI is best for determining pericardial thickness whereas CT is ideal for pericardial calcification.

18% of patients with constrictive pericarditis can have normal pericardial thickness.

Hemodynamic Findings

1. An increase in right atrial pressure and a dip-and-plateau configuration of the right and left ventricular diastolic pressure tracings
2. Because there is no restriction of early ventricular filling, the y descent is quite prominent
3. Ventricular interdependence and the reciprocal pressure changes in the right and left ventricles with respiration which lead to discordant direction of pressure changes with respiration

Treatment: Pericardiectomy

Restriction Versus Constriction

Feature	Constriction	Restriction
Physical exam	Kussumaul's sign, Pericardial knock	No pericardial knock
Echo	Normal wall thickness,Septal bounce, Increased E', Exaggerated respiratory variation of mitral E velocity	Increased wall thickness, Biatrial enlargement, Reduced E', Normal respiratory variation of mitral E velocity
CT/MRI	Thick pericardium	Normal pericardium
Cardiac catheterization	LVEDP=RVEDP RVSP < 50 mmHg RVEDP > 1/3 of RVSP Discordance of LV and RV pressure during respiration	LVEDP > RVEDP RVSP > 50 mmHg RVEDP < 1/3 of RVSP Concordance of LV and RV pressure with respiration

Miscellaneous

Answer: 85. D. Left ventricular reduction surgery

Batista procedure: Partial left ventriculectomy or LV reduction surgery done in patients with end-stage dilated cardiomyopathy refractory to conventional medical therapy.

Found to be not very effective and is not a recommended treatment

Answer: 86. B. Hypercalcemia

Causes of potentially reversible LV systolic dysfunction:

1. Tachy-arrhythmic cardiomyopathy
2. Alcoholic cardiomyopathy
3. Stress induced cardiomyopathy
4. Peripartum cardiomyopathy
5. CAD
6. Hypertension, Pheochromocytoma
7. Infections and Sepsis
8. Acute myocarditis
9. Metabolic causes:
   Hypocalcemia
   Hypophosphatemia
   Thiamine deficiency
   Selenium deficiency (Keshan's disease)
   Vitamin D deficiency

Answer: 87. D. Arrhythmogenic right ventricular dysplasia

RBBB is commonly associated with ARVC

Answer: 88. A. Phenylephrine

Phenylephrine is also the DOC for hypotension in HOCM & SAM

Answer: 89. B. Consumption of more than 80 gm of ethanol per day for at least 5 years

Alcoholic cardiomyopathy:

Acquired dilated cardiomyopathy which is associated with long-term heavy alcohol consumption (defined as >80 g per day over a period of at least five years).

Women develop condition at a lower total dose of alcohol.

It can be reversed with abstinence of alcohol.

7 Deep Venous Thrombosis, Pulmonary Embolism and Pulmonary Artery Hypertension

Deep Venous Thrombosis

1. All of the following conditions produce hypercoagulable state except:
- A. Protein C deficiency
- B. Antithrombin excess
- C. Factor V leiden mutation
- D. Prothrombin gene mutation

2. Pain and tenderness on dorsiflexion of ankle is known as:
- A. Mose's sign
- B. Homan's sign
- C. Traube's sign
- D. Trousseau sign

Pulmonary Thromboembolism

3. Wells criteria is for the diagnosis of:
- A. Acute pulmonary embolism
- B. Right ventricular infarction
- C. Primary pulmonary hypertension
- D. Cardiac tamponade

4. All of the following are characteristics of massive PE except:
- A. Syncope
- B. Cyanosis
- C. RV strain
- D. Hemoptysis

5. Sign of massive pulmonary embolism all except:
- A. Syncope
- B. Pleuritic chest pain
- C. RV strain
- D. Cyanosis

6. Sign of massive pulmonary embolism all except:
- A. Syncope
- B. Pulmonary infarction on CXR
- C. RV strain
- D. Cyanosis

7. All of following are suggestive of massive PTE except:
- A. Pleuritic chest pain
- B. RV dysfunction
- C. Cyanosis
- D. Hypotension

8. A 40 year old male patient without any previous comorbidity presents to emergency department with history of severe respiratory distress. Which of the following is strongly against the diagnosis of pulmonary embolism?
- A. No past history suggestive of deep venous thrombosis
- B. Absolutely normal chest X-ray
- C. Negative D dimer test
- D. No hemoptysis

9. Which of the following statements is false regarding venous thromboembolism?
- A. McConell sign is echocardiographic evidence of right ventricular hypokinesia (free wall) in cases of PE.
- B. Hampton's hump is a peripheral wedge-shaped opacity above the diaphragm seen in cases of PE.

C. Classic Well's criteria is used to assess clinical likelihood of death in pulmonary embolism
D. Alteplase has been approved for massive PE in a dose of 100 mg in continuous infusion during 2 hours without concomitant heparin.

10. $S_1Q_3T_3$ sign in pulmonary embolism is seen in:
A. 20% B. 10%
C. 30% D. 1%

11. A 60-year old male presented to emergency department with sudden onset chest pain and hypotension. He gives history of air travel for 12 hours, two days prior to presentation. The best diagnostic test should be:
A. D-dimer
B. Transesophageal echocardiography (TEE)
C. Invasive coronary angiography
D. Multi-slice CT angiography

12. All of the following are true regarding "D-dimer assay" except:
A. First line investigation in high probability of PE
B. Negative test rules out PE in mild and moderate probability of PE
C. ELISA is highly sensitive for screening
D. Screening procedure of choice in emergency department

13. Window period for thrombolysis in acute pulmonary embolism?
A. 7 days B. 14 days
C. 24 hours D. 21 days

14. Which of the following is fibrin non-specific thrombolytic agent?
A. Alteplase
B. Urokinase
C. Reteplase
D. Tenecteplase

15. Which is the preferred modality to diagnose thromboembolic PH?
A. V/Q scan
B. CT pulmonary angiography
C. Gd-enhanced MR pulmonary angiography
D. Transesophageal echocardiography

16. A 38-year old lady is a known case of CTEPH. CT angiography revealed presence of non-occluding chronic thrombus in right and left proximal pulmonary artery. The treatment of choice should be:
A. IV prostacyclin
B. Switch to heparin in place of warfarin
C. Thrombolytic therapy using tenecteplase
D. Surgical pulmonary thrombo-endarterectomy

Pulmonary Artery Hypertension

17. Which of the following mutations is responsible for the majority of patients with familial PH?
A. BMPR2 mutations
B. BMPR1B mutation
C. SMAD9 mutation
D. None of the above

18. Pulmonary hypertension in chronic lung disease is caused by:
A. Hypercapnia
B. Intracardiac shunt
C. Pulmonary vein in-situ thrombosis
D. Alveolar hypoxia

19. The PA pressure in a 37-year-old patient who had VSD patch closure at the age of 15 years is 60/35 mmHg. Based on the current classification system, which of the following options best describes this patient's condition?
A. No PH B. Group 1 PH
C. Group 2 PH D. Group 3 PH

20. 25 years old female presents with history of syncope and breathlessness on exertion, CXR- PA view and lateral view-prominent right descending PA, and peripheral oligemia. Which of the following is most possible diagnosis?
A. IPAH
B. Valvular PS
C. Scimitar syndrome
D. Sarcoidosis

21. Which of the following statements is untrue about vasoreactivity testing in PH?
A. Vasoreactivity testing is recommended in patients with idiopathic PAH, hereditary PAH, and PAH associated with drugs used to detect patients who can be treated with high doses of a CCB
B. A positive response to vasoreactivity testing is defined as a reduction of mean PA pressure ≥10 mmHg to reach an absolute value of mean PA pressure ≤40 mmHg with an increased or unchanged cardiac output
C. Nitric oxide is recommended for performing vasoreactivity testing.
D. Adenosine can be considered for performing vasoreactivity testing as an alternative
E. The use of oral or IV CCBs in acute vasoreactivity testing is recommended

22. All of the following are used to assess pulmonary vasoreactivity except:
A. Oxygen
B. Adenosine
C. Nitric oxide
D. Isoprenaline

23. One of the following drugs is not useful in Primary Pulmonary hypertension:
A. Bosentan
B. Sildenafil
C. Telmisartan
D. Iloprost

24. Sitaxentan used in primary pulmonary hypertension is a:
A. Prostanoid
B. Phosphodiesterase type 5 inhibitor
C. Endothelin receptor antagonist
D. Calcium channel blocker

25. Bosentan belongs to one of the following group:
A. Endothelin receptor antagonist
B. Phosphodiesterase inhibitors
C. Soluble guanylate cyclase stimulators
D. Prostanoids

26. A 40-year-old female patient is a case of idiopathic pulmonary artery hypertension (IPAH). She is hospitalized with class IV symptoms. The treatment strongly recommended to relieve her symptoms and improve survival is:
A. Bosentan
B. Intravenous epoprostenol
C. Long-acting nifedipine
D. Sildenafil

27. The mechanism of action of Selexipag is:
A. Oral prostacyclin analogue
B. Intravenous prostacyclin analogue
C. Guanylate cyclase stimulator
D. Prostacyclin receptor agonist

Miscellaneous

28. Prothrombinase contains:
A. Va
B. Xa
C. Both of the above
D. None of the above

29. True about Anti-phospholipid antibody syndrome all except:
A. SLE in 80% patients
B. Thrombocytopenia
C. Prolongation of activated partial thromboplastin time
D. Recurrent arterial thrombosis

ANSWERS

Deep venous thrombosis (DVT):

Answer: 1. B. Antithrombin excess

Answer: 2. B. Homan's sign

Pathogenesis of DVT is related to the **Virchow triad**: venous stasis, endothelial injury, and a procoagulant state.

Proximal vein DVT in lower limbs (Iliac and femoral veins) have more propensity of embolize to lungs than calf vein DVT.

Diagnosis of DVT:

Clinical: **Homans sign** (pain and tenderness on dorsiflexion of the ankle) and the **Moses sign** (pain on pressing the calf muscle)

D-dimer

Radiographic investigations: Duplex ultrasonography, Impedance plethysmography, Contrast venography, CT and MR venography

Classification of Hypercoagulable States

Inherited

Loss of function

- Antithrombin deficiency
- Protein C deficiency
- Protein S deficiency

Gain of function

- Factor V Leiden mutation
- Prothrombin factor II G20210A mutation
- Elevated level of factor VIII, IX, or XI

Acquired

Previous venous thromboembolism

Obesity

Cancer

Pregnancy, puerperium

Drug-induced

- Heparin-induced thrombocytopenia
- Prothrombin complex concentrates

L-Asparaginase

Hormonal therapy

Postoperative

Myeloproliferative disorders

Mixed

Hyperhomocysteinemia

- Pregnant women have 5-fold increased risk of VTE.
- DVTs are more common during pregnancy, whereas PEs seem to be more common in the postpartum period
- Active cancer is one of the strongest risk factors for VTE, increasing the risk by 5- to 6-fold.

Thrombophilic Disorders and VTE

In about 25% of patients with VTE, the VTE episodes are unprovoked.

In more than 90%, the identified defect is either a **heterozygous factor V Leiden (most common)** or prothrombin factor II G20210A mutation.

Pulmonary thromboembolism (PTE):

Answer: 3. A. Acute pulmonary embolism

Answer: 4. D. Hemoptysis

Answer: 5. B. Pleuritic chest pain

Answer: 6 B. Pulmonary infarction on CXR

Answer: 7. A. Pleuritic chest pain

Answer: 8. C. Negative D dimer test

Answer: 9. C. Classic Well's criteria is used to assess clinical likelihood of death in pulmonary embolism

→ Well's criteria are used to assess the clinical likelihood of presence of DVT or pulmonary embolism and is not used for prognosis of the patient.

Answer: 10. B. 10%

Answer: 11. D. Multi-slice CT angiography

Answer: 12. A. First line investigation in high probability of PE

Answer: 13. B. 14 days

Answer: 14. B. Urokinase

Answer: 15. A. V/Q scan

Answer: 16. D. Surgical pulmonary thrombo-endarterectomy

Pulmonary thromboembolism:

Hypoxia, tachycardia, dyspnea, chest pain or discomfort, syncope, cough, and fever are all signs and symptoms associated with acute pulmonary embolism.

Hemoptysis and chest pain due to pulmonary infarction may be seen with **small** pulmonary embolisms also.

Hypoxia, Cyanosis, Syncope, Systemic hypotension are suggestive of massive pulmonary embolism.

Diagnosis

Well's criteria for diagnosis of pulmonary embolism

Clinical factors	Points
DVT symptoms or signs	3
An alternative diagnosis is less likely than PE	3
Heart rate > 100 beats/min	1.5
Immobilization or surgery within 4 weeks	1.5
Previous DVT or PE	1.5
Hemoptysis	1
Cancer treated within 6 months or metastatic	1

A score of 4 or more is suggests high probability for pulmonary embolism

Padua prediction score is also for identification of hospitalized patients at risk for pulmonary embolism.

Vienna Prediction Model uses a nomogram to predict the likelihood of recurrence of pulmonary embolism.

Investigations

- CTPA:
  Multidetector CTPA has become the first-line diagnostic test for PE
- Echocardiography:
  Rarely shows thrombus in RA, RV or proximal PAs.
  Most often, it provides indirect evidence by demonstrating RV dilatation or systolic dysfunction with flattening of the intraventricular septum resulting in a D-shaped left ventricle.
  A reduction in RV free wall contractility with preserved RV apical function (McConnell sign)
- Serum markers: D- dimer is highly sensitive but not specific for pulmonary embolism. A negative D dimer can rule out pulmonary embolism in low to moderate risk patients but not in high risk patients.
- Pulmonary angiography
- V/Q scan: Useful in situations such as contrast dye allergy and renal dysfunction, in which contrast nephropathy would be a serious concern
- ECG:
  Tachycardia
  T-wave inversion in the precordial leads (V1 to V4)

The pattern of S wave in lead I, Q wave and deep S wave in III ($S_1Q_3T_3$ pattern) (in 10-15%) Right bundle branch block (in 12%), and left-axis deviation (in 12%)

- Chest Radiography:
  Classic signs such as Westermark's sign (focal oligemia) and Hampton's hump (peripheral wedge-shaped **opacity adjacent to the diaphragm),** Palla's sign **(enlarged right descending pulmonary artery).**

Prognosis

Pulmonary embolism severity index (PESI), the Geneva rule, and the PREP study score

Treatment of Acute pulmonary embolism (PE)

Mortality in massive PTE is approximately 10% within 1 hour and up to 85% in the first 6 hours

1. Submassive PTE without RV strain: Anticoagulation
2. Submassive PTE with RV strain or Positive biomarkers: Thrombolysis if hypotension (SBP <90), hypoxemia (SpO2 < 95%), moderate to severe RV dysfunction on Echo or above borderline positive biomarkers (BNP > 100, NT Pro-BNP > 900)
3. Massive PTE: SBP < 90 mmHg for more than 15 minutes, Thrombolysis

Window period for thrombolysis in pulmonary embolism: **14 days**

If there is contraindication for thrombolysis or if thrombolysis is unsuccessful then surgical pulmonary embolectomy should be considered.

Thrombolytic agents:

Fibrin specific (Preferentially activate fibrin bound plasminogen): Streptokinase; Acylated plasminogen streptokinase activator complex (anistreplase); Urokinase.

Non-fibrin specific (Don't discriminate between fibrin bound and circulating fibrinogen): Recombinant t-PA (rtPA), also known as alteplase or activase; and two recombinant derivatives of rt-PA, Tenecteplase and Reteplase.

These agents act by converting the proenzyme, plasminogen, to plasmin, the active enzyme.

Activation of circulating plasminogen by non-fibrin specific agents result in the generation of unopposed plasmin, which can trigger the systemic lytic state.

Streptokinase

Patients who receive streptokinase can form antibodies against it. These antibodies reduce the effectiveness of streptokinase.

Allergic reactions occur in approximately 5% of patients treated with streptokinase.

Administered as an intravenous infusion of 1.5 million units over a period of 30 to 60 minutes.

Alteplase

Allergic reactions and hypotension are rare, and alteplase is not immunogenic.

Intravenous infusion of alteplase over a 60 to 90 minute period

Tenecteplase

Longer half-life than t-PA and resistant to inactivation by PAI-1.

Tenecteplase is more fibrin specific than t-PA

Administered as a single intravenous bolus

Reteplase

Produced in Escherichia coli

Given as two intravenous boluses separated by 30 minutes.

Optimal Duration of Anticoagulation after acute event:

First provoked PE/ Proximal leg DVT: 3 to 6 months

First provoked upper extremity DVT or isolated calf DVT: 3 months

Second provoked VTE: Uncertain

Third VTE: Indefinite duration

Cancer and VTE: Indefinite duration or until cancer is cured

Unprovoked PE/ Proximal leg DVT: Indefinite duration

- Unprovoked VTE have a higher rate of recurrence than those with provoked VTE after anticoagulation is discontinued.
- Patients with cancer and VTE: Extended duration of anticoagulation is recommended until the cancer is considered cured. LMWH as monotherapy is the standard anticoagulant used under these circumstances.

Indication of IVC filter for prophylaxis of pulmonary embolism:

(1) Major contraindications to full-dose anticoagulation such as active bleeding

(2) Recurrent PE despite well-documented full-dose anticoagulation for an existing VTE

Chronic Thromboembolic Pulmonary Hypertension

Occurs in 3% patients with PE.

Less than 50% of patients with CTEPH have a history compatible with a previous episode of DVT or PE

Ventilation-perfusion scintigraphy (V/Q scan) has high sensitivity for detecting CTEPH and a negative predictive value of nearly 100%. Hence, this is investigation of choice for CTEPH.

Treatment- Pulmonary thromboendarterectomy

Pulmonary artery hypertension

Answer: 17. A. BMPR2 mutations

Answer: 18. D. Alveolar hypoxia

Answer: 19. B. Group 1 PH

Answer: 20. A. IPAH

Answer: 21. E. The use of oral or IV CCBs in acute vasoreactivity testing is recommended.

Answer: 22. D. Isoprenaline

Answer: 23. C. Telmisartan

Answer: 24. C. Endothelin receptor antagonist

Answer: 25. A. Endothelin receptor antagonist

Answer: 26. B. Intravenous epoprostenol

Answer: 27. D. Prostacyclin receptor agonist

Diagnosis of pulmonary hypertension:

Pulmonary artery hypertension is defined as mean pulmonary artery pressure greater than 25 mm Hg.

Precapillary PH is defined as an mPAP of 25 mm Hg or more; a PCWP of 15 mm Hg or less; and a PVR of more than 3 Wood units.

Postcapillary PH is present when the mPAP is 25 mm Hg or more and the PCWP is 15 mm Hg or more. Postcapillary PH is most common in group 2 patients, or those with PH due to left heart disease.

Clinical Classification of Pulmonary Hypertension (Dana Point, 2008)

Group 1: Pulmonary arterial hypertension (PAH)

Idiopathic, Heritable (BMPR2 mutation), Drug and Toxin induced, Connective tissue disease, HIV, Portal hypertension, Congenital heart disease with increased pulmonary blood flow, Schistosomiasis.

Group 1' Pulmonary veno-occlusive disease and/or pulmonary capillary hemangiomatosis

Group 1" Persistent pulmonary hypertension of newborn

Group 2: Pulmonary hypertension owing to left heart disease (Cause PAH due to pulmonary venous hypertension)

LV systolic dysfunction, LV diastolic dysfunction, Valvular disease, Left heart inflow obstruction, Acquired or congenital pulmonary venous stenosis.

Group 3: Pulmonary hypertension owing to lung diseases and/or hypoxia

COPD, ILD, OSA and hypoventilation disorder, Chronic exposure to high altitude.

Group 4: Chronic thromboembolic pulmonary hypertension

CTEPH, Other pulmonary artery obstruction (Angiosarcoma, arteritis, congenital pulmonary artery stenosis, Parasites)

Group 5: Pulmonary hypertension with unclear multifactorial mechanisms

Hematologic disorders: Hemolytic anemias, myeloproliferative disorders, splenectomy

Systemic disorders: Sarcoidosis, pulmonary histiocytosis, lymphangioleiomyomatosis

Metabolic disorders: Glycogen storage disease, thyroid disorders

Others: Chronic renal failure (with or without dialysis), segmental pulmonary hypertension

Pulmonary arterial hypertension associated with congenital heart disease is placed in type 1 PAH group.

It includes:

1. Eisenmenger syndrome
2. PAH associated with systemic-to-pulmonary (left to right) shunts
3. PAH with small or coincidental defects

   Marked elevation in PVR in the presence of small cardiac defects, which themselves do not account for the development of elevated PVR; the clinical picture is very similar to idiopathic PAH; closing the defects is contraindicated.
4. PAH after defect correction

   Congenital heart disease is repaired but PAH either persists or recurs after correction in the absence of significant postoperative haemodynamic lesions

ECG features of PAH: Right atrial enlargement, right axis deviation, and right ventricular enlargement, often with a strain pattern.

CXR features of PAH: Enlarged main and hilar pulmonary arteries with "pruning" of the peripheral vasculature and right ventricular enlargement.

Acute vasodilator testing

Recommended in patients with idiopathic PAH, hereditary PAH or PAH associated with drugs to detect whether they will receive benefit with high doses of CCBs.

Agents: Oxygen, Adenosine, Nitric oxide, Epoprostenol

NB: Calcium channel blockers are **not** used for vasodilator testing.

Positive response is defined as a fall in mPAP of at least 10 mm Hg to an mPAP of 40 mm Hg or less with unchanged or increased CO.

Such patients may be treated with a high dose of calcium channel– blocking agent.

Treatment of idiopathic pulmonary artery hypertension:

General Measures:

Oxygen supplementation to keep the saturation higher than 92%

sodium-restricted diet (<2400 mg/day)

Routine immunizations, such as those against influenza and pneumococcal pneumonia

Avoid pregnancy or terminate early (Maternal mortality rate of 30-50%)

Diuretics

Calcium channel blocking agents:

Treatment of choice for patients who are responsive to acute vasodilator testing.

Long-acting nifedipine, diltiazem, and amlodipine are the most commonly used agents.

Prostacyclin I2 analogues:

Epoprostenol (continuous intravenous), treprostinil (continuous subcutaneous, continuous intravenous, intermittent inhaled and oral), and iloprost (intermittent inhaled)

Improvements in exercise tolerance as measured by 6MW distance, hemodynamics, quality of life, and survival over a 12-week period

Endothelin Receptor Antagonists

Bosentan, Ambrisentan, and Macitentan

Improvement in 6MW distance and the composite endpoint of time to clinical worsening

Side effects: Hepatotoxicity, Anemia, Lower extremity edema and Headache.

Phosphodiesterase Inhibitors

PDE5 inhibitors inhibit the hydrolysis of cyclic GMP and increase level of NO, which causes pulmonary vasodilation.

Sildenafil, Tadalafil

Riociguat

Directly stimulates soluble guanylate cyclase independent of NO

Riociguat should not be used concurrently with PDE5 inhibitors

Selexipag: Oral, selective prostacyclin receptor agonist

NB→ The use of PAH approved therapies is not recommended in patients with pulmonary hypertension due to **left heart disease (group 2) or lung diseases (group 3).**

Miscellaneous:

Answer: 28. C. Both

The prothrombinase complex consists of the serine protein, Factor Xa, and the protein cofactor, Factor Va.

Prothrombinase catalyses conversion of prothrombin to thrombin.

Answer: 29. A. SLE in 80% patients

Antiphospholipid syndrome (Hughes syndrome):

Autoimmune, hypercoagulable state caused by antiphospholipid antibodies; promotes thrombosis in both arteries and veins, frequently associated with pregnancy related complications.

Can occur as primary condition or in association with other immune condition (Secondary APLA). In a cohort of APLA patients, around **36%** were found to have SLE.

Antiphospholipid Antibodies: Lupus anticoagulant, Anti-β2-glycoprotein and Anti-cardiolipin antibodies.

Diagnosis: Thrombocytopenia and raised aPTT.

Dilute Russell's viper venom time (DRVVT), kaolin clotting time (KCT), dilute thromboplastin time (TDT/DTT), silica clotting time (SCT) are used for diagnosis of APLA.

8 Peripheral Vascular Diseases

Atheroembolism

1. Hollenhorst plaque in fundus is seen in:
A. Hypertension
B. Diabetes
C. Takayasu arteritis
D. Atheroembolism

2. All of the following are true about athero-embolism except?
A. Eosinophiluria
B. Thrombocytosis
C. Livedo reticularis
D. Hollenhorst plaque

Aortic Aneurysm

3. Surgery is indicated in ascending aortic aneurysm if diameter of ascending aorta or aortic sinus is:
A. 4.5cm
B. 5.5cm
C. 6.5cm
D. 7.5cm

4. A 60/M patient was diagnosed with infrarenal abdominal aortic aneurysm of 5.5 cm. What should be next line of management?
A. CT every 6–12 months
B. Should undergo repair
C. Monitored by ultrasound every 3–6 months
D. Only A and C

5. BAV with gradient > 45 mm Hg with aortic root dilatation of 46 mm with class II angina treatment:
A. Medical management
B. Bioprosthetic valve
C. Mechanical valve
D. Bentall procedure

6. Drug used to prevent aortic root dilatation:
A. Amlodipine B. Losartan
C. Eplerenone D. Tadalafil

7. Risk factor for abdominal aortic dilatation except?
A. DM B. Smoking
C. HTN D. Dyslipidemia

8. Drugs decreasing progression of size of abdominal aortic aneurysms all except:
A. Doxycycline B. Losartan
C. Beta-blocker D. Colchicine

Aortic Dissection

9. Aortic dissection is an uncommon but potentially catastrophic illness. Which of the following statements is false?
A. Stanford Type A dissections are all dissections not involving the ascending aorta.
B. In a small minority of patients with ascending aortic dissection, the proximal dissection flap may involve ostium of right coronary artery more commonly than left coronary artery.

C. Antihypertensive choice in cases of aortic dissection should include combination of both vasodilator & beta blocker.
D. In cases of aortic dissection associated with cardiac tamponade, pericardio-centesis may sometimes in fact deteriorate the hemodynamics.

10. Which one of the following genetic condition is not associated with aortic dissection?
A. Marfan syndrome
B. Down syndrome
C. Turner syndrome
D. Bicuspid aortic valve

11. Incidence of acute MI due to aortic dissection is:
A. 5% to 10% B. 1% to 2%
C. 20% to 30% D. 40% to 50%

12. Which of the following is true for acute aortic intramural hematoma?
A. It has benign self-limiting course in majority of cases
B. TEE is better than CT angiography for early diagnosis
C. Occurs due to bleeding from the damaged vasa vasorum
D. Usually associated with acute aortic regurgitation

13. A 75-year hypertensive male patient presents with severe chest pain of 2-hours duration. Blood pressure in right upper limb is 160/100 and left upper limb is 100/70. Heart rate is 110 beats/minute. There is 2-mm ST segment elevation in inferior leads. Echo reveals large pericardial effusion. The immediate management should include?
A. Urgent pericardiocentesis
B. Urgent coronary angiography and PCI of culprit vessel
C. Urgent transesophageal echocardiography
D. Urgent contrast-enhanced CT of chest and abdomen

14. All the following statements about aortic dissection are true, except:
A. Aortic regurgitation occurs in up to 70% of Type A (Stanford) dissections
B. Left coronary involvement in the dissection is more common than right coronary artery involvement
C. Majority of type B (Stanford) aortic dissections can be medically managed initially
D. Pulse deficit is more common in ascending aortic dissections

15. Which of the following is incorrect regarding myocardial infarction in ascending aortic dissection?
A. Due to involvement of coronary arteries
B. Incidence rate 1–2%
C. Right coronary more commonly involved than left coronary
D. Thrombolytics are indicated

16. The treatment of choice in a 49 Y/M with acute type III aortic dissection, BP of 200/100 mmHg, severe interscapular pain, pallor, and tachycardia is which of the following?
A. Emergency surgery
B. Endovascular graft implantation with fenestration
C. Intravenous (IV) nitroprusside
D. IV esmolol

Aortic Syndromes

17. In patient with Marfan syndrome pregnancy is contraindicated if diameter of ascending aorta is greater than?
A. 4.5 cm B. 5 cm
C. 6 cm D. 3 cm

18. A bifid uvula is seen in which of the following?
A. Ehlers–Danlos syndrome (EDS)
B. Loeys–Dietz syndrome (LDS)

C. Aneurysms–osteoarthritis syndrome (AOS)
D. Marfan syndrome

19. Which of the following is most prone for acute aortic rupture?
A. Marfan
B. LD syndrome
C. Familial A. dissection
D. EDS-IV

20. All of the following are true for LOEYS DIETZ syndrome except:
A. It is an autosomal dominant disorder
B. Bifid broad uvula is a feature
C. It is associated with arterial tortuosity and aortic aneurysms
D. It has a less aggressive vascular phenotype than Marfan syndrome

Carotid Artery Disease

21. What does the term "bovine" arch refer to?
A. The aortic arch morphology in cattle
B. A shared common origin of the brachiocephalic and left common carotid arteries
C. A shared common origin of the left subclavian and common carotid arteries
D. A shared common origin of the left and right common carotid arteries

22. Carotid artery stenting is preferred over carotid endarterectomy in the presence of?
A. Visible thrombus
B. Contralateral carotid artery occlusion
C. Platelet disorder
D. Tortuous aortic arch

23. Carotid artery stenting is not recommended in patients with the following features except?
A. Heavily calcified aortic arch or protruding atheroma
B. Total occlusion of carotid artety
C. Post-radiation or post-surgical stenosis
D. Contraindication to DAPT

Peripheral Arterial Disease

24. Ankle-Brachial index in critical limb ischemia:
A. <0.5
B. <0.8
C. <0.9
D. <1.0

25. An Ankle Brachial Index (ABI) >1.40 may signify which of the following?
A. Stiff (calcified) arteries
B. May be observed in the case of diabetes, ESRD, and in the very elderly.
C. A substantial proportion of patients with an elevated ABI actually do have occlusive artery disease.
D. All the above

26. Patient with peripheral artery disease who is asymptomatic at rest but is able to walk < 200 m is under?
A. Fontaine class IIa
B. Fontaine class IIb
C. Fontaine class IIIa
D. Fontaine class IIIb

27. Which of the following peripheral revascularization techniques is associated with worst patency rate at 5 years?
A. Femoro-popliteal bypass graft using saphenous venous graft
B. Femoro-popliteal stenting using self-expanding stents
C. Iliac artery stenting
D. Infra-popliteal peripheral angioplasty

28. All are true for mesenteric vein thrombosis leading to mesenteric ischemia except:
A. Associated with oral contraceptives
B. Presents with weight loss, lower GI bleeding
C. Inferior mesenteric vein is more commonly involved than superior mesenteric vein

D. Less common than the mesenteric arterial involvement (as a cause of mesenteric ischemia)

29. All of the following are true regarding carotid duplex ultrasound for measuring the severity of carotid artery stenosis except:

A. It is less precise in determining stenosis of less than 50 percent compared with higher percent stenosis
B. Can accurately distinguish between subtotal and total occlusion of carotid artery
C. Contralateral stenosis results in overestimation of ipsilateral stenosis
D. The measurement is dependent on the cardiac output

30. Clinical situations where the diagnosis of renal artery stenosis should be considered include all except:

A. Onset of hypertension before the age of 30 years
B. Onset of hypertension after 55 years
C. Malignant hypertension (hypertension with coexistent end-organ damage, i.e. acute renal failure, flash pulmonary oedema)
D. White coat hypertension

31. Which of the following is not an indication for percutaneous revascularization of RAS?

A. Patients with hemodynamically significant RAS
B. Recurrent, unexplained congestive heart failure
C. Sudden, unexplained pulmonary edema
D. Treatment naïve hypertension patients

32. Takayasu's arteritis affects which of the following?

A. Aorta
B. Pulmonary arteries
C. Renal arteries
D. All of the above

33. Giant cell arteritis does not involve following artery:

A. Temporal artery
B. Internal carotid artery
C. Subclavian artery
D. Axillary artery

34. All are true about Giant cell arteritis except:

A. Anterior ischemic optic neuropathy can be seen
B. Aortic dissection is seen as a late complication
C. Low complement levels
D. Panarteritis of large and medium sized vessels

35. All of the following are true about Wegener's granulomatosis except:

A. Involves upper airways in 95%
B. Necrotising granulomatous vasculitis
C. Immune complex deposits are seen on renal biopsy
D. Involves small arteries and veins

Miscellaneous

36. A 6.5 cm infrarenal aortic aneurysm was repaired a year ago. The aneurysm has continued to grow by 1 cm on a follow-up CT scan. There is no contrast seen within the sac of the aneurysm. What is this an example of?

A. Type I endoleak
B. Type II endoleak
C. Type IV endoleak
D. Type V endoleak

37. Leriche syndrome is associated with which of the following?

A. Impotence
B. Buttock claudication
C. Atrophy of the lower extremities

ANSWERS

Aortic atheroembolism

Answer: 1. D. Atheroembolism

Answer: 2. B. Thrombocytosis

Atheroembolism is characterized by **livedo reticularis**, blue toes, palpable pulses, hypertension, renal insufficiency, increased erythrocyte sedimentation rate, and eosinophilia (transient).

Hollenhorst plaques are cholesterol emboli seen in retinal arteries, and usually embolize from internal carotid arteries.

Aortic aneurysm

Answer: 3. B. 5.5cm

Answer: 4. B. Should undergo repair.

Answer: 5. D. Bentall procedure

Answer: 6. B. Losartan

Answer: 7. A. DM

Answer: 8. D. Colchicine

Thoracic Aortic Aneurysm

Causes:

Atherosclerosis, Marfan syndrome, bicuspid aortic valve, giant cell arteritis (cranial arteritis) Takayasu arteritis, infections (syphilis), familial aortopathy, and trauma.

Indications for surgical resection:

- Presence of symptoms attributable to the aneurysm
- Aneurysm rapidly enlarging under observation (particularly if the patient has hypertension), Posttraumatic aneurysm
- Pseudoaneurysm
- Aneurysm with a diameter of more than 5.5cm
- In patients with Marfan syndrome and in patients with bicuspid aortic valve, ascending aortic diameter is 5.0 cm or more.
- In patients undergoing other cardiac surgery like aortic valve replacement, diameter of 4.5 cm or more.

Abdominal Aortic Aneurysm

The US Preventive Services Task Force recommends a 1-time screening ultrasonographic examination for men aged 65 to 75 who have ever smoked. For men who are either siblings or offspring of patients with AAA, screening generally begins at age 60.

Rupture aneurysm size: for an AAA diameter of 5.5 to 5.9 cm, the 1-year incidence of rupture is 9.4%; for a diameter of 6.0 to 6.9 cm, 10.2%; and for a diameter of 7.0 cm or more, 32.5%.

Frequency of surveillance:

Surveillance intervals are 3 years for an AAA diameter of 3.0–3.4 cm; 1 year for a diameter of 3.5–3.9 cm; and 6 months for a diameter of 4.0–4.9 cm

Elective surgical or endovascular treatment: Aneurysms with a diameter of 5.5 cm or more.

Surgery is also indicated for AAAs that are symptomatic, traumatic, or infectious in origin or are rapidly expanding (>0.5 cm yearly)

AORTIC DISSECTION

Answer: 9. A. Stanford Type A dissections are all dissections not involving the ascending aorta.

Answer: 10. B. Down syndrome

Answer: 11. B. 1% to 2%

Answer: 12. C. Occurs due to bleeding from the damaged vasa vasorum

Answer: 13. D. Urgent contrast-enhanced CT of chest and abdomen

Answer: 14. B. Left coronary involvement in the dissection is more common than right coronary artery involvement

Answer: 15. D. Thrombolytics are indicated

Answer: 16. D. IV esmolol.

Aortic dissection

DeBakey Classification: type I originates in ascending aorta and progresses to arch ± descending aorta; type II is confined to ascending aorta; type III originates in and is generally localized to the descending aorta.

Stanford Classification: Type A involves ascending aorta regardless of origin; type B is distal to the ascending thoracic aorta

Causes and associations- Marfan syndrome, Ehler-Danlos syndrome, Loeys-Dietz syndrome, Turner syndrome, Bicuspid aortic valve, CoA, Trauma, Syphilis, Iatrogenic, Atherosclerosis, Hypertension.

Acute onset of severe pain (often migratory) in the anterior chest, back, or abdomen is the most suggestive clinical finding in aortic dissection.

Additional findings include hypertension (49% of patients), an aortic diastolic murmur, pulse deficits or blood pressure differential, syncope from cardiac tamponade and neurologic changes.

Pericardiocentesis may sometimes **worsen** the hemodynamic stability in cardiac tamponade caused by aortic dissection.

Aortic regurgitation may be seen in upto 50 to 70% patients with Type A aortic dissection.

Acute myocardial infarction – Incidence is **1 to 2%,** and most commonly it is inferior infarction due to **right coronary artery** ostial dissection. Thrombolytics are absolutely **contraindicated.**

For suspected acute aortic dissection, CT has an overall accuracy of 96%.

15-20% patients may present with acute intramural hematoma.

Treatment:

If untreated, acute aortic dissection has a mortality of 33% within the first 24 hours and rises to 50% mortality by the first 48 hours.

Target systolic blood pressure, unless hypotension is present, should be 100–110 mmHg, with a target heart rate of between 50 and 60 beats per minute.

Intravenous β-blockers are the initial agent of choice

Type A aortic dissection: Mortality rates of 1-2% per hour, hence urgent surgery is required.

Type B aortic dissection: Medical therapy

Type B dissections require surgery if complicated by organ mal-perfusion or rupture.

Bentall procedure: This procedure includes aortic root and valve replacement with either a biologic valve or a mechanical valve and requires coronary artery reimplantation.

In the absence of clinically significant aortic valve regurgitation, a valve-sparing aortic root replacement can be considered

2 kinds of valve sparing operations: 1) Yacoub operation (Remodelling technique) 2) David procedure (Reimplantation technique)

Penetrating aortic ulcer:

Penetrating aortic ulcer occurs when an atherosclerotic plaque undergoes ulceration and penetrates the internal elastic lamina.

Penetrating aortic ulcer most commonly involves the mid or distal descending thoracic aorta and less often the ascending or abdominal aorta

Clinical features: Severe retrosternal pain radiating to back like aortic dissection.

Treatment: Similar to aortic dissection.

Acute intramural hematoma:

Intramural hematoma is contained aortic wall hematoma with bleeding within the media but **without** initial intimal flap formation.

Condition is characterized by blood leaking through the innermost layer of the aortic wall, possibly due to **rupture of vasa vasorum** inside vessel wall. This leakage does not occur due to a tear in the aortic wall and aortic wall is intact.

Patients present with severe chest, back or abdominal pain.

Similar to acute aortic dissection, it is classified as Stanford type A (ascending aorta) or B (exclusive involvement of the descending aorta). Most patients with IMH have Stanford type B (50% to 85%).

IMH may convert into aortic dissection (45%).

CT or MR angiography are better diagnostic tools than ultrasonography or TEE.

Aortic IMH is a life-threatening condition, treatment is usually needed immediately.

Patients with type A IMH should undergo early surgery, whereas patients with type B IMH can be managed conservatively in the absence of complications.

Aortic syndromes

Answer: 17. A. 4.5 cm

Contraindications of pregnancy due to cardiac cause:

PAH of any cause

Severe systemic ventricular dysfunction (EF < 30%, NYHA III-IV)

Previous peripartum cardiomyopathy with residual impairment of LV function

Severe MS, Severe AS or Severe CoA

Marfan syndrome with aortic diameter >45 mm

BAV with aortic diameter > 50 mm

Answer: 18. B. Loeys–Dietz syndrome (LDS).

Answer: 19. D. EDS-IV

Answer: 20. D. It has a less aggressive vascular phenotype than Marfan's syndrome

Marfan syndrome:

Autosomal dominant with high penetrance caused by mutation in fibrillin-1 gene located at chromosome 15q21.

Revised Ghent criteria: Used for the diagnosis of Marfan syndrome

Non-cardiac features: Tall stature, high arched palate, wrist sign, thumb sign, chest wall deformity, dural ectasia, protrusion acetabuli, increased arm span to height ratio, decreased upper segment to lower segment ratio, ectopia lentis (Lens dislocated to upward and lateral side).

Cardiovascular features: Aortic root disease leading to aortic aneurysm and aortic dissection, mitral valve prolapse, tricuspid valve prolapse, pulmonary artery enlargement.

Management:

β-blockade and possibly ARBs should be considered in all patients unless contraindicated.

ARBs (Sartans) slow the growth of aortic aneurysms.

Maintain BP <120/80. Avoid strenuous exercises.

Prophylactic surgery is recommended when the diameter of the aortic sinuses of Valsalva reaches 5.0 cm or the aortic size index is 4.25 cm/m2 or more.

Need for surgery at an aortic sinus dimension of 4.5 cm or less: 1. Family history of aortic dissection, 2. Personal history of descending aortic dissection, 3. Severe aortic valve regurgitation with associated symptoms or progressive ventricular dilatation or dysfunction, 4. the contemplation of pregnancy, and 6. rapid rate of aortic dilatation (aortic root growth >5 mm per year)

Pregnancy in Marfan Syndrome

2 major issues: risk of cardiovascular complications in the affected mother and the 50% risk of transmission of Marfan syndrome to the fetus

Risk of aortic root complication is increased when the aortic root diameter is **more than 4 cm** at the start of pregnancy, and aortic diameter more than 4.5 cm is contraindication for pregnancy.

A planned caesarean delivery is generally preferred for patients who have Marfan syndrome and aortic dilatation

Homocystinuria:

Shares several skeletal features (tall stature, overgrowth of long bones) and ocular features (ectopia lentis) with Marfan syndrome, in addition to mitral valve prolapse

In contrast have, mental retardation, predisposition to thromboembolism. And it is an autosomal recessive disorder. Lens dislocation is to towards medial and downward side in eye.

Loeys-Dietz syndrome:

Unique features of hypertelorism, a **broad bifid uvula,** and vascular involvement characterized by arterial tortuosity and aneurysms with an increased risk of dissection throughout the arterial tree, often at small arteries.

Ehlers-Danlos syndrome:

Type IV EDS has significantly shortened life spans (50% mortality rate by 48 years) due to the spontaneous rupture of visceral organs (colon, uterus) and blood vessels; it affects the entire vascular system and the heart.

Carotid artery disease

Answer: 21. B. A shared common origin of the brachiocephalic and left common carotid arteries.

Answer: 22. B. Contralateral carotid artery occlusion

Answer: 23. C. Post-radiation or post-surgical stenosis

Aortic arch anatomy:

The aortic arch is defined as type I, II, or III depending on the relationship of the innominate artery to the inner and outer aortic arch curvature.

The three types of aortic arch morphologies are determined by the relationship of the brachiocephalic trunk to the aortic arch.

In the type I morphology, the origin of all three great vessels originates from the same linear plane. In type II, the brachiocephalic trunk originates from a plane between the outer and inner curvatures of the aortic arch. In type III, it originates below the inner curvature of the aortic arch.

Bovine aortic arch is a variant of normal arch anatomy in which the brachiocephalic artery and the left common carotid artery share a common origin from the aortic arch.

Term bovine arch is a misnomer.

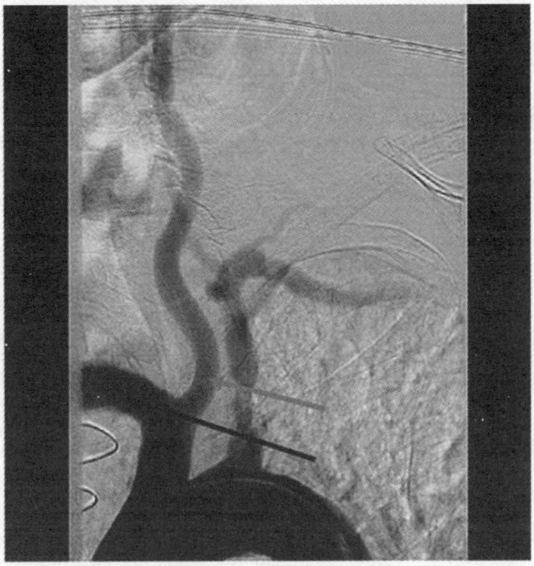

Image showing Bovine arch i.e. left common carotid artery (red arrow) arising from right brachiocephalic artery (black arrow).

Modified Stradness criteria: For diagnosis of carotid stenosis on USG.

Carotid intima media thickness: Measure of subclinical atherosclerosis and usually measured in the common carotid artery.

Associated with a higher risk of myocardial infarction (MI), stroke, and cardiovascular death

Treatment:

All patients with documented carotid disease should receive single antiplatelet drug (clopidogrel or aspirin) and statin for primary prevention of stroke. Aspirin may be combined with dipyridamole. MATCH and CHARISMA were negative trial for DAPT, hence DAPT is not recommended.

Anticoagulation indicated in suspected cardioembolic stroke and it has no role in non-cardioembolic stroke.

Carotid endarterectomy:

Endarterectomy of the carotid artery was first performed by Dr. Michael DeBakey.

For symptomatic >50% (Class I) and asymptomatic >70% carotid artery stenosis (Class IIa).

Not indicated in <50% stenosis (Class III).

Higher risk of periprocedural MI and cranial nerve injury.

It is associated with a lower rate of periprocedural stoke.

Carotid artery stenting:

Risk of stroke is significantly higher; and the risk of periprocedural MI and cranial nerve injury is significantly lower with CAS as compared with CEA.

High risk patients having indication of CEA may be considered for CAS. Symptomatic >50% (Class I) and asymptomatic >70% carotid artery stenosis (Class IIb).

Peripheral arterial disease

Answer: 24. A. <0.5

Answer: 25. D. All the above

Answer: 26. B. Fontaine class IIb

Answer: 27. D. Infra-popliteal peripheral angioplasty

Answer: 28. C. Inferior mesenteric vein is more commonly involved than superior mesenteric vein.

Superior mesenteric vein is more commonly involved than inferior mesenteric vein in thrombosis. Rest all are true.

Answer: 29. B. Can accurately distinguish between subtotal and total occlusion of carotid artery

Answer: 30. D. White coat hypertension

Answer: 31. D. Treatment naïve hypertension patients

Answer: 32. D. All of the above.

Answer: 33. Internal carotid artery

Answer: 34. C. Low complement levels

→ NORMAL levels are seen. Also, in Takayasu & Henoch schonlein purpura.

Answer: 35. C. Immune complex deposits are seen on renal biopsy

→ Wegeners granulomatosis, microscopic polyangitis, and churg strauss syndrome are PAUCI IMMUNE.

Peripheral arterial disease

Rose claudication questionnaire is a simple screening tool for claudication.

Acute limb ischemia, characterized by the "6Ps" of pain, paresthesias, pallor, pulselessness, paralysis, and poikilothermia (or "polar"), is a vascular emergency due to thrombotic arterial occlusion that requires urgent revascularization with thrombolytic therapy and/or thrombectomy

Critical limb ischemia is defined as objectively proven PAD plus ischemic rest pain, nonhealing ulceration, or gangrene that has been present for at least 2 weeks

Fontaine classification of peripheral artery disease:

Stage	Symptoms
I	Asymptomatic
IIa	Claudication distance >200 metres
IIb	Claudication distance <200 metres
III	Rest/Nocturnal pain
IV	Necrosis/Gangrene

Ankle-Brachial Index

Ratio of ankle systolic pressure to brachial systolic pressure.

An ABI of > 1 .4 is not normal and suggests noncompressible vessels either from vascular calcifcation ("medial calcinosis") or from inability to compress arteries due to obesity

ABI value	Interpretation
1-1.39	Normal
0.9-0.99	Borderline ABI, consider exercise ABI testing
<0.9	Abnormal, PAD
<0.4	Severe PAD
>1.4	Noncompressible vessels

Drugs:

Cilostazol: Phosphodiesterase type III inhibitor. Increases cyclic AMP levels, inhibits platelet aggregation and smooth muscle cell proliferation, and has a weak vasodilator eûect

Increase the maximal walk distance by 50%

Cilostazol is contraindicated in patients with congestive heart failure

Pentoxifylline: Methylxanthine derivative, improves blood viscosity. Less effective than cilostazol.

Revascularization of PAD

1. Revascularization is clearly indicated for the patient with acute limb ischemia or critical limb ischemia
2. Significant (i.e., lifestyle- or vocationally limiting) symptoms after a trial of exercise and/or pharmacologic therapy.
   - → Endovascular therapy is first line approach, if unfavourable anatomy is present then open bypass surgery may be necessary.
   - → Favourable anatomy for endovascular therapy: Aortoiliac occlusive disease
   - → Infra-popliteal peripheral angioplasty is associated with worse outcomes.

Indications of Percutaneous revascularization of RAS:

1. Patients with hemodynamically significant RAS Recurrent, unexplained congestive heart failure
2. Sudden, unexplained pulmonary edema
3. Percutaneous revascularization may be considered for patients with RAS and chronic renal insufficiency with unilateral RAS.
4. Accelerated hypertension, resistant hypertension, malignant hypertension, hypertension with an unexplained unilateral small kidney, and hypertension with intolerance to medication.

Takayasu arteritis (Pulseless disease):

It is a form of large vessel granulomatous vasculitis (panarteritis).

Takayasu's arteritis affects the aorta and its branches, the pulmonary arteries, and the renal arteries that can cause renovascular hypertension.

It is characterized by segmental and patchy granulomatous inflammation of the aorta and branches, leading to arterial stenosis, thrombosis, aneurysms, and dissections in late stages.

Most commonly affects young or middle-age women of Asian descent.

Females are about 8–9 times more likely to be affected than males.

Treatment:

Inflammatory phase: Steroids and other immunosuppressants (Mycophenolate, Tocilizumab).

Fibrotic phase: Revascularization for arterial stenosis, either via vascular bypass or angioplasty and stenting.

Giant cell arteritis:

Giant-cell arteritis (GCA), also called temporal arteritis

GCA is frequently associated with polymyalgia rheumatica.

Typically occurs in those **over the age of 50 and females** are more often affected than males.

Involvement of internal carotid vessels is quite rare but has been described in some case reports.

Features: Headache with pain and tenderness over the temples, jaw claudication, blindness.

Sudden vision loss is most commonly due to **acute ischemic optic neuropathy**.

Complements level are normal.

Diagnosis: Biopsy of temporal artery.

Treatment is typically with high doses of steroids, such as prednisone.

Granulomatosis with polyangiitis (Wegener's granulomatosis):

Necrotising granulomatous vasculitis which affects small- and medium-size vessels affecting many organs

Pathogenesis: Inflammation of blood vessels associated with poorly formed granulomas, necrosis, and many giant cells.

Anti-neutrophil cytoplasmic antibodies **(cANCAs)** which react with proteinase 3 are responsible for the inflammation in GPA.

Renal or skin biopsy shows leukocytoclastic vasculitis with necrotic changes and granulomatous inflammation.

Organ involvement:

Nose or sinus involvement: Upper airway is almost always involved; stuffiness, nosebleeds, and saddle-nose deformity.

Eyes: Scleritis and conjunctivitis

Kidney: rapidly progressive glomerulonephritis (75%)

Lungs: pulmonary nodules, infiltrates, cavitary lesions, pulmonary haemorrhage causing haemoptysis

Treatment:

Combination of immunosuppressive medications such as rituximab or cyclophosphamide and high-dose corticosteroids to induce remission and azathioprine, methotrexate, or rituximab to keep the disease in remission.

Plasma exchange is also used in severe cases

Thromboangiitis obliterans (Buerger disease):

Progressive inflammation and thrombosis (clotting) of small and medium arteries and veins of the hands and feet.

Strongly associated with smoking and tobacco consumption, predominantly affects between 20–40 years old males.

Considered as autoimmune disease and high titres of **anti-endothelial antibodies** are present.

Superficial thrombophlebitis may predate the onset of ischemic symptoms due to arterial occlusive disease and frequently parallels disease activity.

Presentation:

Main symptom is pain in the affected areas, at rest and while walking

Peripheral pulses are diminished or absent

Ulcerations and gangrene in the extremities are common complications, often resulting in the need for amputation

Angiogram: "corkscrew" appearance of arteries with occlusions (blockages) or stenosis (narrowings) in multiple areas of both the arms and legs.

Inflammatory markers, such as ESR and CRP, ANCA and cryoglobulins are all negative.

Treatment:

Pharmacologic therapy including immunosuppressants is generally ineffective; abstinence from tobacco is the only measure known to prevent disease progression.

Miscellaneous

Answer: 36. D. Type V endoleak.

Types of aortic leaks

Type I is a leak from either end of the graft due to a gap between the graft and the aorta; type II is filling of the sac via collaterals – most commonly lumbar; type III is a break in the components of the graft; type IV is leak from the fabric of the graft material; type V is no cause.

Answer: 37. D. All of the above.

Leriche syndrome is due to atherosclerotic total occlusion of the terminal aorta. The triad of symptoms are as noted.

9 Arrhythmia and Sudden Cardiac Death

Brugada Syndrome

1. Mutation seen in Brugada syndrome is:
A. Voltage-gated sodium channel
B. L-type calcium channel
C. SCN5A-encoded sodium channel
D. Potassium channel

2. Which of the following is correct about Brugada Syndrome?
A. Functional phase 2 re-entry
B. Female preponderance
C. Autosomal recessive inheritance
D. Exertional syncope

3. False statement about Brugada syndrome:
A. Phase 4 re-entry
B. Mutations in SCN5A
C. Ventricular fibrillation
D. ST elevation in V1-V3

4. Which of the following is correct regarding Brugada syndrome?
A. Female preponderance
B. AR inheritance
C. Exertional syncope
D. Functional phase 2 re-entry

5. What is not correct about Brugada Syndrome?
A. Male preponderance
B. Cardiac events never occur during sleep or rest
C. Concealed forms may be unmasked by provocative drugs like Ajmaline and Flecainide
D. Quinidine may be used as an adjunct to ICD

6. Stimuli for sudden death in Brugada syndrome is:
A. Auditory B. Sleep
C. Swimming D. Visual

7. The antiarrhythmic drug which decreases the frequency of ventricular fibrillation in Brugada Syndrome:
A. Quinidine
B. Sotalol
C. Metoprolol
D. Amiodarone

8. In a patient with type I Brugada syndrome presenting with syncope, the 2-year risk of sudden death is?
A. 2% B. 10%
C. 30% D. 80%

9. Which of the following is correct regarding Brugada syndrome?
A. Genetically determined sodium channelopathy
B. Mortality risk is independent of amount of ST elevation
C. The ECG changes are stable and do not change over time
D. They have underlying LV dysfunction

10. Which of the following is true about Brugada syndrome?
A. More common in females
B. Usually seen in first decade of life
C. Quinidine is the treatment of choice in symptomatic patients
D. ST elevation in V1 – V3 increases with flecainide

11. SCN5A gene mutations are involved in all the following conditions, except:
A. Sick sinus syndrome
B. Familial atrial fibrillation
C. Progressive cardiac conduction defect
D. Short QT syndrome

QT Syndromes

12. Genetic testing is most appropriate for:
A. Long QT syndrome
B. Dilated cardiomyopathy
C. Coronary artery disease
D. Atrial fibrillation

13. Which of the following is true regarding LQT1 syndrome?
A. Resting ECG shows broad T waves
B. Rest and sleep trigger tachyarrhythmias
C. Tachycardia onset always pause dependent
D. QT interval shortens with exercise

14. What is the defect in Long QT3 syndrome?
A. KCNQ1-encoded slow component of the delayed rectifier potassium current (IKs)
B. KCNH2-encoded rapid component of the delayed rectifier potassium current (IKr)
C. SCN5A-encoded sodium channel
D. None of the above

15. The mechanism of medications that prolong QT as a cause for acquired long QT syndrome is which of the following?
A. SCN5A-encoded sodium channel
B. Voltage-gated sodium channel
C. Inhibition of KCNH2-encoded HERG potassium channel
D. Inhibition of calcium channel

16. What is the channel that is most commonly affected in long QT syndrome?
A. Potassium channel
B. Sodium channel
C. Calcium channel
D. Transient outward potassium channel

17. Which of the following drug is least likely associated with TdP?
A. Propafenone
B. Disopyramide
C. Quinidine
D. Dofetilide

18. Which of the following match of Genetic channelopathies with the affected gene is not correct?
A. LQT 1- Loss of function KCNQ1
B. LQT 3- Loss of function SCN5A
C. CPVT 1- Gain of function RyR2 (Ryanodine receptor)
D. Timothy Syndrome -Gain of function CACNA1c

19. Short QT syndrome all true except:
A. QTc < 300 msec
B. QTc < 88 percentile
C. Treated with hydroquinine
D. HERG mutation

20. Which of the following diseases has been linked to mutation in the cardiac sodium channel?
A. Long QT Syndrome
B. Brugada Syndrome
C. Sinus node disease
D. All of the above

Catecholaminergic Polymorphic Ventricular Tachycardia (CPVT)

21. Not true regarding symptomatic catecholamine-induced polymorphic VT (CPVT)?

A. Type 1 CPVT results from mutations in RYR2-encoded cardiac ryanodine receptor
B. Type 2 CPVT results from mutations in CASQ 2-encoded calsequestrin
C. Characterized by stress-induced syncope with structurally normal heart and normal QT interval
D. First line of therapy is amiodarone

22. All of the following drugs may be useful for treatment of catecholaminergic polymorphic ventricular tachycardia (CPVT) except:
A. Quinidine B. Nadolol
C. Verapamil D. Flecainide

AV Block

23. Which of the following is incorrect about Mobitz type I block?
A. Progressive increase of PR interval
B. Progressive increase of RR interval
C. Block occurs at AV nodal level
D. Is less dangerous than Mobitz type II block

SVT and Re-entrant Tachycardias

24. Entrainment is a feature of:
A. Reentry
B. Automaticity
C. Triggered activity
D. All of the above

25. Excitable gap is present in all except:
A. EAT B. WPW
C. VT with scar D. AVNRT

26. Which one of the following are most common accessory pathways?
A. Right lateral
B. Left lateral
C. Left posteroseptal
D. Right anteroseptal

27. Which of the following statements is true regarding persistent junctional reciprocating tachycardia (PJRT)?
A. It is an antidromic variety of AVRT
B. It has short R-P interval
C. The tachycardia rates are usually slower than other tachyarrhythmias
D. It is usually seen in elderly patients

28. All of the following are true regarding multifocal atrial tachycardia (MAT) except:
A. Variable P wave morphologies
B. Variable P-P interval
C. Constant PR interval
D. Variable R-R interval

29. True about multifocal atrial tachycardia (MAT) except:
A. Seen in chronic pulmonary disease
B. Atrial rate is usually > 100/min
C. Varying PP interval but fixed RR interval
D. Commonly seen in critically ill and elderly patients

30. Which of the following is not true about atrioventricular nodal re-entrant tachycardia?
A. It is a cause of short RP supraventricular tachycardia
B. Mostly manifests as incessant tachycardia leading to ventricular dysfunction
C. May be controlled with beta blockers
D. Is quite suitable for radiofrequency ablation

31. A 15-year-old athlete is diagnosed to have Ebstein's anomaly. He has no limitation in his physical activity. There is no cardiomegaly. Recently, he had two episodes of palpitations and dizziness but no syncope. The likely arrhythmia in this patient will be?
A. Atrial fibrillation
B. Atrial flutter

C. AVRT
D. Ventricular tachycardia

32. Identify the correct statement in concealed anomalous pathway:
A. Can present with re-entrant tachycardia
B. There is no retrograde conduction but anterograde conduction is preserved
C. High risk of developing rapid ventricular response to AF
D. Anomalous pathway is manifest in sinus rhythm

33. In patient with atrial fibrillation and fast conduction through accessory pathway, all drugs can be used except:
A. Quinidine B. Flecanide
C. Amiodarone D. Digoxin

34. A 25-year old male presents to OPD with a regular narrow QRS tachycardia at a rate of 80bpm, with P waves following each QRS. During carotid sinus massage, the tachycardia converts to LBBB morphology at a rate of 165bpm. The most likely diagnosis is:
A. AVNRT
B. Orthodromic AVRT using a left-sided bypass tract
C. VT with 1:1 VA conduction
D. AVNRT & VT co-existing

35. A 40/M patient presented to the emergency with 2-hours history of rapid heartbeat associated with dizziness. The blood pressure is 90/60 mmHg; ECG shows atrial fibrillation with ventricular preexcitation. What is the best treatment option?
A. Intravenous (IV) metoprolol
B. IV digoxin
C. Cardioversion
D. IV diltiazem

36. All of the following is a short RP narrow QRS tachycardia except:
A. Orthodromic AVRT
B. Typical AVNRT
C. Junctional ectopic tachycardia
D. Permanent form of junctional reciprocating tachycardia

Radiofrequency Ablation

37. A 65/M patient presents with history of recurrent palpitations associated with near syncope. He has been on metoprolol. The 12-lead ECG is suggestive of AVNRT. Which of the following would you recommend next?
A. Continue metoprolol
B. Flecainide
C. Amiodarone
D. EP study/ablation

38. Complications are least in radiofrequency ablation of which accessory pathway?
A. Left anteroseptal pathway
B. Left posteroseptal pathway
C. Right posteroseptal pathway
D. Left lateral pathway

39. The most common energy source used for catheter ablation for treatment of arrhythmias is:
A. Cryoablation
B. Radiofrequency
C. High frequency ultrasound
D. Laser

40. A 50/M patient with h/o symptomatic supraventricular tachycardia wishes to undergo EP studies and catheter ablation. What is the expected success rate?
A. 70–75% B. 80–85%
C. 90–95% D. 100%

Atrial Fibrillation and Flutter

41. The most common cause of a cerebral embolism is?

A. Cardiac prosthetic valves
B. Dilated cardiomyopathy
C. Endocarditis
D. Atrial fibrillation

42. Which of the following drugs are not recommended for pharmacological conversion of atrial fibrillation?
A. Amiodarone 5mg/kg I/V over 1 hour
B. Metoprolol 5mg I/V over 5 minutes
C. Ibutilide 1mg I/V over 10 minutes
D. Propafenone 2 mg/kg I/V over 10 min or 450-600 mg P/O

43. Out-of-hospital self-treatment of recent-onset atrial fibrillation (Pill-in-the-Pocket approach) can be done by taking:
A. Quinidine B. Amiodarone
C. Sotalol D. Flecainide

44. Drug used in "Pill in pocket" approach in acute atrial fibrillation:
A. Propafenone B. Sotalol
C. Amiodarone D. Disopyramide

45. Mechanism of counterclockwise atrial flutter is:
A. Automaticity in the cavotricuspid Isthmus
B. Triggered activity
C. Reentry using cavotricuspid Isthmus
D. Any of the above

Ventricular Tachycardia

46. Capture beats are characteristic of:
A. Ventricular tachycardia
B. Atrial flutter
C. PSVT
D. Atrial fibrillation

47. Point favouring supraventricular tachyarrhythmia over VT:
A. QRS > 160 msec
B. AV dissociation
C. Irregularly irregular rhythm
D. Northwest axis

48. Which of the following statements is false regarding diagnosis & management of tachyarrhythmias?
A. CHADS2 score assesses risk of stroke in patients with Non valvular AF.
B. Bundle branch re-entry (BBR) tachycardia is a type of sustained monomorphic VT, common in patients with dilated cardiomyopathy.
C. Bidirectional VT can be a manifestation of digitalis excess, typically in older patients & severe myocardial disease.
D. Belhassen's VT or Idiopathic left fascicular VT is due to re-entry & is resistant to Verapamil.

49. All of the following are true about idiopathic left ventricular tachycardia except:
A. β blocker is the treatment of choice
B. Atrial pacing may induce it
C. Arise from infero-posterior part of ventricular septum
D. Mostly associated with false tendons

50. In idiopathic outflow tract VT, all are true except?
A. Typically has a LBBB pattern in V1
B. Vagal maneuvers can terminate VT
C. High risk of sudden cardiac death
D. More common in women

51. Which of the following is correct regarding Bundle branch re-entrant ventricular tachycardia (BBRVT)?
A. RBBB morphology during tachycardia
B. HV interval during VT is typically shorter than during sinus rhythm
C. Patients with no structural heart disease
D. Poor response to pharmacological therapy

Anti-arrhythmic Drugs

52. The following anti arrhythmic drug has no place in Vaughan Williams classification

A. Lignocaine B. Adenosine
C. Ibutilide D. Verapamil

53. Action potential not prolonged by which class of antiarrhythmics?
A. IA B. IB
C. IC D. III

54. All are true for adenosine except:
A. Negative dromotropic effect
B. Depresses automaticity
C. Bronchoconstriction
D. Renal vasodilation

55. All of the following are cardiovascular effects of adenosine except:
A. Depression of automaticity
B. Negative dromotropic
C. Renal vasodilatation
D. Coronary steal phenomenon

56. Which is not a Class IA antiarrhythmic agent?
A. Ajmaline B. Disopyramide
C. Moricizine D. Procainamide

57. Digoxin does not cause:
A. Ventricular extrasystoles
B. Mobitz type 2 block
C. Complete heart block
D. Sinus arrest

58. All are specific for digitalis toxicity except:
A. Parasystole
B. Paroxysmal atrial tachycardia with varying AV block
C. Regularisation of rate in patients of AF
D. Biventricular tachycardia

59. Treatment of choice for digoxin induced ventricular tachyarrhythmias:
A. Amiodarone B. Phenytoin
C. Quinidine D. Sotalol

60. Bidirectional VT in digoxin toxicity is due to?
A. Triggered activity associated with calcium overload
B. Increased automaticity
C. Reentry
D. Suppression of phase-0

61. What is not true regarding amiodarone?
A. Prolongs APD & refractoriness of all cardiac fibres without affecting resting membrane potential.
B. Amiodarone is a peripheral & coronary vasodilator
C. Doses need not be reduced in renal diseases
D. With concomitant use of warfarin with amiodarone, dose of warfarin should be increased.

62. All of the following are true about amiodarone induced pulmonary toxicity except:
A. Young age
B. Serum level of deoxy amiodarone
C. High daily dose
D. Decreased baseline DLCO

63. Which of the following is correct about Amiodarone?
A. QT prolongation is commonly associated with ventricular arrhythmias
B. Warfarin dose needs to be increased due to interaction in patients taking amiodarone
C. Stop amiodarone if patients develop clinical hypothyroidism
D. Pulmonary toxicity is uncommon at maintenance dose of 100 mg/day

64. All of the following are true about antiarrhythmics except?
A. Vernacline is used in AF
B. Dronedarone effective in VT
C. Ranolazine prevents VT in NSTEMI
D. Ivabradine used in Inappropriate sinus tachycardia

65. The management of polymorphic VT in the setting of myocardial infarction in acute phase may include all except?

A. I/V Beta-blockers
B. I/V Amiodarone
C. Urgent angiography when myocardial ischaemia cannot be excluded
D. I/V Sotalol

66. All of the following are correct regarding bidirectional VT except:
A. Digoxin toxicity
B. Anderson's syndrome
C. CPVT
D. Cerebrovasular accident

67. Urinary retention may be seen with:
A. Procainamide B. Disopyramide
C. Amiodarone D. Flecainide

68. Which of the following is anti-arrhythmic drug has β-blocker properties?
A. Ajmaline B. Procainamide
C. Flecainide D. Propafenone

69. Hemorrhagic pericardial effusion can be seen with:
A. Procainamide B. Amiodarone
C. Moricizine D. Dofetilide

ICD

70. AICD-Secondary prevention trial all except?
A. MADIT II B. AVID
C. CIDS D. CASH

71. A 45-year-old male patient is a case of CAD, post CABG, LVEF 28%. He is having class II symptoms (dyspnea) on optimal medical management. His ECG shows sinus rhythm, PR interval 220 msec and QRS duration of 112 msec. There is no history of syncope or pre-syncope or palpitations. The likely management should include:
A. ICD implantation
B. CRT implantation
C. Combo (ICD and CRT implantation)
D. No device therapy (at present)

72. Which among the following is not an indication for AICD implantation?
A. Survivors of cardiac arrest secondary to ventricular fibrillation (VF)
B. Structural heart disease and spontaneous sustained ventricular tachycardia (VT) which is hemodynamically stable
C. Incessant VT or VF
D. Nonischemic dilated cardiomyopathy in patients who have an left ventricular ejection fraction 35% and are in NYHA functional class II or III

73. An ICD implant for primary prevention is indicated for which of the following patients?
A. 50-year-old patient with history of myocardial infarction 6 weeks ago, NYHA class I symptoms, LVEF 30%
B. 40-year-old asymptomatic male with ECG suggestive of Brugada syndrome, whose brother died suddenly
C. 45-year-old asymptomatic patient with history of hypertrophic cardiomyopathy, LV thickness 2.0 cm
D. 18-year-old female with lightheaded spells and QT prolongation on ECG.

74. All of the following are true regarding ICD except:
A. Dual chamber ICD better than single chamber ICD in reducing mortality
B. ICD increases survival in patients with EF < 30%
C. Poor prognosis in patients who receive shock as compared to those who do not
D. Mortality is increased due to progressive heart failure in patients who have an ICD with appropriate shock

Pacemakers

75. False about NASPE Generic code for Antibradycardia pacing is?

A. Position I - Chamber(s) paced
B. Position III - Rate modulation
C. Position II - Chamber(s) sensed
D. Position V - Multisite pacing

76. Which of the following is a Class I indication of pacing as per ACC/AHA guidelines?
A. Patient with inferior wall MI and complete heart block lasting 7 days
B. An asymptomatic 18 year old female with congenital CHB and escape rate of 50/min
C. Recurrent syncope of undetermined etiology with LBBB
D. Symptomatic chronotropic incompetence

77. A 70 years old woman presents with chronic atrial fibrillation and ventricular rate of 30 per minutes. Pacemaker of choice is:
A. DDDR B. AAIR
C. VVIR D. VVI

78. Pacemaker setting with single chamber pacing in asynchronous mode:
A. AAI B. DDI
C. VOO D. DOO

79. In dual chamber pacemakers important feature to prevent endless loop tachycardia:
A. AV interval
B. PVARP
C. Hysteresis interval
D. Automatic interval

80. Which is true regarding different parameters tested during pacemaker testing?
A. In case of lead dislodgement, pacing threshold will be increased
B. In case of insulation failure, lead impedance will be increased
C. In battery depletion, lead impedance will be decreased
D. On loose setscrew, pacing threshold will be decreased

81. A 50 year old male patient on VVI pacemaker for complete heart block has to undergo surgical treatment using cautery. Any of the following perioperative strategy is useful except?
A. Place a magnet over the pacemaker during the procedure
B. Program the pacemaker to VOO mode
C. Switch off the hysteresis
D. Use bipolar electro cautery

82. All of the following are true about pacemaker syndrome except:
A. More common in patients with VA conduction
B. Responds to mode change to VVIR
C. Presents with dizziness and syncope
D. More common in elderly

83. Features of bipolar leads over unipolar leads all except:
A. Increased incidence of cross-talk
B. Decrease in far field sensing
C. Decrease myopotential oversensing
D. Decrease in stimulus artefact of pacemaker

CRT

84. Cardiac resynchronization therapy is indicated in:
A. HOCM B. RCMP
C. DCMP D. CHB

85. In a patient with ischemic cardiomyopathy, ejection fraction (EF) 30%, and New York Heart Association (NYHA) class I, which of the following condition is most optimum for CRT implantation?
A. Left bundle branch block (LBBB) with QRS duration 120–149 ms
B. Non-LBBB with QRS duration 120–149 ms
C. LBBB with QRS duration >150 ms
D. Non-LBBB with QRS duration >150 ms

Syncope

86. A 40 year old female presents with recurrent episodes of syncope. The episodes were preceded by weakness and nausea. Physical examination was unremarkable. ECG, echo and 24 hour Holter monitoring are normal. What is the next investigation of choice?

A. EPS
B. Head up Tilt Table test
C. Signal averaged ECG
D. Implantable arrhythmia monitor

87. Drug which is used for pharmacologic provocation during upright tilt table test includes?

A. Esmolol B. Nifedipine
C. Isoproterenol D. Nicornadil

88. Drugs which have been investigated for pharmacological treatment of neuro-cardiogenic syncope include all of the following except?

A. Midodrine B. Pyridostigmine
C. Diltiazem D. Theophylline

89. Which of the following statement is not true regarding carotid sinus hyper-sensitivity?

A. Elderly patients may present with unexplained falls without loss of consciousness
B. The reflex has a cardio-inhibitory component
C. There is no vasodepressor component
D. Permanent pacing is indicated in patients who develop pause > 3.0 s with carotid sinus massage

90. Which of the following is best treatment for reflex syncope?

A. Isometric counterpressure manoeuvres
B. Tilt training
C. Midodrine
D. β blocker

91. Treatment of choice for Postural syncope:

A. Midodrine
B. B blockers
C. Tilt training
D. Isometric compressive manoeuvre

Cardiac arrest and resuscitation

92. Which of the following is most common cause of SCD?

A. IHD
B. HOCM
C. Brugada syndrome
D. ARVD

93. Most common cause of death in young athletes?

A. Anomalous origin of coronary artery from wrong sinus
B. HOCM
C. Marfan syndrome
D. Congenital aortic valve stenosis

94. Most common game associated with Commotio cordis is?

A. Foot ball B. Baseball
C. Cricket D. Ice hockey

95. The most effective treatment which improves survival for a comatose patient who has been resuscitated from out-of-hospital cardiac arrest is?

A. Therapeutic hypothermia
B. Hyperventilation using mechanical ventilation
C. Immediate coronary angiography and PCI
D. Dobutamine infusion

96. With waveform capnography, what is the normal expected value?

A. 35–45 mmHg
B. 20 mmHg
C. <10 mmHg
D. 0 mmHg

97. With waveform capnography, what is the expected during CPR in a code setting with a dislodged ET tube?

A. 35–45 mHg
B. 20 mmHg
C. <10 mmHg
D. 0 mmHg

98. For witnessed out-of-hospital cardiac arrest due to ventricular fibrillation, what is the appropriate energy level for defibrillation?

A. 120–200 J with a biphasic shock device
B. 360 J with a monophasic shock device
C. 2–4 J/kg body weight for a child
D. All of the above

99. What is the desired depth of chest compression in adult CPR?

A. ≥2 in
B. 1.5–2 in
C. Enough to produce a pulse
D. 2-2.4 inches

100. What is the desired rate of chest compression in adult CPR?

A. At least 100/min
B. 80–100/min
C. 60/min in adult, 100/min in a child, 120/min in an infant
D. 100-120 per minute

101. In two-rescuer CPR, what is the optimal compression-to-ventilation ratio?

A. 15 : 2 B. 30 : 2
C. 5 : 1 D. 10 : 2

102. One of the following statements is false:

A. Sequence of steps in Basic Life Support: "C-A-B" (Chest compression, Airway, Breathing)
B. Ventilations with advanced airway (10 breaths/min)
C. Compression to ventilation ratio of 30:2 in adults if one rescuer is there.
D. Routine use of atropine during asystole is likely to have therapeutic benefit.

103. Immediate therapy for VT with no pulse is:

A. Synchronized cardioversion
B. Defibrillation (nonsynchronized)
C. Lidocaine bolus IV
D. Any of the above

Miscellaneous

104. False statement about Parasystole:

A. Intervals are multiples of basic interval
B. Functions like fixed rate asynchronous pacemaker
C. Functions like fixed rate synchronous pacemaker
D. Can exhibit entrance block or exit block

105. True statement about late potentials:

A. Filtered QRS duration 114-120 msec
B. <20 mV of root mean square signal amplitude in the last 40 msec of filtered QRS complex
C. Terminal filtered QRS complex remains below 40 mV for >38 msec
D. All of the above

106. Arrhythmias causing tachycardia-mediated cardiomyopathy include all of the following except?

A. Ectopic atrial tachycardia
B. Atrial fibrillation
C. Persistent junctional reciprocating tachycardia (PJRT)
D. Bidirectional ventricular tachycardia

107. EPS is least useful in diagnosis of:

A. Brugada syndrome
B. Idiopathic VT
C. LQTS (and TDP)
D. ARVC

108. Defibrillation threshold is raised by all except:

A. Disopyramide B. Flecainide
C. Dofetilide D. Amiodarone

ANSWERS

Brugada syndrome

Answer: 1. C. SCN5A-encoded sodium channel.

Brugada syndrome: Loss of function mutation in the SCN5A-encoded sodium channel.

LQT3 syndrome: Gain of function in the same SCN5A-encoded sodium channel.

Answer: 2. Functional phase 2 re-entry

Answer: 3. A. Phase 4 re-entry

Answer: 4. D. Functional phase 2 re-entry

Answer: 5. B. Cardiac events never occur during sleep or rest

Answer: 6. B. Sleep

Answer: 7. A. Quinidine

Answer: 8. C. 30%.

An ICD is also indicated

Answer: 9. A. It is a genetically determined sodium channelopathy.

Answer: 10. D. ST elevation in V1 – V3 increases with flecainide

Answer: 11. D. Short QT syndrome

Brugada syndrome:

Cause of ventricular arrhythmia in structurally normal heart.

Autosomal dominant genetic disorder.

Loss of function genetic mutation in cardiac sodium channels **(SCN5A and SCN10A).**

Functional phase 2 re-entry leads to ventricular arrhythmias in Brugada.

ECG: Right bundle branch pattern with ST elevation in V1 to V3 leads.

Types of Brugada syndrome:

Type 1: Coved type ST elevation ($\geq$2 mm) with inverted T waves

Type 2: Saddle-back ST-T wave configuration with an upright or biphasic T waves

Image: Types of Brugada syndrome (see next page)

Brugada pattern ECG is more common in **men** as compared to women and in southeast asia.

Arrhythmic events more common during **night and during sleep** (Not during exertion).

The ECG changes can be **dynamic** and come and go and can be provoked with procainamide challenge.

Type I Brugada with ST elevation of **>10 mm has a very high risk** of sudden death.

Image: Types of Brugada syndrome

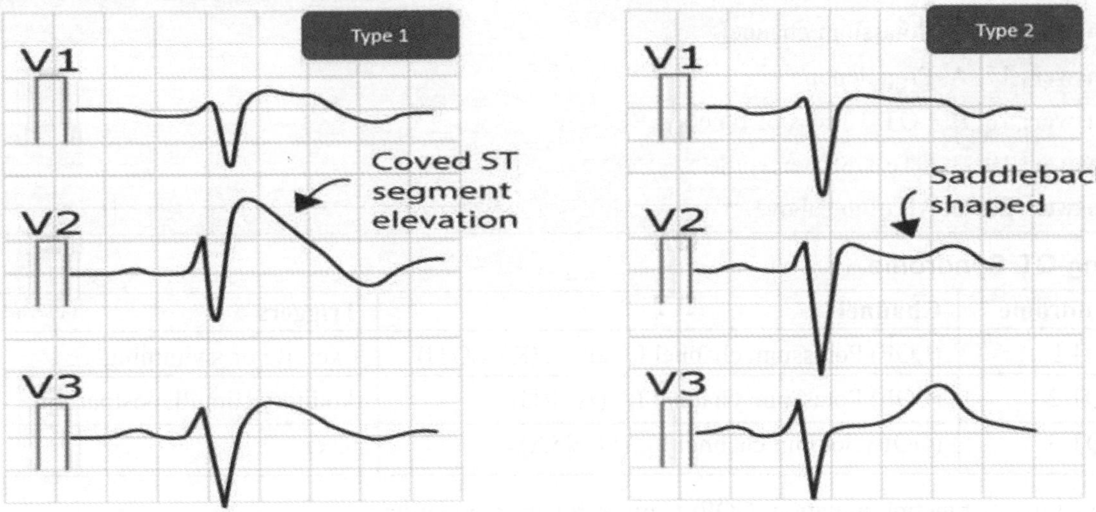

Fever and sodium channel blocker (Flecainide, ajmaline, procainamide) can provoke arrhythmias.

These drugs are also used for **drug challenge test** for diagnosis of Brugada as they unmask the Brugada pattern of ECG.

Treatment: Isoprenaline and Quinidine theoretically might be helpful but have not been found to be much helpful.

ICD insertion is only effective treatment to prevent SCD. The indications include history of syncope (Class I) or sudden cardiac death (Class I); inducible VT on EPS (Class IIa) and family history of sudden cardiac death (Class IIb).

Sodium channelopathies:

1. Brugada syndrome
2. Congenital long QT syndrome
3. Isolated cardiac conduction system disease
4. Congenital sick sinus syndrome
5. Familial AF

QT syndromes

Answer: 12. A. Long QT syndrome

Answer: 13. A. Resting ECG shows broad T waves

Answer: 14. C. SCN5A-encoded sodium channel.

Long QT3 channelopathy occurs due to a mutation in the SCN5A encoded sodium channel (gain of function). Mutation in the KCNQ1 (IKs) channel is associated with long QT1, and mutation in the KCNH2 (IKr) channel is associated with long QT2 syndrome.

Answer: 15. C. Inhibition of KCNH 2-encoded HERG potassium channel.

Answer: 16. A. Potassium channel.

Answer: 17. A. Propafenone

Answer: 18. B. LQT 3- Loss of function SCN5A

Answer: 19. B. QTc < 88 percentile

Answer: 20. D. All of the above

Long-QT Syndrome

Syndrome	Channel	Triggers
LQT 1	(LOF) Potassium channel I_{Ks} alpha (KVLQTl)	Exercise or swimming
LQT 2	(LOF) Potassium channel I_{Kr} (HERG)	Auditory stimuli, postpartum
LQT 3	(GOF) Sodium channel I_{Na} (SCN5A)	Sleep

LOF- Loss of function mutation, GOF- Gain of function mutation

LQT1: LQT1 is usually associated with **broad-based T waves.**

LQT2: **Notching of T waves** is present.

LQT3: Associated with a long isoelectric ST segment with a **normal T wave morphology.**

Increased risk of SCD by polymorphic ventricular tachycardia (PMVT) or TdP.

Abnormal QTc cut-off values are commonly selected as >440 milliseconds in men and >460 milliseconds in women.

The longer the QTc, the higher is the arrhythmic mortality, being about 5% in those with QTc of 450 ms, and 50% in those with QTc >500 ms over lifetime. Syncope in these patients is likely due to runs of polymorphic VT

Jervell and Lange-Nielsen syndrome: Autosomal recessive inherited long QT syndrome and associated with congenital sensorineural deafness caused by mutation in potassium channels.

Romano-Ward syndrome: Autosomal dominant inherited long QT syndrome without deafness, caused by mutation in potassium channels and sodium channels.

Treatment: Beta blocker therapy (First line)

Mexiletine useful in LQT3, blocks SCN5A sodium channels.

If VT or syncope on beta blocker therapy: ICD implantation

Other causes of QT prolongation:

Electrolyte abnormalities:

- Hypokalemia
- Hypocalcemia

- Hypomagnesemia

Drugs:

- Antiarrhythmics: class IA (disopyramide, quinidine, procainamide), class III (sotalol, dofetilide)
- Tricyclic antidepressants (amitriptyline, desipramine)
- Antifungals (itraconazole, ketoconazole)
- Antihistamines (astemizole, terfenadine)
- Antimicrobials (Bactrim, Erythomycin, pentamidine)
- Neuroleptics (phenothiazines, thioridazine)
- Organophosphate insecticides
- Promotility agents (cisapride)
- Oral hypoglycemics (Glibenclamide)

Other conditions

- Bradycardia
- Hypothyroidism
- Subarachnoid hemorrhage

Most of the medications that prolong QT act by inhibiting the KCNH2- **encoded HERG potassium channel**.

Timothy syndrome (Long QT 8 syndrome):

- Long QT syndrome, syndactyly, autism
- Mutation in Calcium channel (CACNA1C), Autosomal dominant pattern of inheritance.

Short-QT syndrome

Characterized by QTc intervals <300 milliseconds and associated with SCD by VT and VF

Gain of function mutation in the gene for **potassium channels** are responsible. **HERG** (or KCNH2) and KCQN1.

Management: Quinidine (prolongs QT and prevents VT), ICD

Catecholaminergic polymorphic ventricular tachycardia

Answer: 21. D. First line of therapy is amiodarone.

Answer: 22. A. Quinidine

Catecholaminergic polymorphic ventricular tachycardia

Arrhythmias seen in **structurally normal heart** typically occur during **exercise** or at times of emotional stress, when chemical messengers like adrenaline, known as catecholamines, are released within the body and typically take the form of **bidirectional ventricular tachycardia** or ventricular fibrillation.

Caused by genetic mutations affecting proteins that regulate the concentrations of calcium within cardiac muscle cells. The most commonly identified gene is **RYR2,** encoding a protein encoding a channel known as the **ryanodine receptor.**

Most common **autosomal dominant** inheritance.

Mutations associated with CPVT have also been identified in the CASQ2 gene which encodes **calsequestrin**, and have **autosomal recessive** inheritance.

Mechanism of VT: Delayed afterdepolarisation

Treatment:

Beta-adrenoceptor blockers (Class I indication): First line drugs

Flecainide: Inhibits cardiac ryanodine receptor mediated Ca release. It is prescribed in addition to beta blockers.

ICD: Who have survived cardiac arrest (Class I), who have sustained syncope or VT while receiving beta blockers (Class IIa).

Left cervical sympathectomy:

When beta blockers are contraindicated and AICD can not be placed or recurrent VT in patients having AICD despite maximal medical treatment.

Type	Gene Code	Inheritance	Protein
CPVT1	RYR2	AD	Ryanodine receptor
CPVT2	CASQ2	AR	Calsequestrin
CPVT3	TECRL	AR	Trans-2,33-enoyl-CoA
CPVT4	CALM1	AD	Calmodulin
CPVT5	TRDN	AR	Triadin

ATRIOVENTRICULAR (AV) BLOCK

Answer: 23. B. Progressive increase of RR interval

First-Degree AV Block

PR interval greater than 200 ms

Second-Degree AV Block

Second-Degree AV Wenckebach Block (Mobitz I)

The block occurs at the level of the AV node

PR interval progressively increases followed by a pause (prolonged RR interval) in which there is a P wave that is not followed by a QRS complex.

As the PR interval increases, each increment is progressively smaller

Each RR interval is progressively smaller

The RR "pause" is longer than the longest P-P interval and shorter than double the shortest P-P interval

Second-Degree AV Type II Block (Mobitz II)

PR interval constant with intermittent absent R waves.

Block is below the level of AV node (infranodal) and within the His Purkinje System

Mostly requires permanent pacemaker.

Third-Degree (Complete) AV Block

Absence of atrioventricular conduction (AV dissociation)

P waves present but no direct relationship with R waves.

If QRS narrow, block is near AV node and if QRS is wide, block is more distal in His purkinje system.

Block is below AV node and at level of His Purkinje System.

Suprahisian vs infrahisian block

	Suprahisian heart block	Infrahisian heart block
Location of heart block	AV node	Infranodal block
ECG	First degree, Mobitz type I, Complete heart block (narrow QRS complex)	Mobitz II, Complete heart block (wide QRS complex)
QRS duration	Normal (Less than 120 msec)	Wide (More than 120 msec)
Origin of escape rhythm	AV node	Ventricular conduction system
Escape rhythm (rate)	≥ 40 bpm	≤ 30 bpm
Prognosis	Good	Poor (Requires urgent temporary or permanent pacemaker)
Associated myocardial infarction	Inferior wall MI	Anterior wall MI
Pathogenesis in MI	Excess parasympathetic activity	Ischemia, extensive necrosis

Sick Sinus Syndrome (SSS)

Also called as sinus node dysfunction or sinoatrial node disease (SND).

It is a group of abnormal heart rhythms caused by malfunction of sinus node; usually causing brady-arrhythmias such as sinus arrest, sinus node exit block and sinus bradycardia.

Tachycardia-bradycardia syndrome is a variant of SSS, in which atrial brady-arrhythmias alternate with tachy-arrhythmias such as AF, AFl, other supraventricular/atrial tachycardias.

Symptoms: Dizziness, palpitations, fatigue, shortness of breath, Stokes-Adams attacks (Syncope due to asystole or ventricular fibrillation)

Treatment: Symptomatic SSS requires permanent pacemaker implantation.

SVT and Re-entrant tachycardias

Answer: 24. A. Re-entry

Answer: 25. A. EAT

Presence of excitable gap and entrainment are features of re-entry.

Answer: 26. B. Left lateral

Answer: 27. C. The tachycardia rates are usually slower than other tachyarrhythmias

Answer: 28. C. Constant PR interval

Answer: 29. C. Varying PP interval but fixed RR interval

Answer: 30. B. Mostly manifests as incessant tachycardia leading to ventricular dysfunction

Answer: 31. C. AVRT

Answer: 32. A. Can present with re-entrant tachycardia

Answer: 33. D. Digoxin

Answer: 34. B. Orthodromic AVRT using a left-sided bypass tract

Answer: 35. C. Cardioversion.

In a patient with Wolff–Parkinson–White (WPW) syndrome and atrial fibrillation, cardioversion is indicated. All other options are contraindicated.

Answer: 36. D. Permanent form of junctional reciprocating tachycardia

Mechanism of Tachyarrhythmias:

1. Enhanced automaticity: Inappropriate sinus tachycardia, Atrial tachycardia, Accelerated idiovenricular rhythm
2. Triggered activity (After depolarization):

EAD (Early After depolarization)- Abnormal depolarization during phase 2 or phase 3.

Examples- Torsades de pointes, Long QT syndrome, Hypokalemia

DAD (Delayed After depolarization)- Abnormal depolarization during phase 4.

Examples- Digitalis toxicity, RVOT-VT, Catecholaminergic polymorphic ventricular tachycardia (CPVT)

3. Re-entry: Atrial flutter, Atrial fibrillation, AVNRT, AVRT, Polymorphic and uniform VT, Bundle branch re-entry, Ventricular fibrillation.

Re-entry occurs due to presence of excitable gap.

Entrainment is a feature of re-entry tachycardia.

Atrio-ventricular nodal re-entrant tachycardia (AVNRT)

Regular narrow QRS tachycardia at rates between 120 and 220 bpm with abrupt onset and offset.

Typical (Slow-Fast) AVNRT: 90% cases

Antegrade conduction (toward the ventricles) proceeds through the slow pathway and retrograde activation through the fast pathway

Causes rapid retrograde activation of the atria, as a result, the P wave occurs at the within or at end of QRS complex (pseudo R prime)

The RP interval is shorter than half of the RR interval of the AVNRT (Short RP tachycardia)

Atypical (Fast-Slow) AVNRT:

Antegrade conduction is via the fast pathway and there is late activation of the atria from retrograde conduction via the slow pathway

The P wave occurs late and within the ST segment, hence it is long RP tachycardia

Atrio-ventricular reciprocating tachycardia (AVRT):

Characterized by presence of accessory pathways that function as part of the tachycardia re-entrant circuit.

Macro-re-entrant circuit between the atria and the ventricles involves conduction via an accessory pathway between the atria and ventricles (e.g. bundle of Kent).

Most common accessory pathway: Left lateral

Least complications during RF ablation: Left lateral pathway

Other accessory pathways:

James fibers – intranodal or paranodal fibers that bypass all or part of the AV node to enter the bundle of His before the bifurcation, resulting in an electrocardiogram with a short PR with normal duration QRS

Lown-Ganong-Levine (LGL) syndrome is the occurrence an ECG with a short PR and normal duration QRS together with tachyarrhythmias

Mahaim fibers -

Mahaim fibers are atriofascicular pathways that are typically associated with left bundle branch block (LBBB) tachycardias in which the atriofascicular fiber (typically RA to right bundle branch (RBB) connection) is used as the antegrade limb and the AV node as the retrograde limb of the re-entrant circuit.

Multiple accessory pathways can be present in Ebstein's anomaly.

Orthodromic AVRT: antegrade through the AV node and retrograde via the accessory pathway, resulting in a narrow-complex tachycardia with retrograde P waves occurring after the QRS complex typically within the ST segment

Antidromic AVRT (less common) – conduction occurs antegrade through the accessory pathway and retrograde via the AV node, resulting in a delta wave, wide-complex QRS, short PR tachycardia

Concealed accessory pathway:

When accessory pathway is able to conduct **only retrogradely** and anterograde conduction is absent, it is called concealed accessory pathway; and it **does not** manifest in sinus rhythm.

Concealed accessory pathways are mostly **left sided**.

There is **no risk** of AF terminating into VF as anterograde conduction over accessory pathway is absent.

Do not generate a delta wave and the WPW pattern on the surface ECG but are still capable of supporting re-entrant tachycardia **(Orthodromic AVRT).**

Wolff-Parkinson-White (WPW) syndrome:

Antidromic tachycardia through accessory pathway (bundle of Kent) causing short PR and wide QRS with a delta wave at the onset of the QRS.

AF in this setting can rapidly terminate into VF and can cause SCD.

Treatment:

Class IA antiarrhythmic agents (procainamide), amiodarone or cardioversion used to terminate arrhythmia.

Verapamil and digoxin are **contraindicated** for termination of pre-excited AF, may result in higher ventricular rates.

Paroxysmal junctional re-entrant tachycardia (PJRT):

Seen in **children** and characterised by an incessant **orthodromic** tachycardia with anterograde conduction over the atrioventricular node and by retrograde conduction via an accessory pathway

Has **long** RP interval, and tachycardia rates are slower than other tachyarrhythmias.

The arrhythmia is commonly incessant from birth or infancy, even though it may not be recognised until adulthood.

Persistence over a long period of time may lead to a **tachycardia induced cardiomyopathy**

Spontaneous resolution of tachycardia is not uncommon

Arrhythmia is considered to be usually refractory to drug treatment

Narrow QRS tachycardia:

1. **Short RP interval:** Typical AVNRT, Orthodromic AVRT, junctional tachycardia
2. **Long RP interval:** Atrial tachycardia, PJRT, Atypical AVNRT, Antidromic AVRT, sinus tachycardia

Radiofrequency ablation:

Answer: 37. D. EP study/ablation.

Answer: 38. D. Left lateral pathway

Answer: 39. B. Radiofrequency

Answer: 40. C. 90–95%.

Catheter ablation of arrhythmias

Common types: Radiofrequency ablation (most common) and cryoablation

Recurrence rates are slightly higher with cryoablation.

It is usually done in SVT, atrial flutter, atrial tachycardia, atrial fibrillation and specific types of ventricular arrhythmias.

High success rates in re-entrant tachycardias such as atrial flutter, AVNRT and AVRT.

Ablation of AVRT having accessory pathways: Success rates of left sided pathways is higher than the right sided pathways; and **left lateral pathway** has the highest success rate for ablation and lowest rate for recurrence.

Success rates: SVT (90-95%), Typical atrial flutter (90-95%), VT without structural heart disease (90%), VT with structural heart disease (70%), Atrial fibrillation (60-70% with one procedure; 80-90% with subsequent procedures).

Ablation procedures for AF

1. Maze procedure:

- Typically done at the time of concomitant valvular or coronary bypass procedures
- Creation of linear lines of block resulting in isolation of the pulmonary veins

2. Catheter ablation for AF

- Involves electrical "isolation" of the sites of arrhythmia origin using ablative energy to block electrical propagation, rather than the primary goal of ablating the site of origin

Indications for catheter ablation of AF:

- Symptomatic paroxysmal or persistent AF resistant to antiarrhythmic drug therapy
- AF associated with hemodynamic compromise and resistant to antiarrhythmic drug therapy

Success rate for catheter ablation: 60–75 % after first procedure and 80–90 % in subsequent procedures

Lower rate of success in persistent AF, older patients, in those with structurally abnormal hearts and hugely dilated LA

Major complications of catheter ablation of AF:

- Thromboembolic stroke or TIA (0.5–1 %)
- Cardiac perforation with tamponade (1 %)
- Local catheter site or retroperitoneal bleeding (1 %)
- Phrenic nerve injury (more common with balloon vs. catheter technologies)
- Atrio-esophageal fistula (<0.1 %)

Atrial fibrillation and flutter

Answer: 41. D. Atrial fibrillation

Answer: 42. B. Metoprolol 5mg I/V over 5 minutes

Metoprolol is used for rate control of AF.

Answer: 43. D. Flecainide

Pill in the pocket therapy for AF: 1. Flecainide 2. Propafenone

Answer: 44. A. Propafenone

Answer: 45. C. Re-entry using cavotricuspid isthmus

ATRIAL FIBRILLATION (AF)

AF is the most common sustained arrhythmia

Prevalence increases with age, 10% of persons over the age of 80 have AF.

Classification of AF:

Paroxysmal AF: 2 or more episodes that terminate spontaneously within 7 days

Persistent AF: Persisting beyond 7 days

Permanent AF: More than 12 months duration and decision have been made not to restore sinus rhythm.

Lone AF: AF in the absence of other heart disease, occurs in younger individuals (<60 years of age).

ECG:

Absence of organized atrial activity, associated with an irregularly irregular ventricular rhythm.

Rate control:

Agents: Beta blocker, CCB, digoxin

Amiodarone can be used for rate control if other agents fail and also useful to maintain sinus rhythm.

Rhythm control:

Agents: Class Ic drugs (Flecainide, Propafenone), Class III drugs (Amiodarone, sotalol, dofetilide, dronedarone, ibutilide)

DC cardioversion and catheter ablation.

AFFIRM trial: Survival not different between rhythm and rate control strategies.

Antithrombotic therapy:

CHA_2DS_2-VASc score: CHF (1 point), HTN (1 point), Age >75 years (2 points), DM (1 point), Stroke/ TIA (2 points), Vascular disease (1 point), 65-74 years (1 point), Sex category, female (1 point)

Score of zero: Aspirin or no therapy, score of 1: Aspirin or OAC, Score of >1: OAC.

Atrial flutter (AFL):

Regular atrial cycle length, (F-F interval) in AFL with rate in the range of 250-320 bpm.

Type I or typical AFL:

Single **re-entrant** circuit circulating around the tricuspid annulus in RA **(cavotricuspid isthmus).**

Negative F wave in lead II and positive F wave in aVL and aVR.

Most often counterclockwise in direction (90%)→ positive F waves in V1, rarely clockwise (10%)→ negative F waves in V1.

ECG: Saw tooth appearance (most visible in V1-2 or inferior leads).

Type II or atypical AFL: Different location and re-entrant circuits than cavotricuspid area, isthmus independent.

Treatment: Cardioversion, if unsuccessful then EP study and ablation of flutter.

Ventricular tachycardia

Answer: 46. A. Ventricular tachycardia

Answer: 47. C. Irregularly irregular rhythm

Answer: 48. D. Belhassen's VT or Idiopathic left fascicular VT is due to re-entry & is resistant to Verapamil.

Answer: 49. A. β blocker is the treatment of choice

→ CCB's are used and RFA is treatment of choice.

Answer: 50. C. High risk of sudden cardiac death

Answer: 51. D. Poor response to pharmacological therapy

Features favouring VT in wide complex tachycardia:

Brugada's algorithm:

1. Absence of RS complex in all precordial leads.
2. R to S interval >100 ms in any precordial lead (Brugada sign)
3. AV dissociation
4. Morphologic criteria

Additional features:

- QRS duration >160 ms
- Right superior QRS axis (north-west axis, extreme axis deviation)
- Capture beats
- Fusion beats
- Josephson's sign: Notching near the nadir of S-wave
- Vereckei sign: A dominant initial R wave in aVR

Outflow tract ventricular tachycardia:

Mechanism: cAMP mediated delayed afterdepolarizations, triggered activity

Not associated with risk of syncope or sudden cardiac death.

Most often from RVOT- Inferior axis with LBBB morphology.

Vagal maneuvers, Adenosine, CCB or Beta blocker sensitive; drug of choice is beta blocker.

Easily treatable with catheter ablation

Bundle branch re-entrant ventricular tachycardia (BBR VT):

The arrhythmia is usually seen in patients with an **acquired heart disease** such as DCMP, ICMP or valvular heart disease.

Symptoms: Presyncope, syncope or sudden cardiac death

QRS morphology during VT: Usually **LBBB pattern** (as anterograde conduction over RBB and retrograde conduction over LBB).

Prolonged His-ventricular (HV) interval in majority of patients with BBR VT.

Pharmacologic antiarrhythmic therapy is usually **ineffective**.

RF ablation of a bundle branch (usually right bundle branch) can cure BBR VT and is first line therapy.

Idiopathic left ventricular tachycardia (Fascicular VT or Verapamil sensitive VT or Belhassen's tachycardia)

Most idiopathic VTs arise in RV while rest 10-20% arise from LV, specially from left posterior fascicle.

Types:

1. Posterior fascicular VT:
   Most common subtype, accounts for 90-95% of cases.
   Arise from posterior fascicle, hence characterized by RBBB with left axis deviation.
2. Anterior fascicular VT:
   Second variant in terms of frequency.
   RBBB with right axis deviation
3. Upper fascicular VT:
   Rare, RBBB with normal frontal axis.

Patients are young and healthy, without any structural heart disease; VT precipitated by exercise, excitement, and infection.

VT is typically hemodynamically stable and sudden death is rare. QRS is relatively narrow.

Intravenous verapamil successfully terminates this VT and RF ablation also has high success rate for permanent termination.

Polymorphic VT (Torsades de pointes):

Associated with long QT interval

Can be caused by any of condition predisposing to long QT or by certain drugs. (See the long QT syndrome)

Treatment: IV magnesium or isoproterenol or temporary pacing at 100 to 110 pulses per minute

ANTIARRHYTHMIC DRUGS

Answer: 52. B. Adenosine

Answer: 53. B. IB

Answer: 54. D. Renal vasodilation

Answer: 55. C. Renal vasodilation

Answer: 56. C. Moricizine

Answer: 57. B. Mobitz type 2 block

Answer: 58. A. Parasystole

Answer: 59. B. Phenytoin

Answer: 60. A. Triggered activity associated with calcium overload

Answer: 61. D. With concomitant use of warfarin with amiodarone, dose of warfarin should be increased.

Answer: 62. A. Young age

Answer: 63. D. Pulmonary toxicity is uncommon at maintenance dose of 100 mg/day

Answer: 64. B. Dronedarone effective in VT

Answer: 65. D. I/V Sotalol

→ Mortality was increased with Sotalol in VT after acute MI in SWORD trial.

Answer: 66. D. Cerebrovasular accident

Answer: 67. B. Disopyramide

Answer: 68. D. Propafenone

Answer: 69. A. Procainamide

Vaughan Williams classification

Class I: predominantly sodium channel blockers.

IA: Additional K channel blocking action. Reduce Vmax and prolong the action potential duration. E.g: Procainamide, Disopyramide, Quinidine, Ajmaline.

IB: Additional K channel opening action. Does not reduce Vmax and **shortens** the action potential duration. E.g: Mexiletine, Phenytoin, Lignocaine

IC: No action on K channel. E.g: Moracizine, Propafenone, Flecainide

Class II: β-adrenergic receptor blockers. E.g: Propranolol, Metoprolol, Nadolol.

Class III: potassium channel blockers (I_{kr}) and prolong repolarization (all clinically used agents block I_{Kr} and prolong the QT interval).

Eg: Sotalol, Amiodarone, Dofetilide, Ibutilide, Dronedarone

Class IV: calcium channel blockers (I_{CaL}). Verapamil, Diltiazem

Class I drugs bind to the sodium channel in such a way that the drug effect is increased at faster heart rates. This phenomenon is known as use-dependent action.

Class III drugs show reverse-use dependency (i.e., greater efficacy at slower heart rate)

Class IA and III drugs increase QT interval by blocking K channels, hence have the tendency for Torsades de pointes.

All class I drugs can increase QRS duration by blocking Na channels.

Amiodarone:

Contains 37% iodine by weight, and is used in the treatment of atrial and ventricular arrhythmias.

Highly lipid soluble, accumulates extensively in body organs, prolonging its elimination half life.

Metabolized in **liver** by cytochrome P450 enzyme to desethylemiodarone (DEA).

Increases QT but tendency for Torsades de pointes is very low

Amiodarone has class I (blocks I_{Na}), class II (antiadrenergic), and class IV (blocks $I_{Ca.L}$) actions in addition to its predominant class III effects (blocks I_K)

Half life: 53 days

Side effects:

Pulmonary toxicity

Hypo and hyperthyroidism

Hepatotoxicity

Photosensitivity

Discoloration of the skin

Corneal microdeposits

→ **Pulmonary toxicity** is most serious adverse event. Correlates better with total cumulative dose rather than daily dose or plasma concentration.

Can occur at any time after treatment is initiated, risk is more in those who have received daily 400 mg or daily for more than 2 months.

Incidence- 2%

Risk: Males, advanced age, pre-existing lung disease, decreased baseline DL_{CO} higher daily dose.

Reduced diffusing capacity of the lung for carbon monoxide (DL_{CO}) is typically seen along with restrictive pattern on PFT.

→ **Thyroid abnormalities:** Amiodarone induced thyrotoxicosis (AIT) is seen in 1-2% patients whereas amiodarone induced hypothyroidism (AIH) is seen in 2-4% patients. Hypothyroidism occurs because amiodarone inhibits conversion of T4 to T3 in peripheral tissues. Amiodarone need not be stopped in case of AIH and levothyroxine can be externally supplemented.

Amiodarone induced thyrotoxicosis (AIT):

Two forms

Type 1: Caused by iodine induced excess thyroid hormone synthesis and release (Jod-Basedow phenomenon).

Affects patients with latent or pre-existing thyroid disorders and is more common in areas of low iodine intake.

Type 2: Caused by destructive thyroiditis which leads to release of preformed thyroid hormones from damaged thyroid follicular cess.

Occurs in patients with a previously normal thyroid gland.

→ **Drug interactions:**

Amiodarone decreases the clearance of digoxin leading to **increase** in serum levels. Hence, dose of digoxin should be decreased in these patients.

Amiodarone potentiates the action of warfarin by inhibition of CYP2C9 coenzyme and P-glycoprotein system.

Amiodarone increases statin concentration and increases risk of statin induced myopathy because of inhibition of CYP3A4.

It decreases clearance of lidocaine and potentiates the effect of beta and calcium channel blockers.

Dronedarone

Dronedarone **does not contain iodine** and therefore does not cause iodine-related adverse reaction and adverse effects.

For patients with **atrial fibrillation and flutter**, but not approved for ventricular arrhythmias

Contraindicated in symptomatic CHF patients

Side effects: Liver toxicity and QT prolongation

ANDROMEDA study: Dronedarone was associated with an approximate doubling of mortality rate in patients with moderate to severe CHF

Sotalol:

SWORD trial: d-Sotalol was associated with an increased mortality rate compared with placebo in patients with LV dysfunction and recent MI.

Dofetilide

Approved for treatment of atrial fibrillation and flutter

DIAMOND study: Dofetilide does not affect the mortality rate of patients with prior MI and LV dysfunction

Adenosine:

Endogenous nucleoside, indicated to treat SVTs (such as AVNRT and AVRT)

Activates K^+ channels, shortens atrial APD and decrease atrial contractility.

Half-life: 1 to 6 seconds

Side effects: Flushing, dyspnea and chest pressure.

Renal vasoconstriction is caused by A_1 receptors.

Adenosine receptors and functions:

Receptor	**Functions**
A1	Decreased heart rate Bronchoconstriction Afferent arteriolar **constriction** in kidneys
A2a	Coronary artery **vasodilation** Decreased dopaminergic activity in CNS (**Regadenoson** is specific agonist of A2a receptors)
A2b	Bronchospasm
A3	Cardiac muscle relaxation Smooth muscle contraction Cardioprotective in cardiac ischemia Inhibition of neutrophil degranulation

Digoxin:

Used for ventricular rate control during AF.

Mechanism: Na-K ATPase channel inhibitor, increases Ca concentration in cell leading increased myocardial contractility. Also enhances central and peripheral vagal tone leading to slowing of sinus node discharge rate and AV nodal refractoriness.

Half-life: 36 to 48 hours

Side-effects:

Digoxin has narrow therapeutic index. Therapeutic range: 0.5 to 1.0 ng/ml. Toxic level >2.0 ng/ml

Headache, nausea and vomiting, altered color perception, halo vision.

Digitalis-related arrhythmias: Bradycardias related to a greatly enhanced vagal effect (e.g., sinus bradycardia or arrest, AV node block) and tachyarrhythmias that may be caused by DAD-mediated triggered activity (e.g., atrial, junctional, and fascicular or ventricular tachycardia).

Arrhythmia **most specific** for digoxin toxicity: Paroxysmal atrial tachycardia with AV block.

Three characteristic arrhythmias seen in digoxin toxicity: PAT with AV block, Bidirectional VT, and AF/AFl with regular ventricular rate.

Arrhythmias **not seen** in digoxin toxicity: New onset Atrial flutter, Atrial fibrillation, and **Mobitz type II AV block**.

Worsening renal function, advanced age, hypokalemia, hypomagnesemia, hypercalcemia, hypothyroidism, and amyloidosis increase digitalis toxicity.

Life-threatening arrhythmias can be treated with digoxin-specific antibody fragments. Electrical DC cardioversion should be avoided in a digitalis-toxic patient because life-threatening VT or VF can result and can be difficult to control

Important: Causes of **bidirectional ventricular tachycardia** → 1. Digoxin toxicity, 2. CPVT, 3. Aconite poisoning, 4. Anderson syndrome

Important points about antiarrhythmic drugs:

→ Disopyramide is a class Ia antiarrhythmic drug which also has anticholinergic properties and therefore causes side effects such as urinary retention, constipation, dry eyes and dry mouth.

→ Ajmaline (Class Ia) also inhibits platelet activity, more potently that aspirin.

Effects:

1. Delta wave disappearance in WPW syndrome (suggesting higher refractory period of accessory pathway)
2. ST abnormalities and IVCD in patients with occult Chagas disease.
3. Right precordial ST elevation in patients of suspected Brugada syndrome with normal resting ECG.

→ Procainamide (Class Ia) can produce SLE like manifestations causing arthralgia, fever, pleuropericarditis, hepatomegaly, and hemorrhagic pericardial effusion with tamponade.

However, unlike classical SLE, brain and kidneys are spared and there is no predilection of women.

The syndrome occurs more commonly in slow acetylators of procainamide.

Antinuclear antibodies (ANA) develop in 60-70% patients receiving long term procainamide therapy but clinical symptoms develop in 20-30% only. Symptoms improve when procainamide is stopped or with the help of steroids.

Development of ANAs is not an indication to stop procainamide but development of symptoms or a positive anti-DNA antibody indicates that drug should be discontinued.

→ Propafenone is a class Ic antiarrhythmic drug but differs from other agents of similar class by have beta blocker properties by which it can cause bradycardia and bronchospasm.

Intra-cardiac cardioverter defibrillator

Answer: 70. A. MADIT II

Answer: 71. A. ICD implantation

Answer: 72. C. Incessant VT or VF

Answer: 73. A. 50-year-old patient with history of myocardial infarction 6 weeks ago, NYHA class I symptoms, LVEF 30%.

Answer: 74. A. Dual chamber ICD better than single chamber ICD in reducing mortality

ICD trials:

1. For Primary prevention: MADIT I and II, CABG- Patch, MUSTT, DEFINITE, DINAMIT, SCD-HeFT
2. For Secondary prevention: AVID, CASH, CIDS

Indications of ICD:

Class I recommendations

- Cardiac arrest due to VT/VF without a reversible cause
- Structural heart disease and spontaneous sustained VT
- Syncope of undetermined origin with inducible VT/VF at EPS
- LVEF ≤35 % due to prior MI ≥40 days ago with NYHA class II or III symptoms
- LVEF ≤35 % due to nonischemic cardiomyopathy with NYHA class II or III symptoms
- LVEF ≤30 % due to prior MI ≥40 days ago with NYHA class I symptoms
- LVEF ≤40 % due to prior MI and nonsustained VT with inducible VT/VF at EPS

Class III recommendations (Contraindicated)

- Expected survival < 1 year with poor functional status
- Incessant VT/VF
- NYHA Class IV heart failure with drug-refractory symptoms who are not candidates for cardiac transplantation or cardiac resynchronization and defibrillator therapy

- Syncope of undetermined cause in a patient without inducible ventricular tachyarrhythmias and without structural heart disease
- When VF or VT is amenable to surgical or catheter ablation
- Ventricular tachyarrhythmias due to a completely reversible disorder

Dual versus Single Chamber ICDs

In addition to providing dual-chamber bradycardia pacing, dual-chamber ICDs provide atrial electrograms (EGMs).

It enhances physician interpretation of stored EGMs and permit both diagnostics for AF and dual-chamber algorithms to discriminate SVT from VT. So, Dual chamber discrimination is superior when overlap in VT and SVT rates.

In randomized trials, there is no benefit of dual chamber over single chamber in terms of reduction of mortality or hospitalizations.

Dual chamber ICDs are associated with higher risk of device related complication.

The present consensus recommends reserving dual-chamber ICDs for patients who need dual chamber pacing or have SVT and monomorphic VT at overlapping ventricular rates.

Pacemakers

Answer: 75. B. Position III - Rate modulation

Answer: 76. D. Symptomatic chronotropic incompetence

Answer: 77. C. VVIR

Answer: 78. C. VOO

Answer: 79. B. PVARP

Answer: 80. A. In case of lead dislodgement, pacing threshold will be increased

Answer: 81. C. Switch off the hysteresis

Answer: 82. B. Responds to mode change to VVIR

Answer: 83. A. Increased incidence of cross-talk

Pacemaker coding:

Positions	Category	Options
I	Chamber paced	O- None, A-Atrium, V- Ventricle, D-Dual
II	Chamber sensed	O- None, A-Atrium, V- Ventricle, D-Dual
III	Response to sensing	O- None, T- Triggered, I- Inhibited, D-Dual
IV	Rate modulation	O- None, R- Rate modulation
V	Multisite pacing	O- None, A-Atrium, V- Ventricle, D-Dual

Commonly used modes of pacemaker:

1. **VVIR mode:** It is also called ventricular demand pacing, used in single chamber ventricular lead devices. There is single lead which is in right ventricle and right ventricle is paced, sensed and inhibited in response to a sensed beat. It is commonly used in chronic AF patients with slow ventricular rate.

Disadvantages:

(i) AV synchrony is not maintained and chronic RV pacing is associated with increased risk of heart failure and atrial fibrillation due to ventricular dyssynchrony.

(ii) Some patients may develop pacemaker syndrome.

2. **DDDR mode:** It represents dual chamber pacing in which one lead is in RA and other in RV. It is programmed to maximize appropriately timed and intact native A-V conduction (i.e., through self-inhibition), add ventricular paced beats in the presence of significant AV delay or block (after allowing for native atrial depolarization), or synchronously add paced atrial and ventricular beats (in the setting of SND or asystole).

3. **VOO or DOO mode:** These are asynchronous pacing modes in which device will pace without respect to native conduction. These modes are used for limited period during surgeries in which there is high risk of interference with cautery resulting in errors in sensing.

Bipolar versus unipolar leads in pacemaker:

	Unipolar leads	**Bipolar leads**
Advantages	• Smaller diameter • Easier to implant • Exhibit large pacing artefact on surface ECG	• Less susceptible to oversensing of non-cardiac signals (e.g. myopotentials, EMI etc) • Programming flexibility present
Disadvantages	• No programming flexibility • Causes pectoral muscle stimulation • Far field oversensing and increased cross-talk	• Larger diameter • Small pacing spike • Higher impedance • Voltage threshold is higher

Complications of pacemaker:

Pacemaker syndrome:

Loss of AV synchrony in some of the pacemaker patients results in simultaneous contraction of atrium and ventricle; i.e. atria contracts against the closed AV valves. Usually occurs in single chamber pacing patients and requires intact VA conduction.

There is loss of atrial contribution to ventricular filling, fall in cardiac output and generation of abnormal pressure waves.

Symptoms: Neurological (Dizziness, presyncope), Heart failure (dyspnea, orthopnea), Hypotension, Low cardiac output (fatigue, weakness), Pulsations in the neck (cannon A waves).

Management: Change pacemaker to dual chamber, to maintain the AV synchrony.

Pacemaker mediated tachycardia (Endless loop tachycardia):

Classically seen in double chamber pacemaker, in which retrogradely conducted P wave is labelled as atrial sensed event which leads to pacing of ventricle and this generates incessant re-entrant arrhythmia circuit.

Management: Increase post ventricular atrial refractory period (PVARP), so that retrogradely conducted P wave will fall in atrial refractory period and will not be sensed.

Twiddler syndrome:

There is twisting of pulse generator in long axis in subcutaneous region which leads to lead dislodgement or lead fracture; may occur following patient manipulation of pulse generator.

Risk factors: obese women with loose, fatty subcutaneous tissue; Small size of implanted generator with a large pocket.

Lead related complications

	Pacing impedance	**Pacing threshold**
Lead dislodgement	Decreased	Increased
Microdislodgement	Normal	Increased
Insulation failure (Current leak)	Decreased	Increased
Loose setscrew	Increased	Increased
Battery depletion	Normal	Normal
Lead fracture	Increased	Increased

Cardiac resynchronization therapy (CRT)

Answer: 84. C. DCMP

Answer: 85. C. LBBB with QRS duration >150 ms

CRT is the use of biventricular pacemaker with three electrical leads for better co-ordination of atrial and ventricular contractions.

Total 3 leads are placed: 2 endocardial leads, one in RA, one in RV; and 1 lead in tributary of coronary sinus for LV stimulation.

Indications:

NYHA Class II, III, ambulatory class IV with LVEF ≤ 35 % along with

LBBB morphology and QRS width ≥ 150 ms (Class I)

LBBB morphology and QRS width ≥ 120 ms (Class IIa)

Non-LBBB morphology and QRS width ≥ 150 ms (Class IIa)

Not indicated when

- Non LBBB pattern QRS duration ≤ 150 ms

- Expected survival with good functional capacity is less than 1 years.

Syncope

Answer: 86. B. Head up Tilt Table test

Answer: 87. C. Isoproterenol

Answer: 88. C. Diltiazem

Answer: 89. C. There is no vasodepressor component.

In 10–20% of patients a vasodepressor component is present.

Answer: 90. A. Isometric counterpressure manoeuvres

Answer: 91. D. Isometric compressive manoeuvre

Tilt-Table Testing

Most common cause of syncope and neutrally mediated syncope is vasovagal

Tilt-table test may provoke a vasovagal response by venous pooling and orthostatic distress.

Protocol: Duration of 20 to 45 minutes at 60° to 70° tilt.

Pharmacologic agents may be used to provoke a positive response. Most common are Intravenous infusion of **isoproterenol** and sublingual **nitroglycerin**. It increases sensitivity at the cost of specificity.

Positive response to tilt table testing:

Type 1—Mixed i.e. Coexisting bradycardia and hypotension

Type 2—Cardioinhibition i.e. persistent bradycardia or prolonged pauses and an absence of significant hypotension. Cardioinhibition can occur without (type 2A) or with asystole (type 2B).

Type 3—Vasodepressor i.e. significant hypotension in the absence of bradycardia

Treatment of reflex (vasovagal syncope)

Behavioral training

- Education on warning signs and need to lay horizontal when symptoms to prevent injury
- Techniques for avoiding syncope
- Liberalize salt intake and maintain hydration
- Avoidance of triggers for situational syncope

Physical counter-pressure maneuvers (PCM)

- Squatting, arm-tensing, leg-crossing and leg-crossing with lower body muscle tensing
- Shown to reduce total burden and recurrence rate of syncope in patients with recognizable warning symptoms when compared with conventional treatment

Medications

Few randomized clinical trials so insufficient evidence to support or refute use of ANY specific agents

Potential classes

- Volume expanders – e.g. fludrocortisone
- Beta blocker – theoretically lessen impact of adrenergic surge
- Vaso/venoconstrictors – e.g. Midodrine
- Theophylline

Carotid sinus hypersensitivity:

There is an exaggerated response to carotid sinus baroreceptor stimulation. Stimulation to the neck results in marked bradycardia and a drop in blood pressure.

Usually seen in elderly males.

Symptoms: Dizziness or syncope during turning of neck to one side such as shaving, crossing the roads due to transient diminished cerebral perfusion.

3 types:

1. Cardioinhibitory type (70-75%): The predominant manifestation is a decreased heart rate, which results in sinus bradycardia, atrioventricular block, or asystole due to vagal action on sinus and atrioventricular nodes. This response can be abolished with atropine.
2. Vasodepressor type (5-10%): The predominant manifestation is a vasomotor tone decrease without a change in heart rate. This response is not abolished with atropine.
3. Mixed type (20-25%): A decrease in heart rate and vasomotor tone occurs.

Diagnosis:

Carotid sinus massage is the diagnostic maneuver of choice.

Carotid sinus massage should not be performed if there is presence of carotid bruit or there is history of TIA/stroke in preceding 3 months.

Place the patient in the supine position with the neck slightly extended. The patient should lie supine for a minimum of 5 minutes before carotid sinus massage is applied.

Massage over the point of maximal carotid impulse, medial to the sternomastoid muscle at the upper border level of the thyroid cartilage.

Massage for 5-10 seconds on each carotid sinus consecutively, with a 1-minute interval between massages.

Continuously monitor surface ECG and blood pressure. Phasic, noninvasive, beat-to-beat blood pressure monitoring is preferred over using a cuff measurement.

A massage is considered to have a positive result if any of the following 3 criteria are met:

Asystole exceeding 3 seconds (indicates cardioinhibitory CSH)

Reduction in systolic blood pressure exceeding 50 mm Hg independent of heart rate slowing (indicates vasodepressor CSH)

Combination of the above (indicates mixed CSH)

Treatment: Symptomatic CSH is a class I indication for permanent pacemaker implantation.

Cardiac arrest and resuscitation

Answer: 92. A. IHD

Answer: 93. B. HOCM

Cause of sudden cardiac death:

<35 years of age: Most commonly associated with hypertrophic cardiomyopathy (HCM).

>35 years of age: Most commonly associated with coronary artery disease or ischemic heart disease (IHD).

Answer: 94. B. Baseball

Commotio cordis:

Lethal arrhythmia (Ventricular fibrillation) which occurs as a result of blow to the area over precordial region at critical time during cardiac cycle.

It is associated with sudden cardiac death.

Mostly occurs in boys and young med during sports, most frequently **baseball.**

Answer: 95. A. Therapeutic hypothermia

Answer: 96. A. 35–45 mmHg.

Answer: 97. D. 0 mmHg.

Answer: 98. D. All of the above.

Answer: 99. D. 2-2.4 inches

Answer: 100. D. 100-120 per minute

Answer: 101. A. 15 : 2

Answer: 102. D. Routine use of atropine during asystole is likely to have therapeutic benefit.

Answer: 103. B. Defibrillation (nonsynchronized).

New CPR guidelines (2015)

- Initiate chest compressions before giving rescue breaths (C-A-B rather than A-B-C) to reduce delay to first compression.
- In adult CPR, **100 to 120** chest compressions per minute (updated from at least 100 per minute).
- Chest compression depth for adults is **at least 2 inches (5 cm) but not greater than 2.4 inches (6 cm)** (updated from at least 2 inches).
- Untrained lay rescuers should provide compression-only (Hands-Only) CPR.
- If the trained lay rescuer is able to perform rescue breaths, he or she should add rescue breaths in

a ratio of 30 compressions to 2 breaths. If two rescuers are there, then ratio of 15 chest compressions to 2 breaths should be maintained.

- Pauses in compressions should be as short as possible and allow full recoil after each compression.
- Criteria for minimizing interruptions is clarified with a goal of chest compression fraction as high as possible, with a target of at least 60%.
- In patients with an advanced airway, **one breath every six seconds** (10 breaths per minute) should be given with continuous chest compressions.
- Compression depth in children should be one-third or more of anterior-posterior diameter, or about 1.5 inches in infants and 2 inches in children.
- Bystander-administered naloxone may be considered for suspected life-threatening opioid-associated emergencies.
- Shock First vs CPR First: For witnessed adult cardiac arrest when an AED is immediately available, it is reasonable that the defibrillator be used as soon as possible. For adults with unmonitored cardiac arrest or for whom an AED is not immediately available, it is reasonable that CPR be initiated while the defibrillator equipment is being retrieved and applied and that defibrillation, if indicated, be attempted as soon as the device is ready for use.
- The combined use of vasopressin and epinephrine offers no advantage to using standard-dose epinephrine in cardiac arrest. Also, vasopressin does not offer an advantage over the use of epinephrine alone. Therefore, vasopressin has been removed from the Adult Cardiac Arrest Algorithm.
- Low end-tidal carbon dioxide (ETCO2) in intubated patients after 20 minutes of CPR is associated with a very low likelihood of resuscitation. Providers may consider low ETCO2 (less than 10mmHg) after 20 minutes of CPR in combination with other factors to help determine when to terminate resuscitation.
- All comatose (ie, lacking meaningful response to verbal commands) adult patients with ROSC after cardiac arrest should have targeted temperature management (TTM), with a target temperature **between 32°C and 36°C** selected and achieved, then maintained constantly **for at least 24 hours**.
- The routine prehospital cooling of patients with rapid infusion of cold IV fluids after ROSC is not recommended
- **Intravenous lipid emulsion (ILE)** may be considered for treatment of **local anesthetic systemic toxicity.**
- The **C-A-B sequence** as the preferred sequence for paediatric CPR is re-affirmed.

See Table on next page

Miscellaneous

Answer: 104. C. Functions like fixed rate synchronous pacemaker

Parasystole:

Arrhythmia caused by the presence and function of a **secondary pacemaker** in the heart, which works in parallel with the SA node and functions like **fixed rate asynchronous pacemaker.**

Component	Adults and Adolescents	Children (Age 1 Year to Puberty)	Infants (Age Less Than 1 Year, Excluding Newborns)
Scene safety	Make sure the environment is safe for rescuers and victim		
Recognition of cardiac arrest	Check for responsiveness No breathing or only gasping (i.e., no normal breathing) No definite pulse felt within 10 seconds (Breathing and pulse check can be performed simultaneously in less than 10 seconds)		
Activation of emergency response system	In you are alone with no mobile phone, leave the victim to activate the emergency response system and get the AED before beginning CPR Otherwise, send someone and begin CPR immediately; use the AED as soon as it is available	***Witnessed collapse*** Follow steps for adults and adolescents on the left ***Unwitnessed collapse*** Give 2 minutes of CPR Leave the victim to activate the emergency response system and get the AED Return to the child or infant and resume CPR; use the AED as soon as it is available	
Compression-ventilation ratio without advanced airway	***1 or 2 rescuers*** 30:2	***1 rescuer*** 30:2 ***2 or more rescuers*** 15:2	
Compression-ventilation ratio with advanced airway	Continuous compressions at a rate of 100-120/min Give 1 breath every 6 seconds (10 breaths/min)		
Compression rate	100-120/min		
Compression depth	**At least 2 inches (5 cm)***	At least one third AP diameter of chest About 2 inches (5 cm)	At least one third AP diameter of chest About 1½ inches (4 cm)
Hand placement	12 hands on the lower half of the breastbone (sternum)	2 hands or 1 hand (optional for very small child) on the lower half of the breastbone (sternum)	***1 rescuer*** 2 fingers in the center of the chest, just below the nipple line ***2 or more rescuers*** 2 thumb–encircling hands in the center of the chest, just below the nipple line
Chest recoil	Allow full recoil of chest after each compression; do not lean on the chest after each compression		
Minimizing interruption	Limit interruptions in chest compressions to less than 10 seconds		

Parasystolic pacemakers can exist in both the **atrium or the ventricle**. Atrial parasystoles are characterized by narrow QRS complexes

Types: Fixed parasystole and modulated parasystole

Fixed parasystole occurs when it is not influenced by surrounding tissue and its activity is completely independent of sinus node pacing. It is insulated because of complete exit or entrance block.

Modulated parasystole occurs when extra pacemaker activity is affected by surrounding tissue.

Electrocardiographic criteria used to recognize the fixed form of parasystole are:

1. Presence of variable coupling intervals of the manifest ectopic beats
2. Inter-ectopic intervals that are multiples of a basic interval
3. Fusion beats.

Answer: 105. D. all of the above

Late potentials:

Late potentials are thought to be caused by early afterdepolarizations of myocardial cells.

Their amplitude is often too small to show up on a normal ECG. However, when multiple QRS recordings (typically 250 consecutive QRS complexes) are averaged, random noise is filtered out and late potentials can show up. Such a recording is called a Signal Averaged ECG (SAECG).

Imply a higher risk of potentially dangerous ventricular tachyarrhythmias.

Used for the risk stratification of sudden cardiac death in people who have had a myocardial infarction, as well as in people with known coronary heart disease, cardiomyopathies, or unexplained syncope.

Criteria for late potentials on a signal averaged ECG:

1. Filtered QRS duration > 114ms
2. Terminal (last 40ms) QRS root means square (RMS) voltage < 20 μV
3. Low amplitude (<40 μV) signal (LAS) duration > 38ms

Answer: 106. D. Bidirectional ventricular tachycardia

Answer: 107. C. LQTS (and TDP)

Answer: 108. C. Dofetilide

Drug	Pacing threshold	Defibrillation threshold
Quinidine	Increase	Increase
Procainamide	Increase	No change
Lidocaine	No change	Increase
Mexiletine	Slight increase	Increase
Flecainide	Increase	Increase
Propafenone	Increase	No change

Beta blockers	Variable	No change
Sotalol	No change	**Decrease**
Dofetilide	No change	**Decrease**
Ibutilide	No change	**Decrease**
Amiodarone	Variable	Increase
Verapamil	Increase	No change
Digitalis	Decrease	No change or decrease

10 Valvular Heart Diseases

Mitral Stenosis

1. **One of the following disease become symptomatic early in the course of disease:**
   A. Mitral regurgitation
   B. Aortic stenosis
   C. Mitral stenosis
   D. Aortic regurgitation

2. **All of the following are echocardiographic indicators of severe Mitral stenosis except:**
   A. Mean gradient at rest of > 10 mm Hg across mitral valve
   B. MVA < 1 cm^2
   C. PHT of > 240 msec
   D. Mean gradient after exercise of > 15 mm across mitral valve

3. **Criteria for Severe mitral stenosis:**
   A. MVA <1 cm2
   B. PHT>220 msec
   C. Mean gradient > 10 mmHg
   D. All of the above

4. **Which of the following is not an auscultatory finding of Severe mitral stenosis?**
   A. Loud S1 B. Opening Snap
   C. Loud P2 D. LV S3

5. **Absolute contraindications to percutaneous mitral commissurotomy includes?**
   A. Mild mitral regurgitation
   B. Unicommissural calcification
   C. Left atrial thrombus
   D. Moderate tricuspid regurgitation

6. **Wilkin score is used for:**
   A. Mitral stenosis
   B. Pulmonary stenosis
   C. Aortic stenosis
   D. Tricuspid stenosis

7. **Cross sectional area of normal mitral valve is:**
   A. 1 to 2 cm square
   B. 2 to 4 cm square
   C. 4 to 6 cm square
   D. 6 to 8 cm square

8. **Mechanism of balloon mitral valvuloplasty is:**
   A. Chordal separation
   B. Commissural separation
   C. Leaflet stretch
   D. Papillary muscle separation

9. **Contraindications to percutaneous balloon mitral valvotomy include all, except:**
   A. Bilateral calcific mitral valve commissure
   B. Left atrial body clot
   C. Subvalvar disease
   D. Moderate or more mitral regurgitation

Mitral Regurgitation

10. **19 year old student presents with chest pain and shortness of breath on exertion. On examination, patient has mid systolic click**

at apex on auscultation. Likely diagnosis is:

A. Bicuspid aortic valve
B. MVP
C. PAH
D. PS

11. All of the following may be seen in acute severe MR except:

A. Increase pulmonary vascular resistance
B. Decreased cardiac output
C. Displaced hyperdynamic impulse
D. Short systolic murmur

12. All are causes of acute MR except:

A. Spontaneous chordal rupture
B. Cleft mitral valve
C. Infective endocarditis with leaflet perforation
D. AML tear following balloon mitral valvotomy

13. False statement about mitral valve prolapse syndrome:

A. Female B. Malignant course
C. Click D. Thin leaflets

14. Which one of the following echo finding is suggestive of severe MR?

A. Effective regurgitant orifice 0.40 cm square
B. Vena contracta 0.30 cm
C. Central jet MR area > 50% la area
D. Regurgitant fraction 40%

15. Rupture of chordae tendineae to posterior mitral leaflet produces prominent murmur over following area:

A. Apex B. Axilla
C. Base of heart D. Left scapular

16. The underlying lesion in rheumatic mitral regurgitation is due to:

A. Retractile fibrosis of leaflets and chordae with loss of coaptation
B. Dilatation of the mitral annulus
C. Posterior mitral leaflet prolapse
D. Ruptured chordae

17. What are the echocardiographic indices of severe MR?

A. Central jet with the jet occupying >40% LA area
B. Holosystolic eccentric MR jet, which is wall hugging reaching posterior LA wall
C. Vena contracta >0.7 cm, or regurgitant volume >60 mL, or regurgitant fraction >50%
D. ERO area >0.40 cm2
E. Systolic flow reversal in pulmonary vein or veins
F. Any of the above

18. Which of the following are clear indications for surgical repair of primary severe MR?

A. Symptomatic patients with chronic severe primary MR (stage D) and LVEF >30%
B. Asymptomatic patients with chronic severe primary MR and LV dysfunction (LVEF 30 60% and/or LVESD >40 mm, stage C2)
C. Patients with chronic severe primary MR undergoing cardiac surgery for other indications
D. All of the above

19. Which type of anatomy is most suitable for mitral valve repair?

A. Flail P2
B. Flail A2
C. Bileaflet MV prolapse
D. Barlow's disease

Aortic Stenosis

20. Mechanism of syncope in severe aortic stenosis:

A. Systemic vasodilatation
B. Abnormal baroreceptor mechanism
C. Vasodepressor response
D. All of the above

21. Low flow low gradient aortic stenosis:
A. Valve area <1.0 cm
B. LV ejection fraction <40%
C. Mean pressure gradient <30 mmHg
D. All of the above

22. Which of the following is true about aortic stenosis?
A. Surgical valvulotomy is treatment of choice for bicuspid aortic valve in child
B. Rheumatic AS is the commonest cause of AS in child
C. LV diastolic dysfunction is common in severe AS
D. Annulo-aortic ectasia is found in 20% of patients with rheumatic AS

23. Bicuspid aortic valve:
A. AD B. AR
C. XD D. XR

24. All are features of low flow, low gradient Aortic Stenosis except:
A. Aortic valve area < 1 cm2
B. LV EF < 40%
C. AV mean gradient < 30-40 mmHg
D. LV EF <50%

25. Hemodynamic response to dobutamine infusion suggestive of requirement of aortic valve replacement in patient with low gradient, low flow stenosis is:
A. Increase in calculated aortic valve area with same mean gradient
B. Increase in mean gradient with same calculated aortic valve area
C. Increase in calculated aortic valve area with decrease in vascular resistance
D. None

Aortic Regurgitation

26. Which of the following is not a cause of AR due to aortic root dilatation?
A. Ankylosing spondylitis
B. Marfan's syndrome
C. Sub pulmonic VSD with AR
D. Osteogenesis imperfecta

27. Patients with chronic aortic regurgitation are likely to have (as compared to acute aortic regurgitation):
A. Normal pulse pressure
B. Elevated left ventricular end-diastolic pressure
C. Dilated left ventricle
D. Sinus tachycardia

28. In severe aortic regurgitation:
A. Vena contracta width <0.3 cm
B. Regurgitant orifice area >0.3 cm2
C. Regurgitant fraction 40%
D. Regurgitant volume 50 ml

29. To define severe AR, vena contracta on echo should be more than:
A. 0.5cm B. 0.4cm
C. 0.6cm D. 0.7 cm

30. Echocardiographic criteria for severe AR includes all except:
A. Effective regurgitant orifice area > 30 mm2
B. Vena contracta width > 3 mm
C. Regurgitant volume > 60 ml/beat
D. Pressure half time < 200 ms

31. Which one of following pressure half time of AR Doppler signal is suggestive of severe AR?
A. >800 ms
B. 400 to 800 ms
C. 251 to 399 ms
D. < 250 ms

32. Severe AR is suggested by which of the following echocardiographic measures?
A. Doppler jet width ≥65% of LVOT
B. Vena contracta >0.6 cm
C. Holodiastolic flow reversal in the proximal abdominal aorta

D. Regurgitant volume ≥60 mL/beat, or regurgitant fraction ≥50%, or effective regurgitant orifice (ERO) area ≥0.3 cm2
E. All of the above

33. In a patient with chronic severe AR, which of the following constitute a definite indication for AVR?
A. Symptomatic patients with severe AR regardless of LV systolic function, even if EF is <30%
B. Asymptomatic patients with chronic severe AR and LV systolic dysfunction (LVEF <50%)
C. Patients with severe AR (stage C or D) while undergoing cardiac surgery for other indications
D. All of the above

Tricuspid Valve

34. All are true about tricuspid stenosis except:
A. Almost always rheumatic in origin
B. A mean diastolic gradient of 2 mmHg is sufficient to establish the diagnosis
C. Generally accompanies mitral valve disease
D. In severe TS, dyspnea, orthopnea and PND are common symptoms

35. Carcinoid heart disease manifest as:
A. Tricuspid regurgitation
B. Pulmonic stenosis
C. Both of the above
D. None of the above

36. Indicators of severe tricuspid stenosis include which of the following:
A. Mean diastolic gradient >5 mmHg
B. PHT >190 ms
C. Valve area by continuity equation <1.0 cm2
D. All of the above

37. Severe tricuspid stenosis is diagnosed at a mean gradient of:
A. > 2 mm Hg
B. > 5 mm Hg
C. > 10 mm Hg
D. > 20 mm Hg

38. Latent TS may be unmasked by all except:
A. Intravenous atropine
B. Leg raising
C. Isometric exercise
D. Slow IV fluids

39. Latent tricuspid stenosis is detected by all of the following except:
A. IV atropine
B. Isometric exercise
C. Passive leg raising
D. Slow IV fluid infusion

40. Normotensive TR occurs in all except:
A. Ebstein's anomaly
B. Right sided EMF
C. Pulmonary embolism
D. Trauma

41. Which of the following is not a cause of organic Tricuspid Regurgitation (primary TR)?
A. Carcinoid syndrome
B. Right ventricular MI
C. Endomyocardial Fibrosis
D. Infective endocarditis in IV drug users

42. All of the following findings suggest severe tricuspid regurgitation on echocardiography except:
A. Vena contracta width >7 mm
B. Systolic flow reversals in hepatic veins
C. Jet velocity > 4 m/s
D. None of the above

43. If TR jet velocity is 3 m/sec, RA pressure is 8 mm Hg, then RVSP is:
A. 9 mm Hg
B. 13 mm Hg
C. 36 mm Hg
D. 44 mm Hg

44. Criteria for severe tricuspid regurgitation (TR) include which of the following?
A. Central jet area >10 cm2

B. Vena contracta width >0.70 cm
C. Continuous-wave (CW) jet density and contour: dense, triangular with early peak
D. Hepatic vein flow: systolic reversal
E. All of the above

Prosthetic Heart Valves

45. Transcatheter AVR (TAVR) is reasonable in which of the following situations?
A. Severe AS patients who meet an indication for AVR who have a prohibitive surgical risk and a predicted post-TAVR survival >12 months
B. As an alternative to surgical AVR in patients who meet an indication for AVR and who have high surgical risk
C. Both A and B
D. Neither A nor B

46. Which of the following statements is not true about balloon aortic valvuloplasty?
A. It is a good treatment for many forms of congenital AS
B. Percutaneous aortic balloon dilation may be considered as a bridge to surgical AVR or TAVR in severely symptomatic patients with severe AS
C. It is helpful to predilate the aortic valve just before TAVR
D. It is a good definitive treatment for calcific AS of the elderly

47. Absolute contraindications for transcatheter aortic valve implantation include all except:
A. Estimated life expectancy >1 year
B. Annulus size <18 mm
C. Annulus size>29 mm
D. Thrombus in the left ventricle

48. Example for Single tilting disc valve:
A. CarboMedics valve
B. Medtronic Hall valve
C. St. Jude valve
D. Hancock valve

49. Normal finding in Bileaflet tilting disc mitral prosthesis:
A. Diastolic murmur
B. Systolic murmur
C. Both systolic and diastolic murmur
D. No murmur

50. Ross procedure is:
A. Aortic homograft
B. Aortic autograft
C. Pulmonary autograft
D. Pulmonary homograft

51. True statement for Ross procedure:
A. Preferred in elderly patients requiring AVR
B. Suitable in patients with rheumatic valvular involvement
C. Long term anticoagulation not required
D. Aortic reconstruction is done using pulmonary homografts

52. Which of the following factor does not favour choosing mechanical prosthesis over bioprosthesis?
A. Patients at risk of accelerated structural valve deterioration.
B. Age > 65 years
C. For whom future redo valve surgery would be at high risk
D. Patients already on anticoagulation as a result of having a mechanical prosthesis in another valve position

53. Bioprosthetic valve is most preferred in the which of the following patient?
A. 40 years old female with severe calcified MS
B. 60 years old male with severe MS and long standing AF
C. 30 years old male with severe MS and hemophilia
D. 18 years old male with severe AR

54. Which one of the following is not used for the surgical treatment of tricuspid regurgitation?
A. Metallic valve
B. Bioprosthesis
C. Suture annuloplasty
D. Ring annuloplasty

55. Which one of following is not true for mechanical prosthetic valve?
A. Bileaflet valve
B. Trileaflet valve
C. Ball & cage valve
D. Tilting disc valve

56. Which one of following is true for oral anticoagulation after bioprosthetic mitral valve surgery?
A. It is not required
B. It is required for the first 1 year
C. It is required for the first 3 months
D. It is required lifelong

57. Ross procedure is used for:
A. Diseased aortic valve
B. Diseased mitral valve
C. Diseased tricuspid valve
D. Diseased pulmonary valve

58. Which one of following is recommended after mechanical valve replacement?
A. Only Vitamin K antagonist anticoagulant
B. Aspirin + clopidogrel
C. Vitamin K antagonist anticoagulant + aspirin
D. Vitamin K antagonist anticoagulant + dipyridamole

59. All of the following are true for Ross procedure except?
A. Preferred in younger patients
B. Suitable for patients with rheumatic valve disease
C. Long-term systemic anticoagulation is not required
D. Pulmonary reconstruction is performed using pulmonary homograft

60. Which of the following is an abnormal finding in a patient who had undergone mitral valve replacement with bileaflet valve?
A. Opening Click
B. Closing click
C. Diastolic murmur
D. Systolic murmur

61. The recommended period of oral anticoagulant therapy in a patient who had a bioprosthetic valve implantation in sinus rhythm after surgery is:
A. 2 months
B. 3 months
C. 6 months
D. 12 months in rheumatic etiology

62. "Melody valve" implantation is used for percutaneous treatment of
A. Aortic valve
B. Pulmonary valve
C. Mitral valve
D. Tricuspid valve

ANSWERS

Mitral stenosis:

Answer: 1. C. Mitral stenosis

Answer: 2. C. PHT of > 240 msecs

Answer: 3. D. All

Answer: 4. D. LV S3

Answer: 5. C. Left atrial thrombus

Answer: 6. A. Mitral stenosis

Answer: 7. C. 4 to 6 cm square

Answer: 8. B. Commissural separation

Answer: 9. C. Subvalvar disease

Most common cause of mitral stenosis (MS) is rheumatic heart disease.

Rheumatic MS involves mitral valve leaflet thickening and calcification, commissural fusion, chordal fusion, and ultimate obstruction.

Symptoms:

Dyspnea

Orthopnea

Paroxysmal nocturnal dyspnea

Palpitations (if atrial fibrillation develops)

Hemoptysis

Signs:

Loud S1

Opening snap

Mid-diastolic rumbling murmur, which may have pre-systolic accentuation if the patient is in sinus rhythm

In advanced cases, signs of pulmonary hypertension.

Echocardiography

In rheumatic MS, echocardiography characteristically reveals a "hockey-stick" deformity of the anterior mitral leaflet (also described as a "doming" pattern),

Mitral valve area is calculated from the empiric formula:

MVA = 220 / PHT

PHT > 220ms is suggestive of severe MS.

Severity of MS:

	MILD	MODERATE	SEVERE
Mean gradient	<5	5–10	>10
MVA (cm2)	>1.5	1.0–1.5	<1.0
PASP (mmHg)	<30	30–50	>50
PHT			>220 ms

Gorlin formula for mitral valve area:

MVA = CO / 37.7 × HR × DFP √MVG

(MVA- Mitral valve area, CO- Cardiac output, HR- Heart rate, DFP- Diastolic filling period, MVG- Mean valve gradient)

Hakki equation for mitral valve area:

MVA = CO / √MVG

Hemodynamic rate of progression results in a decrease in mitral valve area of approximately 0.1 cm2/ year.

Rate of progression is rapid in developing countries than developed ones because of recurrent episodes of acute rheumatic fever and relative lack of primary and secondary prophylaxis.

Percutaneous mitral valvuloplasty (PMV) or commissurotomy (PTMC)

PMV is the procedure of choice for severe or symptomatic MS, provided the valve morphology is favourable. Improves symptoms by commissural separation.

Wilkins scoring system:

Based on leaflet thickening, leaflet mobility, leaflet calcification and sub-valvular involvement on echo (with each component given a score of 1–4, based on increasing severity)

Allows identification of patients suitable for PTMC

Score of **8 or less** suggests favourable outcome from PTMC

Absolute contraindications of PTMC:

1. LA thrombus
2. Bicommissural calcification
3. More than mild mitral regurgitation

MITRAL REGURGITATION

Answer: 10. B. MVP

Answer: 11. C. Displaced hyperdynamic impulse

Answer: 12. B. Cleft mitral valve

Answer: 13. B. Malignant course

Answer: 14. A. Effective regurgitant orifice 0.40 cm square

Answer: 15. C. Base of heart

Answer: 16. A. Retractile fibrosis of leaflets and chordae with loss of coaptation

Answer: 17. F. Any of the above.

Answer: 18. D. All of the above.

Answer: 19. A. Flail P2.

MVP is the most common structural cause of MR, affecting 2–3 % of the population.

More common in women

MR due to ischemic heart disease is the second most common cause, and is typically due to left ventricular and/or mitral annular dilation.

Midsystolic click is characteristically heard in MVP syndrome.

Mitral valve prolapse (MVP) syndrome:

Myxomatous degeneration of valve, may cause mitral regurgitation, also k/a **Barlow syndrome.**

Prevalence: **2-3%** of general population, more common in **females.**

Mid systolic click followed by late systolic murmur.

Murmurs of MVP is accentuated by standing and valsalva maneuver (earlier systolic click and longer murmur) and diminished with squatting (later systolic click and shorter murmur)

Pathophysiology:

Acute severe MR: Although total stroke volume increases, a percentage of the stroke volume is transmitted to the left atrium, resulting in a decrease in forward stroke volume. The increase in left atrial pressure results in acute, often severe, dyspnea due to pulmonary edema.

Apical impulse is usually normal in location (not displaced) and hyperdynamic.

Murmur may be quite subtle if "wide open" regurgitation is present

Causes of acute MR: Infective endocarditis with leaflet perforation, Post PTMC, Chordal rupture, Acute MI, Trauma.

Chronic MR: End-diastolic volume increases due to chronic volume overload. Eccentric LVH occurs. Left atrial enlargement allows accommodation of regurgitant volume at a lower pressure, with a reduction in symptoms.

The apical impulse may be displaced because of LV dilatation.

Relatively soft first heart sound, followed by a holosystolic blowing murmur.

Causes of chronic MR: RHD, MVP, Cleft mitral valve, Ischemic secondary MR due LV dilatation, DCMP

Radiation of the MR murmur is dependent on the vector of regurgitation.

Central MR: the murmur is typically heard to radiate to the back or clavicular area

Anterior leaflet pathology: Radiation to the axilla

Posterior leaflet pathology: Radiation to the base, sometimes masquerading as AS

Carpentier classification of MR:

Carpentier class	Feature	Pathophysiology	Etiology
Type 1	Normal leaflet mobility	Annular enlargement, perforate leaflet, congenital cleft, annular calcification	Dilated cardiomyopathy, Infective endocarditis
Type 2	Increased mobility (prolapse), includes flail leaflet	Elongated cords, ruptured cords, excessive leaflet tissue	Degenerative valve disease (Fibroelastic deficiency, Barlow's disease, Marfan disease), Endocarditis, Trauma, Ischemic cardiomyopathy
Type 3A	Restricted mobility during diastole	Thickened, rigid leaflets; calcification of leaflets; commissural fusion; shortened or fused tendinous cords	Rheumatic heart disease, Carcinoid disease
Type 3B	Restricted leaflet motion during systole	LV dilatation/ aneurysm, Papillary muscle displacement, Chordae tethering	Ischemic/ Dilated cardiomyopathy

Severity of MR:

PARAMETER	MILD	MODERATE	SEVERE
Color Doppler jet area	<20 %	LA area	>40 % of LA area
Vena contracta (cm)	<0.3	0.3–0.7	>0.7
Regurgitant volume (mL)	<30	30–60	>60
Regurgitant fraction (%)	<30	30–60	>60
Regurgitant orifice area (cm2)	<0.20	0.2–0.4	>0.40

SELLER'S GRADE OF REGURGITATION ON ANGIOGRAPHY

1 Small amount contrast enters LA in diastole and is cleared with each beat

2 More contrast fills LA with faint opacification of the entire LA; contrast does not clear with each beat

3 LA is well opacified with contrast density equal to the LV within 2–3 beats

4 Complete and dense opacification of the LA on the first beat; contrast refluxes into pulmonary veins

Surgical treatment:

Acute severe MR is a surgical emergency.

MV repair is preferred to MV replacement.

Anterior mitral leaflet is divided into 3 segments A1, A2, A3 and posterior mitral leaflet is also divided into 3 segments, P1, P2 and P3. Out of these, **flail P2 repair is easiest**. Repair of anterior leaflet is more difficult.

Indications for surgery:

Symptomatic acute severe MR

Symptomatic chronic severe MR

Asymptomatic chronic severe MR with LVEF <50%, new onset AR or pulmonary hypertension (PASP >50mmHg)

MitraClip: First **transcatheter mitral valve repair** technology to receive FDA approval for patients with primary (degenerative) MR and prohibitive surgical risk. Studied in **EVEREST trial**.

AORTIC STENOSIS

Answer: 20. D. All

Answer: 21. D. All

Answer: 22. C. LV diastolic dysfunction is common in severe AS

Answer: 23. A. AD

Answer: 24. D. LV EF <50%

Answer: 25. B. Increase in mean gradient with same calculated aortic valve area

Most common cause of aortic stenosis is calcific degeneration.

Other causes: Bicuspid aortic valve (Most common cause of AS in child), RHD.

Symptoms: Angina, Syncope, Dyspnea, Pedal edema.

Rheumatic AS is **not** associated with dilatation of aortic root where as it is seen in BAV disease.

BAV is autosomal dominant disorder.

Severity of AS:

	MILD	MODERATE	SEVERE
Aortic jet velocity (m/s)	2.6–2.9	3.0–4.0	>4.0
Mean gradient (mmHg)	<20	20–40	>40
AVA (cm2)	>1.5	1.0–1.5	<1.0
Indexed AVA (cm2/m2)	>0.85	0.60–0.85	<0.6

Examination:

Reduction in the amplitude and velocity of the carotid upstrokes

Loss of the second heart sound

Mid-to-late peaking nature to the systolic murmur (radiates to bilateral carotids)

Murmur increases with squatting, decreases with standing and handgrip.

Gorlin formula:

AVA = CO / (44.3 × HR × SEP √MVG)

(AVA- Aortic valve area, CO- Cardiac output, HR- Heart rate, SEP- Systolic ejection period, MVG- Mean valve gradient)

Hakki equation:

AVA = CO / √MVG

Prognosis:

With the development of angina, syncope, or heart failure, only 50 % of patients will survive 5, 3, and 2 years respectively.

LV diastolic dysfunction is common in aortic stenosis because of LVH.

Treatment:

AVR is treatment of choice, balloon aortic valvuloplasty (BAV) may be successful in children but not in adults and older patients.

BAV may be used as a bridge to surgical or transcatheter AVR in unstable patients with severe AS.

Patients at high-risk for surgical AVR, transcatheter aortic valve replacement (TAVR) has recently been approved.

Indications for AVR:

Symptomatic severe AS (Class I)

Asymptomatic severe AS undergoing cardiac surgery (Class I)

Asymptomatic severe AS and LV systolic dysfunction (LV EF <50 %) (Class I)

Moderate AS undergoing cardiac surgery (Class IIa)

Low flow low gradient AS (LFLG AS):

Presence of severe AS (AVA $\leq$1 cm^2 with AVA indexed to body surface area $\leq$0.6 cm^2/m^2) with stroke volume indexed to surface area $\leq$35 mL/m^2 **and** mean pressure gradient $\leq$40 mmHg.

Usually low gradient is due to LV systolic dysfunction. However, low flow can occur in presence of normal LV function which is known as **paradoxical low flow low gradient AS.** The causes in this case may be LV diastolic dysfunction (due to hypertension), RV dysfunction, associated MR or MS. All these conditions can cause low stroke volume.

True severe versus pseudo-severe AS

True severe AS

In patients with true severe AS, the primary lesion is severe AS and low gradient is caused by a low stroke volume. When true severe AS is accompanied by LV systolic dysfunction, the LV dysfunction may be secondary to AS or caused by a concurrent condition.

Valve replacement is likely to be beneficial in these patients.

Pseudosevere AS

In patients with pseudosevere AS, a low transvalvular pressure gradient is caused by the combination of mild to moderate AS and low stroke volume. The low stroke volume can occur in the context of reduced LVEF or preserved LVEF.

The low stroke volume reduces the valve opening forces, resulting in limited opening of a valve that is not severely diseased. And, estimated valve area comes less than 1 cm^2.

These patients with pseudosevere AS are unlikely to benefit from valve replacement and face considerable risk of operative death.

Low-dose dobutamine stress echocardiography (DSE) is used to differentiate true severe from pseudosevere AS in patients with classical LFLG AS.

- True severe AS: DSE shows an AVA $\leq$1 cm^2 (with AVA indexed to BSA $\leq$0.6 cm^2/m^2) with transvalvular mean gradient $\geq$40 mmHg (or Vmax $\geq$4 m/s). Aortic valve surgery is useful in these patients.
- Pseudosevere AS: DSE shows an AVA >1 cm^2 (or AVA indexed to BSA >0.6 cm^2/m^2) with transvalvular mean gradient <40 mmHg.

AORTIC REGURGITATION

Answer: 26. C. Sub pulmonic VSD with AR

Answer: 27. C. Dilated left ventricle

Answer: 28. B. Regurgitant orifice area >0.3 cm2

Answer: 29. C. 0.6cm

Answer: 30. B. Vena contracta width > 3 mm

Answer: 31. D. < 250 ms

Answer: 32. E. All of the above.

Answer: 33. D. All of the above.

Acute Aortic Regurgitation:

Causes: Infective endocarditis, Aortic dissection, Trauma, Iatrogenic.

LV diastolic pressure rises sharply as LV cavity is non-compliant, leading to elevation of left atrial pressure and pulmonary edema.

Features: Manifestations of cardiogenic shock (tachycardia and peripheral vasoconstriction) and pulmonary edema usually dominate. The pulse pressure is normal or may be reduced, but the arterial pulsation is usually low amplitude and rapid. The cardiac apex is generally not displaced and is not hyperdynamic. The peripheral manifestations of chronic AR, associated with an increased pulse pressure, may be entirely absent with acute AR.

Auscultation: Soft or absent S1, Soft A2 and loud P2 due to pulmonary hypertension. Murmur of acute AR is low pitched early diastolic unlike holodiastolic high pitched murmur of chronic AR.

Chronic Aortic Regurgitation:

Causes: Rheumatic heart disease (most common), congenital bicuspid aortic valve, degenerative aortic valve disease and aortic root dilation.

Features: LV enlargement and eccentric hypertrophy are able to maintain total stroke volume and cardiac output; LV end diastolic pressure is not elevated; and patient may remain asymptomatic for long.

Peripheral manifestations associated with wide pulse pressure are present. Cardiac apex is displaced laterally and inferiorly; and is diffuse and hyperdynamic.

Auscultation: S1 and A2 are soft, early decrescendo holodiastolic murmur is heard in chronic severe AR. A low pitched mid to late diastolic rumble may be appreciated at apex known as Austin Flint murmur.

AR due to dilatation of aortic root:

Acute: Aortic dissection,

Chronic: Hypertension, Marfan syndrome, Syphilitic aortitis, Cystic medial necrosis, Osteogenesis imperfecta, Ankylosing spondylitis, Ehlers-Danlos syndrome.

Severity of AR:

PARAMETER	MILD	MODERATE	SEVERE
Jet width/LVOT (%)	<25	25–65	>65
Vena contracta (cm)	<0.3	0.3–0.6	>0.6
Pressure half-time (ms)	>500	200–500	<200
Regurgitant volume (mL)	<30	30–60	>60
Regurgitant fraction (%)	<30	30–50	>50
Regurgitant orifice area	<0.10	0.1–0.3	>0.30

Seller's criteria for severity of AR on angiography:

GRADE	Criteria
1	Small amount contrast enters LV in diastole and is cleared with each beat
2	More contrast fills LV with faint opacification of the entire LV
3	LV is well opacified with contrast density equal to the ascending aorta
4	Complete and dense opacification of the LV on the first beat with contrast density greater than the ascending aorta

Treatment of choice: AVR

Indications of AVR:

Symptomatic severe AR (Class I)

Asymptomatic severe AR and LV systolic dysfunction (LV EF <50 %) (Class I)

Asymptomatic severe AR undergoing cardiac surgery (Class I)

Asymptomatic severe AR with severe LV dilatation (EDD >75 mm or ESD >55 mm) (Class IIa)

Patients with moderate AR undergoing cardiac surgery (Class IIb)

Indications of Aortic surgery in bicuspid aortic valve:

Diameter of the aortic sinuses or ascending aorta is greater than 5.5 cm. (Class I)

Diameter of the aortic sinuses or ascending aorta is greater than 5.0 cm and a risk factor for dissection is present (family history of aortic dissection or if the rate of increase in diameter is ≥0.5 cm/year). (Class IIa)

Diameter of the ascending aorta is greater than 4.5 cm and patient undergoing aortic valve surgery for severe AS or AR. (Class IIa)

TRICUSPID VALVE DISEASES

Answer: 34. D. In severe TS, dyspnea, orthopnea and PND are common symptoms

Answer: 35. C. Both

Answer: 36. D. All of the above.

Answer: 37. B. > 5 mm Hg

Answer: 38. C. Isometric exercise

Answer: 39. B. Isometric exercise

Answer: 40. C. Pulmonary embolism

Answer: 41. B. Right ventricular MI

Answer: 42. C. Jet velocity > 4 m/s

Answer: 43. D. 44 mm Hg

Answer: 44. E. All of the above

TRICUSPID STENOSIS (TS)

Most common cause: RHD, often coexistent with MS.

Symptoms of right sided heart failure such as pedal edema, ascites, prominent neck veins.

Diagnosis of TS: MDG of 2 mmHg, Severe TS: MDG of 5 mmHg

The TS murmur and opening snap are increased by maneuvers that increase right sided flow, such as inspiration, leg raising, right lateral decubitus position, Müller's maneuver, amyl nitrate inhalation, squatting, intravenous fluids and isotonic exercises **(not isometric exercises).**

Severe TS:

Mean gradient >5 mmHg

Peak velocity approaching 2 m/s

Valve area by continuity equation ≤1.0 cm 2

Pressure half time ≥190 ms

TRICUSPID REGURGITATION

Most common cause of TR: Functional

Severe TR

Regurgitant jet area >10 cm2

Vena contracta width >0.7 cm

Systolic flow reversal in the hepatic vein

Normotensive TR: Ebstein anomaly, Endomyocardial fibrosis, Trauma, Carcinoid syndrome, infective endocarditis of TV.

Hypertensive TR: Pulmonary embolism, Primary pulmonary artery hypertension, Eisenmenger, Severe pulmonic stenosis.

PROSTHETIC HEART VALVES

Answer: 45. C. Both A and B.

Answer: 46. D. It is a good definitive treatment for calcific AS of the elderly.

The results are only transient in calcific AS.

Answer: 47. A. Estimated life expectancy >1 year

Answer: 48. B. Medtronic Hall valve

Answer: 49. A. Diastolic murmur

Answer: 50. C. Pulmonary autograft

Answer: 51. C. Long term anticoagulation not required

Answer: 52. B. Age > 65 years

Answer: 53. C. 30 years old male with severe MS and hemophilia

Answer: 54. A. Metallic valve

Metallic valve is not usually used for tricuspid valve replacement because of very high risk of thrombosis.

Answer: 55. B. Trileaflet valve

Answer: 56. C. It is required for the first 3 months

Answer: 57. A. Diseased aortic valve

Answer: 58. C. Vitamin k antagonist anticoagulant + aspirin

Answer: 59. B. Suitable for patients with rheumatic valve disease

Answer: 60. D. Systolic murmur

Answer: 61. B. 3 months

Answer: 62. B. Pulmonary valve

Two major types of prosthetic valves:

1. **Mechanical valves:** three main types
   A. Bileaflet: St. Jude's medical, CarboMedics and On-X valves
   Most commonly used
   B. Tilting disc: Bjork-Shiley, Omniscience and Medtronic Hall valves
   C. Ball in cage: Starr- Edwards
2. **Bioprosthetic valves:**
   A. Heterografts: Carpentier-Edwards, Hancock I and II, Medtronic Intact
   B. Homografts: Harvested from human cadavers, Useful in infective endocarditis of valves.

Valve selection:

Bioprosthetic valves are less durable and need for re-operation is higher than mechanical valves.

Age: Less than 60 years prefer mechanical valves, More than 70 years prefer bioprosthetic valves

Mechanical valves have higher thrombogenicity, require life-long anticoagulation, which in turn increases bleeding complications.

Patients unwilling or unable to take warfarin or less likely to comply with INR monitoring should receive tissue valves.

Mechanical valves are preferred if patient requires long term anticoagulation for any reason like AF.

In patient with high risk of bleeding such as haemophilia, bioprosthetic valves are preferred.

Anticoagulation therapy:

Bioprosthetic valves: Aspirin + Warfarin for 3 months followed by life long aspirin only.

Mechanical valve: Aspirin + Warfarin life long

INR goals:

2 to 3: Low risk AVR

2.5 to 3.5: High risk AVR, MVR (All)

High risk conditions for thrombogenicity include: AF, Prior thromboembolism, severe LV dysfunction (EF <30%), require INR between 2.5 and 3.5.

Ross Procedure:

Aortic valve reconstruction is done using pulmonary valve **autograft** (not homograft) i.e. pulmonary valve of the patient (pulmonary autograft) is placed in aortic position and another homograft is placed in pulmonary position.

Done in children and adolescents

Not done in elderly or rheumatic aortic valve disease.

Advantages: No need for anticoagulation, growth of the valve and root in children

Transcatheter valve replacement:

Medtronic Melody valve is approved for transcatheter **pulmonary valve** replacement in patients with dysfunctional right ventricular outflow tract conduits.

Transcatheter aortic valve replacement (TAVR):

Two main types of stent design: balloon-expandable and self-expanding.

The Edwards Sapien Valve (Edwards Lifesciences, Irvine, California) is a cobalt chromium balloon-expandable valve with the valve leaflets made of treated bovine pericardium.

The CoreValve (Medtronic, Minneapolis, Minnesota) is the most common self-expanding nitinol valve

PARTNER 1A: TAVR found to be non-inferior to surgical AVR (SAVR) in high surgical risk patients.

PARTNER 1B: Demonstrated superiority of TAVR to medical therapy in inoperable patients, with an absolute survival advantage of 23% at 5 years

PARTNER 2A: TAVR was non-inferior to SAVR in intermediate surgical risk patients.

Complications of TAVR: Increased risk of stroke, paravalvular leaks, requirement of permanent pacemaker

11 Congenital Heart Diseases

Atrial Septal Defects

1. **Crochetage sign in ECG is seen in:**
   A. ASD B. VSD
   C. PDA D. Coronary AV fistula

2. **Which type of atrial septal defects are associated with partial or complete connection of pulmonary veins to right side of heart:**
   A. Secundum ASD
   B. Superior sinus venosus defect
   C. Primum ASD
   D. Inferior sinus venosus defect

3. **Cleft mitral valve is common in:**
   A. Ebstein's anomaly
   B. Cor triatriatum
   C. Atrioventricular septal defects
   D. Congenital mitral stenosis

4. **Which one of following type ASD is suitable for device closure ?**
   A. Ostium primum
   B. Ostium secundum
   C. Sinus venosus
   D. Unroofed coronary sinus

5. **Sinus venosus ASD is commonly associated with which of the following?**
   A. Cleft mitral valve
   B. Partial anomalous pulmonary venous drainage
   C. Persistent left superior vena cava (SVC)
   D. Goose-neck deformity

6. **Ostium secundum ASDs make up what proportion of ASDs?**
   A. 90% B. 25%
   C. 80% D. 75%

7. **A 26-year-old patient is referred to you for a murmur. A transthoracic echocardiogram (TTE) is performed which fails to show any valvular pathology or a shunt lesion. The TTE is remarkable for dilatation of right atrium and right ventricle. What would the next step be?**
   A. Reassure the patient; no further test is needed
   B. Cardiac catheterization
   C. Transesophageal echocardiogram (TEE)
   D. Cardiac magnetic resonance imaging (MRI)

8. **A primum ASD is associated commonly with which of the following?**
   A. Left axis deviation on surface electrocardiogram (ECG)
   B. Cleft of the anterior mitral leaflet
   C. Left axis deviation and cleft mitral leaflet
   D. Persistent left SVC

9. **All are seen in Ostium Primum ASD with left to right shunt greater than 2:1 except:**
   A. Early systolic murmur in pulmonary area
   B. Wide and fixed split of S2
   C. Right QRS axis with RBBB
   D. Tricuspid mid diastolic murmur

Ventricular Septal Defects

10. Commonest ventricular septal defect is:
A. Perimembranous VSD
B. Muscular VSD
C. Inlet VSD
D. Subpulmonic VSD

11. Spontaneous closure of VSD occurs up to?
A. 1 year age B. 4 year age
C. 8 year age D. 15 year age

12. A 6 month old child with recent pneumonia undergoes echocardiogram which shows 3 mm perimembranous VSD with maximum velocity of 4M/sec of VSD jet. Appropriate management includes:
A. PA banding
B. Medical follow up with diuretics
C. Patch closure of VSD
D. Cardiac catheterization to decide need of surgery

13. The type of VSD which will have the highest incidence of surgically induced atrio-ventricular block during closure:
A. Perimembraneous VSD
B. Outflow VSD
C. Mid-muscular VSD
D. Apical muscular VSD

14. What is the chamber that dilates in a patient with a significant VSD?
A. Right atrium
B. Right ventricle
C. Left atrium and left ventricle
D. Left ventricle

15. What is the most common lesion that is associated with supracristal VSD?
A. AS
B. Aortic regurgitation
C. Pulmonary regurgitation (PR)
D. PS

16. A patient has a small restrictive peri-membranous VSD. The velocity across the defect is 5 m/s. Blood pressure (BP) recorded at the time of the echocardiogram is 125/75 mmHg. What is the right ventricular (RV) systolic pressure?
A. 40 mmHg B. 25 mmHg
C. 100 mmHg D. 125 mmHg

17. A patient, with a small perimembranous VSD, is undergoing dental work. His dentist recommends him to see you regarding endocarditis prophylaxis. What would your recommendation be?
A. Amoxicillin 2 g prior to commencement of dental work
B. Vancomycin 1 g IV prior to dental work
C. Clindamycin 600 mg prior to dental work
D. No antibiotic prophylaxis is indicated at this time

Patent Ductus Arteriosus

18. Syndromic associations with PDA:
A. Rubella syndrome
B. Trisomy 18
C. Char syndrome
D. All of the above

19. A patient is diagnosed with a PDA. The peak systolic gradient across the defect is 105 mmHg. No other abnormality is noted on the echocardiogram. The BP recorded at the time of the echocardiogram is 130/77 mmHg. Based on the data given, what does the patient have:
A. Suprasystemic RV pressure
B. Normal RV pressure.
C. Systemic RV pressure
D. Cannot tell

20. Device closure can be done in all except?
A. 20 mm OS - ASD with good rims
B. 5 mm tubular PDA

C. PFO R->L shunt with paradoxical embolism
D. 5 mm supracristal VSD

21. Krichenko classification is used for:
A. ASD B. VSD
C. PDA D. TOF

Eisenmenger Syndrome

22. Which of the following disease is not associated with Eisenmenger syndrome?
A. Large PDA
B. TGA
C. TOF
D. Complete AVSD

Anomalous Pulmonary Venous Connection

23. Which one of the following is not true for total anomalous pulmonary venous connection?
A. Right atrium &ventricle are significantly dilated
B. ASD with left to right shunt
C. Snowman appearance is common on X-ray
D. Pulmonary hypertension is common

24. Most common variant of partially anomalous pulmonary venous connection (PAPVC):
A. Right pulmonary vein draining into right superior vena cava
B. Right pulmonary vein draining into inferior vena cava
C. Left pulmonary vein draining into coronary sinus
D. Left pulmonary vein draining into left innominate vein connection

25. Which feature is not seen in total anomalous pulmonary venous connection?
A. Continuous murmur
B. 'Figure of 8 appearance' on chest X-ray in infracardiac type of TAPVC
C. Right axis deviation on the ECG
D. Similar oxygen saturation in all the chambers

Left Ventricular Obstructive Diseases

26. Prevalence of bicuspid aortic valve in general population is:
A. 4–6% B. 20%
C. 1–2% D. 10%

27. Inheritance of BAV is:
A. AD
B. AR
C. X linked dominant
D. X linked recessive

28. Most common cardiac association of coarctation of aorta is?
A. Pulmonary valve stenosis
B. Bicuspid aortic valve
C. Cleft mitral valve
D. Ebstein's anomaly

29. One of the following is not a feature of Williams syndrome:
A. Supravalvular aortic stenosis
B. Tall stature
C. Coanda effect
D. Pulmonary artery stenosis

30. Williams syndrome does not include:
A. Supravalvular aortic stenosis
B. Pulmonary artery stenosis
C. Elfin faces
D. Hyperuricemia

31. Supravalvular aortic stenosis accounts for nearly 7% of all fixed forms of LVOT obstruction. Which of the following is not true regarding Supravalvular AS?

A. Its occurrence has been associated with a loss-of-function mutation of the elastin gene on chromosome 7q11.23.
B. It frequently occurs as part of the Williams-Beuren syndrome, and may be associated with stenosis of major branches of the aorta or pulmonary arteries
C. Due to a preferential jet of blood flow from a SupraAS into the left brachiocephalic artery, there might be marked increase in the left upper extremity systolic pressure relative to the right.
D. Since the coronary arteries are under high pressure, surgery might be considered earlier than in patients with valvular AS, particularly when no valve substitute is required.

32. Coarctation of aorta is common in:
A. Marfan's syndrome
B. Turner's syndrome
C. Down's syndrome
D. All of the above

33. Most common associated anomaly with coarctation of aorta:
A. Cleft mitral valve
B. Bicuspid aortic valve
C. VSD
D. PDA

34. All of the following statements are true regarding coarctation of aorta, except:
A. Only 25% of untreated patients survive their 5th decade
B. Pressure gradient of 20 mm Hg across the segment is class I indication for treatment
C. Patients with Turner's syndrome has higher risk of aortic dissection
D. Balloon angioplasty is the treatment of choice in adults with coarctation

35. Which of the following is the best echocardiographic view to diagnose coarctation of aorta?
A. Suprasternal view
B. Subcostal view
C. Parasternal short axis view
D. Parasternal long axis view

36. Which ONE of the following statements about a 40-year-old man presenting with upper limb hypertension and rib notching is TRUE?
A. Narrowing of the aorta is most likely to be proximal to the left subclavian artery
B. An association with pulmonary stenosis would be an expected finding
C. Marfan's syndrome is a recognized association
D. There is likely to be an increased risk of cerebrovascular accidents

37. Regarding hypertension and coarctation of aorta, which of the following is the true statement?
A. Hypertension is not a problem after repair
B. The prevalence of hypertension is lower regardless of age of repair
C. The prevalence of hypertension is similar to people with no coarctation
D. The prevalence of hypertension is higher with later repair

38. Which of the following is true about coarctation of aorta?
A. Successful repair in adults leads to normal life expectancy
B. Persistence of hypertension is commonly seen after successful repair
C. Risk of re-coarctation more common in adults compared to children
D. Adults with successful repair should be encouraged to do static exercises

39. Which one of the following is not a part of shone's complex?
A. Subaortic stenosis
B. Coarctation of aorta

C. Parachute mitral valve
D. Atretic aortic valve

40. Steidele's complex refers to:
A. Coarctation of aorta
B. Aortopulmonary window
C. Interruption of the aortic arch
D. Truncus arteriosus

41. One of the following is not a component of Shone's complex:
A. Parachute mitral valve
B. Coarctation of aorta
C. Supra mitral stenosing ring
D. Supravalvular aortic stenosis

42. All of the following true about Shone complex except?
A. Cor-triatriatum
B. Subvalvular AS
C. Congenital MS
D. Supravalvular mitral membrane

Tetralogy of Fallot

43. Which of the following is correct about Trilogy of Fallot?
A. VSD + PS + RVH
B. ASD + PS + RVH
C. Pink TOF
D. Adult TOF

44. What is incidence of right aortic arch in Tetralogy of Fallot?
A. 5% to 10 % B. 10 % to 20%
C. 20% to 30% D. 30% to 40%

45. The following statements regarding tetralogy of Fallot (TOF) are true, except:
A. Left axis deviation on the ECG suggests associated AV canal defect
B. Severity is determined by size of VSD
C. Jugular venous pressure is usually not elevated in children with TOF
D. Good surgical outcome is primarily decided by the pulmonary anatomy

46. Which of the following coronary anomalies can interfere with the corrective surgery for Tetralogy of Fallot?
A. LAD artery arising from the right aortic sinus
B. Separate origin of LAD and LCx from left aortic sinus
C. Separate origin of conus artery from right aortic sinus
D. High origin of right coronary artery form right aortic sinus

47. One of the following is a Palliative venous shunt:
A. Potts shunt
B. Central shunt
C. Glenn shunt
D. Blalock Taussig shunt

48. Which of the following is not part of tetralogy of Fallot?
A. Overriding of the aorta
B. RV hypertrophy
C. PS
D. VSD
E. ASD

49. Which of the following is a surgically important anomaly that should be sought out in a patient with TOF being referred for surgical repair?
A. Anomalous origin of left anterior descending (LAD) artery from right coronary artery (RCA)
B. Anomalous RCA from LAD
C. Anomalous left circumflex artery from RCA
D. None of the above

50. The classic Blalock–Taussig shunt is a connection between which of the following?
A. Ascending aorta to PA

B. Subclavian artery to PA
C. Descending aorta to left PA
D. SVC to right PA

Transposition of Great Arteries

51. Aorto-tricuspid continuity seen in:
A. Holmes heart
B. TGA (complete)
C. DORV with transposition
D. Normal heart

52. What is the surgical procedure of choice for the correction of D-TGA?
A. Senning procedure
B. Mustard procedure
C. Jatene arterial switch
D. Rastelli procedure

53. What is the position of the aorta in D-TGA?
A. Central
B. Anterior and rightward
C. Anterior and leftward
D. Posterior

54. Which of the following is true regarding D-transposition of the great arteries (d-TGA)?
A. Infants with d-TGA and VSD are susceptible to early development of pulmonary vascular disease
B. Atrial switch is the most commonly performed definitive repair
C. The aorta arises left and anterior to the pulmonary artery
D. Admixture physiology is common in d-TGA

55. What is a Rastelli repair?
A. Closure of VSD and placement of right ventricle–PA conduit
B. Balloon atrial septostomy
C. Repair of VSD
D. Repair of ASD

56. L loop is seen in:
A. DTGA
B. Isolated ventricular inversion
C. TOF
D. DORV

57. Which one of following is not true for corrected transposition of great arteries?
A. Atrio ventricular discordance present
B. Ventriculo arterial discordance present
C. Cyanosis is common
D. It produces loud second sound at left basal area

58. What is incidence of complete heart block in patients with Corrected transposition of great arteries?
A. 10% B. 5%
C. 30% D. 50%

59. ECG features of corrected transposition of great arteries:
A. Heart blocks
B. Left axis deviation
C. Septal Q wave inversion
D. All of the above

60. Which of the following congenital condition is associated with increased risk of complete heart block?
A. Supravalvar Aortic stenosis
B. TOF with absent pulmonary valve
C. c-TGA (corrected transposition of great arteries)
D. Ebstein's anomaly

61. What is the position of the aorta in levo (L)-TGA?
A. Anterior and rightward
B. Anterior and to the left
C. Central
D. Posterior

62. In what percentage of patients with L-TGA is complete heart block seen?
A. 90% B. 30%
C. 50% D. 10%

63. Taussig-Bing anomaly is:
A. DORV with subpulmonary VSD
B. DTGA
C. LTGA
D. TAPVC

64. Which one of following is not a component of Taussig-Bing anomaly ?
A. Double outlet right ventricle
B. Subpulmonic VSD
C. Pulmonary stenosis
D. Severe PAH

65. Which of the following conditions can have the oxygen saturation of blood in pulmonary artery higher than that in the aorta?
A. Corrected transposition of great arteries
B. Infracardiac TAPVC with patent foramen ovale
C. Taussig Bing anomaly
D. Right pulmonary artery to left atrial fistula

Ebstein's Anomaly

66. The triad of cyanosis, cardiomegaly and ischemic lung fields on chest X-ray suggests:
A. ASD Eisenmenger
B. TOF physiology
C. Ebstein's anomaly
D. Transposition physiology

67. The commonest associated anomaly seen in a patient with Ebstein's anomaly include?
A. Patent ductus arteriosus
B. Atrial septal defect
C. Coarctation of aorta
D. Pulmonary stenosis

68. How much apical displacement of septal leaflet of tricuspid valve is used as a cut off limit for diagnosing Ebstein's anomaly in adults:
A. 25 mm B. 10 mm
C. 15 mm D. 20 mm

69. Cone repair is the surgical technique for:
A. Interrupted aortic arch
B. Fibro muscular subaortic obstruction
C. Supra valvar aortic stenosis
D. Ebstein's anomaly of tricuspid valve

70. Which one of following is not common in ECG of patient with Ebstein's anomaly?
A. Himalayan P wave
B. Type-A WPW syndrome
C. RBBB
D. Prolonged PR interval

71. Most common congenital heart disease associated with pre-excitation:
A. Tricuspid atresia
B. Glycogen storage disorders
C. HOCM
D. Ebstein's anomaly

72. Ebstein's anomaly is characterized by abnormally apical displacement of tricuspid valve leaflets. Which of the following statements is true in this context?
A. The septal leaflet is characteristically described as being sail-like.
B. The most frequently associated anomaly is pulmonary atresia
C. Echocardiography is the key diagnostic technique with apical distal displacement of the septal or posterior leaflet of 8 cm/ m2 BSA.
D. ECG shows prolonged PR interval, RBBB & bizarre "second" QRS attached to preceding normal QRS.

Fontan Procedure

73. Choussat's criteria are operability criteria for which operation?
A. Norwood's procedure
B. Glenn's Shunt

C. Fontan's operation
D. BT Shunt

74. Total cavo-pulmonary connection is the preferred surgical treatment for:
A. Tricuspid atresia with pulmonary stenosis
B. Corrected transposition of great arteries
C. Isolated ventricular inversion
D. Scimitar syndrome

75. The following factors contribute to failure of Fontan repair, except:
A. Progressive right ventricular outflow obstruction
B. Atrioventricular valve regurgitation
C. Pulmonary arteriovenous fistula
D. Left ventricular dysfunction

76. Recurrent palpitations are due to which long term complication of Fontan procedure?
A. Torsade des pointes
B. Ventricular tachycardia
C. Atrial flutter
D. Junctional tachycardia

77. A patient with a h/o Fontan surgery presents with complaints of edema. On examination he has ascites, and his serum chemistry is significant for a low albumin level. What may be the possible cause in this patient?
A. Celiac disease
B. Pericardial constriction
C. Renal failure
D. Protein-losing enteropathy

Heterotaxy

78. True statement in Asplenia syndrome:
A. IVC interruption
B. Females
C. PAPVC
D. Bilocular heart

79. Which of the following cardiac malpositions is associated with highest chances of congenital heart disease?
A. Dextrocardia with situs solitus
B. Dextrocardia with situs inversus
C. Levocardia with situs solitus
D. Levocardia with situs inversus

Other Congenital Heart Diseases

80. Pulmonary atresia with intact ventricular septum is associated with all except:
A. Fistulous communication in RPA to right ventricular sinusoids
B. Atresia and stenosis of LAD
C. Tricuspid valve abnormalities
D. Right to left shunting at atrial level

81. A 19 year old male with mild infundibular pulmonary stenosis was found to have double aortic arch on CT angiography. On Retrospective questioning he reported dysphagia. Recommended treatment:
A. Reassurance and no therapy
B. Division of non-dominant arch
C. Surgery is indicated only when life-threatening symptoms are present in view of the high risk of surgery
D. Prokinetics like Itopride

82. Most common vascular ring:
A. Double aortic arch
B. Right aortic arch with Kommerell's diverticulum
C. Pulmonary sling
D. Retroesophageal descending aorta

83. ALCAPA refers to:
A. Scimitar syndrome
B. Bland-White-Garland syndrome
C. Halfman syndrome
D. Golden har syndrome

84. Not a feature of Kawasaki Syndrome:
A. Strawberry tongue
B. Vesicular eruptions
C. Coronary artery aneurysms
D. Cervical lymphadenopathy

85. Kawasaki disease criteria includes all except:
A. Fever > 5 days
B. Lymphadenopathy
C. Suppurative conjunctivitis
D. Skin desquamation

86. In kawasaki disease, incidence of coronary aneurysms is?
A. Up to 50% B. Up to 25%
C. Up to 70% D. Up to 90%

87. Which one of the following is not true for Uhl's anomaly?
A. Aplasia or hypoplasia of RV myocardium
B. Ventricular arrhythmias
C. RV is enlarged
D. Pulmonary edema

Common Syndromes

88. What are the most common lesions associated with Noonan syndrome?
A. Ventricular septal defect (VSD)
B. Patent ductus arteriosus (PDA)
C. Coarctation of aorta and aortic stenosis (AS)
D. Pulmonary stenosis (PS) and atrial septal defect (ASD)

89. Most common lesion associated with William's syndrome is:
A. VSD
B. Valvular AS
C. Supravalvular AS
D. ASD

90. What are the most common anomalies seen in DiGeorge syndrome (22q11)?
A. Pulmonary valve stenosis
B. ASD
C. VSD and arch anomalies
D. Supravalvular AS

91. CATCH 22 due to deletion at chromosome 22q11.2 is characterised by all except:
A. Cardiac defect
B. Abnormal genitalia
C. Thymic hypoplasia
D. Cleft palate

92. Most common congenital heart lesion seen in Holt–Oram syndrome is:
A. Arch anomalies
B. Coarctation of aorta
C. ASD
D. AS

93. Most common cardiac anomaly seen in Turner syndrome?
A. Coarctation of aorta
B. Tetralogy of Fallot (TOF)
C. VSD
D. Partial anomalous pulmonary venous drainage

94. Which of the following may 45, XO be associated with?
A. Brachiofemoral delay
B. Bicuspid aortic valve
C. Impaired glucose tolerance
D. All of the above

95. What is the incidence of congenital heart disease in Down syndrome?
A. 20% B. 30%
C. 70% D. 50%

96. First trimester maternal rubella infection makes fetus vulnerable for?
A. Supravalvar pulmonary stenosis
B. Pulmonary artery stenosis
C. Infundibular pulmonary stenosis
D. Pulmonary atresia stenosis

97. Which cardiac condition is not associated with left axis deviation?
A. AV canal defects
B. Single ventricle
C. Tricuspid atresia
D. Ebstein's anomaly

98. Right aortic arch is associated with which of the following?
A. TOF
B. Truncus arteriosus
C. Pulmonary atresia
D. All of the above

99. Peripheral pulmonary artery stenosis is seen in all except:
A. Poland syndrome
B. William's syndrome
C. Rubella syndrome
D. Alagillae syndrome

100. LEOPARD syndrome results from:
A. Mutation of 7q11
B. Deletion of 22q11
C. Mutation in FBNI gene
D. Deletion of PTPN 11 gene

Miscellaneous

101. Regarding cyanotic congenital heart diseases select the true statement:
A. Hyperviscosity that occurs by the virtue of erythrocytosis may be aggravated by iron deficiency
B. The total cholesterol levels of these patients is higher than that of general population
C. Glenn shunt is a palliative shunt connecting ascending aorta to right pulmonary artery.
D. Right aortic arch exists in more than 70% of patients with tricuspid atresia.

102. Stereotyped QRS complexes are seen in:
A. Tricuspid atresia
B. Single ventricle
C. VSD
D. Pulmonary atresia

103. Most commonly truncal valve is:
A. Quadricuspid
B. Bicuspid
C. Tricuspid
D. Pentacuspid

104. Surgical treatment for DTGA + VSD + LVOT obstruction:
A. Mustard operation
B. Senning operation
C. Jatane operation
D. Rastelli operation

105. RACHS scoring system is used in surgical risk stratification of:
A. Aortic aneurysm.
B. Aortic valve replacement
C. Congenital heart surgery
D. Heart and lung transplantation

106. Which of the following is wrongly matched?
A. Single ventricle with PS with interrupted IVC – Kawashima operation
B. TOF with severe PS with spells – BT shunt
C. ALCAPA – Takeuchi repair
D. Tricuspid atresia – Rev procedure

107. Which of the following is wrong match?
A. Truncus arteriosus – Total cavo-pulmonary connection
B. TOF with severe PS with spells – BT shunt
C. ALCAPA – Takeuchi repair
D. TGA – Arterial switch operation

108. Which of the following is a wrong match?
A. ALCAPA- Takeuchi
B. Truncus arteriosus- REV
C. Single ventricle with interrupted IVC-Kawashima procedure

D. TOF with VSD with PS- Blalock-Taussig shunt

109. True about DORV with restrictive VSD are all except:

A. PSM on examination
B. LVSP > RVSP on cardiac catheterization
C. RVH on ECG
D. Cyanosis is always present independent of pulmonary obstruction

110. Cyanosis is not found in:

A. TOF with severe PS/single ventricle with PS
B. D-TGA with restrictive VSD
C. DORV with PS/Taussig-Bing anomaly
D. Sinus venosus ASD with PAPVC

111. All are ductus dependent lesions in neonate except:

A. Pulmonary atresia with intact ventricular septum
B. TAPVC
C. Interrupted aortic arch
D. Hypoplastic left heart syndrome

112. All are cyanotic congenital heart diseases with increased pulmonary blood flow except:

A. Double outlet right ventricle with pulmonary stenosis
B. Truncus arteriosus
C. Common atrium
D. Taussig bing anomaly

113. Pulmonary artery dilatation is not a feature in:

A. TOF with absent pulmonary valve
B. ASD with large L-R shunt
C. VSD with severe PH
D. Noonan's syndrome with sever PS due to dysplastic PV

114. All are seen in Pulmonary Stenosis except:

A. Balloon valvotomy can be offered as a permanent cure
B. RVH on ECG is proportional to severity of PS
C. Grade of pulmonic ejection murmur is proportional to severity of PS
D. 50% valvular stenosis have dysplastic valves

115. All are present in sub aortic stenosis except:

A. AR
B. Aortic ejection click
C. LVH
D. Coexistent coarctation of aorta

116. AV canal defects associated with ECG changes all except:

A. Short PR interval
B. rSR' pattern
C. RA enlargement
D. Left axis deviation

117. Identify the moderate severity congenital heart disease in an adult:

A. Pulmonary atresia
B. VSD with AR
C. Eisenmenger syndrome
D. Double outlet right ventricle with subpulmonic VSD

ANSWERS

ATRIAL SEPTAL DEFECT (ASD):

Answer: 1. A. ASD

Answer: 2. B. Superior sinus venosus defect

Answer: 3. C. Atrioventricular septal defects

Answer: 4. B. Ostium secundum

Answer: 5. B. Partial anomalous pulmonary venous drainage.

Answer: 6. D. 75%.

Answer: 7. C. Transesophageal echocardiogram (TEE).

TEE should be performed to look for sinus venosus ASD or partial anomalous pulmonary venous drainage that can be easily missed on a TTE.

Answer: 8. C. Left axis deviation and cleft mitral leaflet.

Answer: 9. C. Right QRS axis with RBBB

Atrial septal defects

Most common congenital heart lesion in adults, **female** predominance

Types:

1. Secundum (65-70%%): Most common
2. Primum (10–15 %): Associated with cleft anterior mitral leaflet with MR, left axis deviation on ECG.
   AV valves are at the same level and the left ventricular outflow tract is elongated and narrow, giving the characteristic "gooseneck" deformity. Primum ASDs constitute a partial AV canal defect.
3. Sinus venosus (10–15 %): Associated with partial anomalous pulmonary venous drainage (superior sinus venosus defect- right upper pulmonary venous anomaly; inferior sinus venosus defect- right lower pulmonary venous anomaly: Scimitar syndrome)
4. Coronary sinus septal defects (rare)

Progressive RA and RV dilatation is seen in ASDs. They eisenmengerize very late in the fourth decade.

ECG:

Incomplete RBBB

Primum defects typically have **left axis deviation**, sinus venosus and secundum generally have a **rightward axis**

Sinus venosus may have a low ectopic atrial rhythm (negative p waves in leads II, III, aVF)

Treatment: Closure of an ASD either percutaneously or surgically is indicated for RA or RV enlargement with or without symptoms in predominantly left-to-right shunts. Closure should not be done in irreversible pulmonary hypertension (Eisenmenger syndrome).

Percutaneous closure: Only for ostium secundum ASDs

Surgical closure: Very large secundum ASD, all sinus venosus, primum and coronary sinus ASDs.

For **sinus venosus** defects with anomalous pulmonary venous drainage, a **Warden technique** is sometimes used.

VENTRICULAR SEPTAL DEFECTS (VSD)

Answer: 10. A. Perimembranous VSD

Answer: 11. C. 8 year age

Answer: 12. B. Medical follow up with diuretics

Answer: 13. A. Perimembranous VSD

Answer: 14. C. Left atrium and left ventricle.

A significant ASD, PAPVC or TAPVC cause enlargement of RA and RV whereas significant VSD and PDA lead to dilatation of LA and LV due to volume overload.

Answer: 15. B. Aortic regurgitation.

The most common associated finding seen in a supracristal VSD is AR, which occurs due to valve distortion.

Answer: 16. B. 25 mmHg.

The left ventricle–right ventricle pressure gradient across the VSD = 4 v2, (where v is velocity across the VSD), that is, 4 × 5 × 5 = 100 mmHg. LV systolic pressure will be equal to systolic BP ie 125 mmHg. Right ventricular systolic pressure is then equivalent to 125–100 mmHg, which calculates to 25 mmHg.

Answer: 17. D. No antibiotic prophylaxis is indicated at this time.

Ventricular septal defects

Most common congenital heart defect at birth and in early childhood.

2/3 close by early school age (by 8 years of age)

Types:

1. Perimembranous: 60–70%, most common
2. Muscular: single or multiple: 10%
3. Supracristal: (5%) Usually small defects located beneath the aortic annulus, frequently associated with progressive aortic leaflet prolapse and insufficiency (right and noncoronary cusp)
4. AV canal defect (Inlet type): common in Down's syndrome, typically involves anterior mitral cleft and occasionally cleft tricuspid septal leaflet; primum ASD may coexist

Clinical presentation:

If small isolated restrictive defect, typically asymptomatic with a murmur

If large defect uncorrected in childhood → Congestive heart failure in childhood and Eisenmenger syndrome later on.

Progressive LA and LV volume overload is seen.

Management:

Closure of a VSD is indicated when there is a Qp/Qs (pulmonary-to-systemic blood flow ratio) of 2.0 or more and clinical evidence of LV volume overload

Closure is contraindicated in irreversible pulmonary artery hypertension (Eisenmenger)

Muscular and perimembranous VSDs may be closed **percutaneously** with device if anatomy permits. Perimembranous VSDs have high incidence of AV block during surgical or device closure.

PATENT DUCTUS ARTERIOSUS (PDA)

Answer: 18. D. All

Answer: 19. B. Normal RV pressure.

The peak gradient across the PDA is 105 mmHg and systolic BP is 130 mmHg.

Gradient across PDA = LVSP- RVSP.

Right ventricular systolic pressure is 130-105 which is 25 mmHg, which is in the normal range.

Answer: 20. D. 5 mm supracristal VSD

Answer: 21. C. PDA

Typically closes early in infancy, with a higher incidence of PDA in premature infants and those living at high altitudes.

Associated with **Congenital Rubella Syndrome** as is branch pulmonic stenosis.

Other associations: Trisomy 18, Char syndrome

Clinical Presentation: varies according to size, from asymptomatic (incidentally noted), to LA and LV volume overload or Eisenmenger syndrome when large and unrepaired

Physical Exam:

Small PDA: soft **continuous** infraclavicular, left sternal border or left upper back murmur, enhanced with isometric exercise.

Moderate PDA: ventricular enlargement and a displaced point of maximal impulse on palpation

Large PDA: LA and LV enlargement; If pulmonary hypertension, there will be a prominent pulmonic component to the second heart sound and RV heave with cyanosis and clubbing [Eisenmenger individual: may have **differential cyanosis**: cyanosis of feet (clubbing of toes) and perhaps left hand with normal right hand pulse oximetry]

Differentials for continuous murmur: PDA, coronary AV fistula, aortopulmonary window, pulmonary AV malformation (Peutz Jaeger syndrome) or the systolic/diastolic murmur of aortic stenosis (AS)/AR

Management:

Closure of PDA either percutaneously or surgically is indicated if there is LA and or LV enlargement, if pulmonary hypertension is present in the presence of net left-to-right shunting or prior endarteritis.

Surgical closure is most appropriate when PDA is too large for percutaneous closure device, or if PDA is aneurysmal, or there is endarteritis.

Closure is not indicated if pulmonary hypertension with net right-to-left shunt (Eisenmenger)

The **Krichenko classification of PDA** is based on angiography and includes type A (conical), type B (window), type C (tubular), type D (complex), and type E (elongated) PDA

EISENMENGER SYNDROME

Answer: 22. C. TOF

Eisenmenger syndrome:

Seen in unoperated large left-to-right shunt lesions (without pulmonic stenosis).

Not seen in congenital heart diseases with significant pulmonic stenosis such as TOF; because PS decreased pulmonary blood flow and prevents development of pulmonary vascular disease.

It is defined as progressive increase in PVR which leads to reversal of shunting (right-to-left) and ultimately right ventricular failure and death.

Clinical Exam:

Cyanosis, clubbing, jugular venous a wave

Prominent RV heave, loud P2

Often no murmur, but occasionally the holosystolic murmur of TR or diastolic murmur of functional PR from elevated PVR

CXR: Large main PA and central PA with oligemic periphery (pruning)

Complications:

Systemic emboli or abscess from right-to-left shunting

Erythrocytosis as a response to chronic hypoxemia, thrombocytopenia from splenic sequestration; neurologic events may occur due to hyperviscosity syndrome

Hemoptysis may occur

Arrhythmia and sudden cardiac death

Management: Pulmonary arterial vasodilators may prolong survival and the only surgical option is heart-lung transplant.

Pregnancy is contraindicated.

ANOMALOUS PULMONARY VENOUS CONNECTION:

Answer: 23. B. ASD with left to right shunt

Answer: 24. A. Right pulmonary vein draining into right superior vena cava

Answer: 25. B. 'Figure of 8 appearance' on chest X-ray in infra-cardiac type of TAPVC

Partial anomalous pulmonary venous connection

The most common form of PAPVC is one in which a right upper pulmonary vein connects to the right atrium or the superior vena cava. This form is almost always associated with a sinus venosus type of atrial septal defect (ASD).

Scimitar syndrome (right pulmonary vein to inferior vena cava with lung sequestration)

The pulmonary abnormality: Sequestered lobe of the lung that is separated from the bronchial tree and has nonfunctioning lung tissue. It is associated with hypoplastic or aplastic right pulmonary artery segments, hypoplastic or absent bronchi, hypoplasia of the right lung.

The venous anomaly: PAPVC, usually with the right pulmonary veins draining into the inferior vena cava

Total anomalous pulmonary venous connection

All the pulmonary veins drain into right atrium and left atrium is supplied by RA through ASD by right to left shunt.

Saturations are similar in all 4 chambers due to mixing at right atrial level.

RA and RV are grossly dilated and patients develop pulmonary hypertension early in life.

Four anatomic forms-

Supracardiac: Most common type, CXR- Classic **snowman sign** (Figure of 8 sign)

Cardiac

Infracardiac: Most commonly associated with obstruction in common pulmonary vein, causing severe pulmonary venous hypertension and pulmonary edema.

Mixed: Least common

LV OBSTRUCTIVE DISEASES

Answer: 26. C. 1–2%.

Answer: 27

Answer: 28. B. Bicuspid aortic valve.

Bicuspid aortic valve is present in 50-65% of cases with coarctation of the aorta.

Answer: 29. B. Tall stature

Answer: 30. D. Hyperuricemia

Answer: 31. C. Due to a preferential jet of blood flow from a SupraAS into the left brachiocephalic artery, there might be marked increase in the left upper extremity systolic pressure relative to the right.

Answer: 32. B. Turner's syndrome

Answer: 33. Bicuspid aortic valve

Answer: 34. D. Balloon angioplasty is the treatment of choice in adults with coarctation

Answer: 35. A. Suprasternal view

Answer: 36. D. There is likely to be an increased risk of cerebrovascular accidents

Answer: 37. D. The prevalence of hypertension is higher especially with later repair.

Answer: 38. B. Persistence of hypertension is commonly seen after successful repair

Answer: 39. D. Atretic aortic valve

Answer: 40. C. Interruption of the aortic arch

Answer: 41. C. Supravalvular aortic stenosis

Answer: 42. A. Cor-triatriatum

Bicuspid aortic valve (BAV):

Most common congenital heart lesion, male predominance, Autosomal dominant, estimated 1–2 % of population.

Most common association in CoA is BAV, should be ruled out in Turner's Syndrome.

Important association with medial connective tissue abnormalities of the ascending aorta.

Regurgitation is less common than stenosis.

Williams Syndrome:

Supravalvular Aortic Stenosis, hypercalcemia, elfin facies, peripheral pulmonary artery stenosis.

Facial features frequently include a broad forehead, short nose and full cheeks, an appearance that has been described as **"elfin facies".**

Autosomal dominant, Chromosome 7.

Coanda effect: In patients with **supravalvular AS**, the high-velocity stream is along the right aortic wall, causing disproportionately **high pressure in the right arm** than the left arm.

Coarctation of the aorta (CoA)

Narrowing in the region of the ligamentum arteriosum distal to the origin of the left subclavian artery is the most common site.

Male predominance

Associated with BAV (50–65 %) and circle of Willis aneurysm (Berry's aneurysm) which increases risk of intracranial bleeding.

Presence of large collaterals may reduce the gradient across the coarctation site.

High prevalence of systemic hypertension which may persist in some individuals even after repair of CoA. Prevalence of HTN is higher with later repair.

Shone's complex: Coarctation associated with left heart obstructions (Supramitral ring, Parachute mitral valve, subaortic stenosis, Coarctation of aorta).

Systolic bruit over the upper left back

Radial-femoral delay

CXR findings:

Aortic indentation at the coarctation site "3 sign"

Notching on the underside of the ribs from collateral vessels

Echocardiography:

Best viewed from suprasternal notch

May see collateral vessel flow

Indications for surgical or percutaneous intervention:

Peak to peak catheterization gradient of 20 mmHg or greater regardless of presence or absence of hypertension OR lesser gradient in the presence of imaging evidence of significant coarctation with significant collateral flow.

- Percutaneous approach may be considered if narrowed site is amenable.
- Surgical intervention for complex anatomy, long segment tubular lesions, prior aneurysm, calcification or poorly compliant arterial system.
- Hypertension may persist even after successful repair of coarctation.

Steidele's complex: Steidele's complex is an eponym to interrupted aortic arch (IAA), which is characterised by complete anatomic discontinuity between the aortic arch and the descending aorta (DA).

TETRALOGY OF FALLOT (TOF)

Answer: 43. B. ASD+PS+RVH

Answer: 44. C. 20% to 30%

Answer: 45. B. Severity is determined by siaze of VSD

Answer: 46. A. LAD artery arising from the right aortic sinus

Answer: 47. C. Glenn shunt

Glenn shunt is a venous shunt, rest three are palliative arterial shunts.

Answer: 48. E. ASD.

Answer: 49. A. Anomalous origin of left anterior descending (LAD) artery from right coronary artery (RCA).

Answer: 50. B. Subclavian artery to PA.

Tetralogy of Fallot

Most common cyanotic congenital heart lesion after infancy.

RV out flow obstruction (valvular and subvalvular/infundibular with generally small pulmonary arteries), large VSD with an overriding aorta and RV hypertrophy.

JVP not elevated, no cardiac enlargement

Severity of cyanosis and symptoms is not determined by size of VSD but by degree of pulmonic stenosis.

Right aortic arch is associated in 25 % of cases.

Approximately ~ 5 % of TOF patients have aberrant course of the left anterior descending (LAD) arising from the proximal right coronary artery (RCA) or right sinus of Valsalva, traversing the RVOT which may be inadvertently cut during RVOT reconstruction.

Palliative interventions:

1. Blalock-Taussig shunt (subclavian artery to branch PA): Most common, in modified BT shunt a PTFE graft is placed between subclavian artery and pulmonary artery.
2. Potts shunt (descending aorta to left PA window)
3. Waterston shunt (ascending aorta to right PA window)
4. Central shunt (Ascending aorta to main PA)

Complete repair (VSD closure, RVOT augmentation): Usually performed in infancy or early childhood is the treatment of choice. Most patients undergo repair between 3 months and 12 months of age.

Significant PR may occur post operatively. **Pulmonic valve replacement** is indicated for severe PR with any of the following: (1) symptoms of decreased exercise tolerance, (2) moderate to severe RV dysfunction or enlargement (3) sustained atrial or ventricular arrhythmias or (4) moderate to severe TR.

Trilogy of Fallot- 1. Pulmonic stenosis 2. RVH 3. ASD

VSD is not part of Trilogy of Fallot.

Tetralogy of Fallot- 1. Pulmonic stenosis 2. RVH 3. Overriding of Aorta 4. VSD

Pentalogy of Fallot- 1. Pulmonic stenosis 2. RVH 3. Overriding of Aorta 4. VSD 5. ASD

TRANSPOSITIONS OF GREAT ARTERIES

Answer: 51. B. TGA (complete)

Answer: 52. C. Jatene arterial switch.

Answer: 53. B. Anterior and rightward.

Normally aorta is posterior and to right of pulmonary artery.

D-TGA: Aorta is anterior and to right of pulmonary artery.

L-TGA: Aorta is anterior and to left of pulmonary artery.

Answer: 54. A. Infants with d-TGA and VSD are susceptible to early development of pulmonary vascular disease

Answer: 55. A. Closure of VSD and placement of a right ventricle–PA conduit.

Answer: 56. B. Isolated ventricular inversion

Answer: 57. C. Cyanosis is common

Answer: 58. C. 30%

Answer: 59. D. all

Answer: 60. C. c-TGA (corrected transposition of great arteries)

Answer: 61. B. Anterior and leftward.

Answer: 62. B. 30%.

Answer: 63. A. DORV with subpulmonary VSD

Answer: 64. C. Pulmonary stenosis

Answer: 65. C. Taussig Bing anomaly

D-TGA:

Great vessels arise from the incorrect ventricle (i.e., **ventriculoarterial discordance**: aorta arises from the morphologic RV and PA arises from the morphologic LV) resulting in parallel circulations.

Most common cause of cyanotic CHD **in neonates.**

Aorta is located **anterior and to right** of pulmonary artery.

Aorto-tricuspid continuity is seen in TGA. (Aorto-mitral continuity: Normal heart; Aorto-mitral discontinuity: Double outlet right ventricle)

Infants with d-TGA and VSD without pulmonic stenosis have increased pulmonary blood flow and pressures and hence are susceptible to early development of pulmonary vascular disease (Eisenmenger syndrome).

Rashkind's balloon atrial septostomy enables early survival.

Atrial switch: Senning and Mustard procedures, not done nowadays.

Arterial switch: Jatene Procedure, procedure of choice.

Rastelli repair: Used for repair of TGA or DORV with VSD with RVOT obstruction.

Aorta is connected to LVOT with gore tex patch, VSD is closed, and an artificial conduit is placed between RV and pulmonary artery.

Congenitally corrected Transposition of the Great Arteries (CC-TGA, L-TGA, ventricular inversion):

Atrioventricular and ventriculoarterial discordance.

L-loop of ventricles is seen due to malrotation during embryogenesis.

Aorta is located **anterior and to left** of pulmonary artery.

Cyanosis is absent since systemic blood goes to aorta and venous blood goes to pulmonary artery for oxygenation, unless additional cardiac defect is present.

Most common associated anomaly is **ASD**. Other associated anomalies include VSD, pulmonic stenosis, or systemic AV valve (tricuspid) insufficiency (occasionally Ebstein-like valve) and complete heart block.

CHB may be seen in upto **30%** patients of corrected TGA.

Incidence of CHB increases by **2% per year**.

Classic ECG is diagnostic: **Q wave in right precordial leads** (septal depolarization direction is altered) with varying degrees of heart block

Taussig-Bing anomaly:

Double outlet right ventricle (DORV) and subpulmonic ventricular septal defect (VSD).

Since VSD is subpulmonic, LV blood flows preferentially to pulmonary artery and RV blood flows mainly to aorta.

Therefore, clinical manifestations of Taussig-Bing anomaly are like D-TGA and treatment involves arterial switch operation.

Oxygen saturation will be more in pulmonary artery than aorta as seen in TGA.

Patient develops Eisenmenger in early life since there is no pulmonic stenosis.

EBSTEIN ANOMALY

Answer: 66. C. Ebstein's anomaly

Answer: 67. B. Atrial septal defect

Answer: 68. D. 20 mm

Answer: 69. D. Ebstein's anomaly of tricuspid valve

Answer: 70. B. Type- A WPW syndrome

Answer: 71. D. Ebstein's anomaly

Answer: 72. D. ECG shows prolonged PR interval, RBBB & bizarre "second" QRS attached to preceeding normal QRS.

→ There is displacement of septal or posterior tricuspid leaflet by 8mm/m^2 (not 8 cm/m^2)

Ebstein's anomaly:

"Apical displacement" of the septal and posterior leaflets of TV, compromising size of the portion of the RV below the TV and enlargement of the RA by portion of the RV above the TV ('atrialized' RV).

Anterior leaflet is largest leaflet and is described as "sail like".

20 mm or 8 mm/m^2 displacement of septal tricuspid leaflet with large redundant anterior leaflet.

From asymptomatic with a nearly silent clinical exam to marked right heart failure, cyanosis, and early death.

Most common associated abnormality **interatrial communication** (ASD or stretched patent foramen ovale [PFO]).

Accessory conduction pathways which can be multiple are present leading to **Wolff-Parkinson-White syndrome (WPW)** in 25 % of patients and presents with palpitations or SVT.

"Sail sound" of a loud systolic sound created by the large anterior leaflet may be heard.

ECG: wide and **splintered QRS complex** (right precordial leads), Peaked P wave due to RA enlargement (described as **Himalayan P waves**), first degree AV block and **Type B** WPW pattern.

CXR: Gross cardiomegaly with oligemic lung fields (described as **Box type** heart)

Echo:

GOSE score (Great Ormond Street Score): Defined as ratio of RA and atrialized RV to the combined area of functional RV, LA and LV. Greater the ratio, worse is the prognosis.

Treatment:

Biventricular repair is procedure of choice.

Cone procedure is done for repair of TV in Ebstein's disease.

FONTAN PROCEDURE

Answer: 73. Fontan's operation

Answer: 74. A. Tricuspid atresia with pulmonary stenosis

Answer: 75. A. Progressive right ventricular outflow obstruction

Answer: 76. C. Atrial flutter

Answer: 77. D. Protein-losing enteropathy.

Fontan surgery is type of **single ventricular repair** required for some complex congenital heart diseases. It is a **multistaged** procedure.

Also known as **Total cavopulmonary connection (TCPC).**

It separates systemic and pulmonary circulation.

1st stage procedure is done to normalize pulmonary blood flow (BT shunt in case of decreased pulmonary blood flow situations like PS and PA band in case of increased pulmonary blood flow situations). 2nd stage is called bidirectional glenn shunt (BDG) or Hemifontan which is done at the age of 4-6 months and final stage is completion of Fontan.

Advantages:

Near normalization of systemic saturation

Abolishment of chronic volume overload on single ventricle

Disadvantages:

Chronic systemic venous hypertension and congestion

Cardiac output is no longer determined by heart, but by transpulmonary flow (in turn regulated by PVR)-> leads to decreased cardiac output both at rest and during exercise

Indications:

Cardiac malformation and a **single functional ventricle** resulting from

- Dysfunctional heart valve
- Absent or inadequate pumping chamber

Most common CHDs palliated with Fontan circulation:

- Tricuspid or mitral atresia
- Pulmonary atresia with intact ventricular septum
- Hypoplastic left or right heart syndrome
- Double-inlet single ventricle

Perioperative mortality now is less than 5% and survival at 10 years has been shown to be around 80-85%.

Original **Ten commandments** by Fontan (Ideal candidate for surgery)

1. Age ≥ 4 and < 15 years
2. Normal sinus rhythm
3. Normal systemic venous connections
4. Normal right atrial volume
5. Mean PA pressure **≤ 15 mmHg**
6. Pulmonary vascular resistance **< 4 Woods units/m^2**
7. Adequate-sized PA (PA to aortic diameter ratio ≥ 0.75)
8. Left ventricular ejection fraction ≥ 60%
9. Competent mitral valve (absence of mitral valve insufficiency)
10. Absence of PA distortion

Fontan Fenestration:

Small opening or fenestration may be created between the conduit and the right atrium at the time of surgery.

It improves cardiac output and decreased venous congestion. Fenestration decreased post-operative pleural effusion. But, it comes at the cost of arterial desaturation.

Complications of Fontan:

Atrial arrhythmias (such as atrial flutter, intra-atrial re-entrant tachycardia)

LV failure causing exercise intolerance

Increased pressure in IVC causing cirrhosis, portal hypertension

Pulmonary AV malformation

Lymphatic system: Protein losing enteropathy, plastic bronchitis, chylothorax

Blood clot and embolism

Heterotaxy (Isomerism of atrial appendages)

Answer: 78. D. Bilobular heart

Answer: 79. D. Levocardia with situs inversus

Right atrial isomerism:

Two right sides with bilateral right atria and atrial appendages and absence of left sided structures such as coronary sinus

Bilateral SVC, Total anomalous pulmonary venous connection

Pulmonary stenosis or atresia

Double SA node

Lungs: Bilateral trilobed lungs with short eparterial bronchi

Abdomen: Asplenia

More common in males

Left atrial isomerism:

Bilateral left atria and atrial appendages

Interrupted IVC, Partial anomalous pulmonary venous drainage

Sinus node dysfunction or atrial fibrillation

Lungs: Bilateral bilobed lungs with longer hyparterial bronchi

Abdomen: Polysplenia

More common in females

Cardiac malposition with least chance of CHD: Situs inversus with dextrocardia

Cardiac malposition with highest chance of CHD: Situs inversus with levocardia

Kartagener's syndrome:

Bronchiectasis, sinusitis, ciliary dysmotility, infertility, dextrocardia.

Other congenital heart diseases

Answer: 80. A. Fistulous communication in RPA to right ventricular sinusoids

Answer: 81. B. Division of non-dominant arch

Answer: 82. Double aortic arch

Answer: 83. B. Bland white garland syndrome

Answer: 84. B. Vesicular eruptions

Answer: 85. C. Suppurative conjunctivitis

Answer: 86. B. Up to 25%

Answer: 87. D. Pulmonary edema

Pulmonary atresia with intact ventricular septum:

Pulmonary valve is atretic, so pulmonary circulation is dependent on PDA.

Patients usually present with cyanosis early in neonatal age at the time of closure of PDA.

RV and tricuspid valve are also usually hypoplastic.

There is obligatory right to left shunting at the atrial level, through ASD or PFO.

Blood flow to pulmonary arteries is through PDA and aortopulmonary collaterals (APCs).

Ventriculo-coronary connections or coronary sinusoids (Fistulous connections between RV and coronary arteries) are present in 45% of cases and correlate directly with severity of RV hypoplasia.

Some of these patients have coronary artery stenosis or atresia, in them coronary artery circulation is dependent on right ventricle (RV dependent coronary circulation). These patients are at particular risk of sudden cardiac death due to ischemia or arrhythmia.

Surgical outcomes depend upon degree of RV hypoplasia and presence of ventriculo-coronary connections.

Double aortic arch:

Double aortic arch is **most common** vascular ring.

Two aortic arches form a **complete vascular ring** that can compress the trachea and/or esophagus.

Two aortic arches, in which one is dominant, join to form descending aorta.

Treatment is surgical (**division of non-dominant arch**) and is indicated in all symptomatic patients.

ALCAPA:

Anomalous left coronary artery origin from the PA

Also known as Bland-White-Garland syndrome

Most die in infancy, if survive may have MI, MR and LV failure in childhood.

Surgery: Takeuchi repair

Kawasaki disease (mucocutaneous lymph node syndrome):

One of the most common vasculitides of childhood

Diagnosis:

Presence of fever (>38.5 C) lasting ≥5 days, combined with at least four of the five following physical findings

1. Bilateral bulbar conjunctival injection (Suppurative conjunctivitis is not seen)
2. Oral mucous membrane changes, including injected or fissured lips, injected pharynx, or strawberry tongue
3. Peripheral extremity changes, including erythema of palms or soles, edema of hands or feet (acute phase), and periungual desquamation
4. Polymorphous rash (vesicular and bullous lesions are not seen)
5. Cervical lymphadenopathy

Cardiovascular findings:

Coronary artery aneurysms occur in approximately 25% patients.

Aneurysms are located in the proximal coronary arteries, most commonly in the proximal left anterior descending and proximal right coronary arteries.

Infants <6 months old with KD have the highest risk of developing cardiac complications.

Coronary aneurysms do not develop until day 10 of illness.

Risk of complications is highest among patients with a history of large or giant aneurysms.

Laboratory: Elevation of acute phase reactants (ESR, CRP), leucocytosis, thrombocytosis, anemia

Treatment:

IVIG + Aspirin

Kobayashi score is for risk assessment and prognosis of Kawasaki disease

Uhl's anomaly:

Very rare congenital heart disease characterized by partial or total loss of the myocardial muscle in the right ventricle with preserved myocardium in left ventricle.

RV is enlarged, patient may present with RV failure or ventricular arrhythmias.

Treatment: Cardiac transplant.

COMMON SYNDROMES WITH CARDIAC DEFECTS

Answer: 88. D. Pulmonary stenosis (PS) and atrial septal defect (ASD).

Answer: 89. C. Supravalvular AS.

The second common associated defect is supravalvular PS.

Answer: 90. C. VSD and arch anomalies.

The most common anomaly seen in DiGeorge syndrome is VSD, followed by arch anomalies. ASD and supravalvular AS are seen in this syndrome.

Answer: 91. B. Abnormal genitalia

Answer: 92. C. ASD.

Answer: 93. A. Coarctation of aorta.

Answer: 94. D. All of the above.

Answer: 95. D. 50%

Answer: 96. B. Pulmonary artery stenosis

Answer: 97. D. Ebstein's anomaly

Answer: 98. E. All of the above.

Answer: 99. A. Poland syndrome

Answer: 100. D. Deletion of PTPN 11 gene

Noonan syndrome:

Autosomal dominant congenital disorder, **PTPN 11 gene** mutation on chromosome 12.

Referred to as a male version of Turner's syndrome

Congenital heart defect **(Pulmonary valve stenosis with dysplastic pulmonary valve**, also atrial septal defect and **hypertrophic cardiomyopathy**), short stature, learning problems, and a characteristic configuration of facial features including a webbed neck and a flat nose bridge.

Turner syndrome:

Known as 45, X or 45, X0, is a condition in which a female is partly or completely missing an X chromosome

Short and webbed neck, low-set ears, low hairline at the back of the neck, short stature, and swollen hands and feet (due to lymphedema) are seen at birth and later have widely spaced nipples, sterility, amenorrhea, shortened 4th metacarpal.

Cardiac: **Bicuspid aortic valve** (most common), **Coarctation of aorta** (2nd most common), ASD and AS.

Have moderately high risk of development of diabetes.

Cognition is normal and intellectual disabilities are absent.

Down's syndrome:

Trisomy 21, Most common chromosomal abnormality in humans.

Characteristic facial features, intellectual disability, single crease of palm.

Cardiac:

Rate of CHD in Down's is 40-50%.

Most common cardiac defect is **atrioventricular septal defect**. Others are VSD, TOF, PDA.

Williams Syndrome:

Supravalvular Aortic Stenosis, hypercalcemia, elfin facies, peripheral pulmonary artery stenosis.

Facial features frequently include a broad forehead, short nose and full cheeks, an appearance that has been described as **"elfin facies".**

Autosomal dominant, Chromosome 7.

Congenital Rubella Syndrome:

Classical triad: Sensorineural deafness, Cataract, CHD (specially Pulmonary artery stenosis and PDA)

DiGeorge syndrome (CATCH-22):

Autosomal dominant, Deletion of chromosome 22q11.2

Defects in palate (Velopharyngeal insufficiency)

Recurrent infections (due to absent or hypoplastic thymus leading to T cell mediated immune deficiency)

Hypocalcemia (due to malfunctioning parathyroid glands)

Features summarized as CATCH-22

- Cardiac abnormality (commonly interrupted aortic arch, truncus arteriosus and tetralogy of Fallot)
- Abnormal facies
- Thymic aplasia

- Cleft palate
- Hypocalcemia/hypoparathyroidism

LEOPARD syndrome:

Lentigines

Electrocardiographic conduction defects

Ocular hypertelorism

Pulmonary stenosis

Abnormalities of genitalia

Retarded growth

Deafness

Hypertrophic cardiomyopathy **(HCM)** is seen in 85% cases which may be clinically silent

Autosomal dominant trait, occurs due to **PTPN11 gene mutation** (Noonan syndrome is also caused by same mutation)

Holt Oram syndrome:

Autosomal dominant, ASD with congenital **abnormality of the hand and radius**.

Important associations:

Supravalvular PS: Occurs in Congenital Rubella syndrome, Williams syndrome and Takayasu arteritis.

Peripheral pulmonary artery stenosis: Rubella, Williams, Allagille. Takayasu, Behcets, Post cardiac surgery

Left axis deviation in CHD: 1. Ostium primum ASD, 2. AVSD, 3. Tricuspid atresia, 4. Single ventricle

Right aortic arch common in: 1. Pulmonary atresia (40%), 2. Truncus arteriosus (35%), 3. TOF (25%).

Miscellaneous

Answer: 101. A. Hyperviscosity that occurs by the virtue of erythrocytosis may be aggravated by iron deficiency

Answer: 102. B. Single ventricle

Answer: 103. C. Tricuspid

Answer: 104. D. Rastelli operation

Answer: 105. C. Congenital heart surgery

Risk prediction in surgery for congenital heart diseases:

1. Aristotle Basic Complexity (ABC) score
2. Risk Adjustment for Congenital Heart Surgery (RACHS)

Answer: 106. D. Tricuspid atresia – Rev procedure

Answer: 107. A. Truncus arteriosus – Total cavopulmonary connection

Answer: 108. B. Truncus arteriosus-REV

Some important surgical procedures:

Single ventricle with PS with interrupted IVC: Kawashima surgery

TGA with VSD with PS: Rastelli, Lecompte, Rev, and Nikaidoh procedures

ALCAPA: Takeuchi repair

Answer: 109. C. RVH on ECG

DORV with restrictive VSD behaves like a subaortic stenosis and causes LVH.

Answer: 110. D. Sinus venosus ASD with PAPVC

Sinus venosus ASD with PAPVC behaves as left to right shunt lesion and cyanosis is not seen until patient develops eisenmengerization.

Answer: 111. B. TAPVC

Ductus dependent lesions:

Ductus dependent systemic circulation: Hypoplastic left heart syndrome, Critical Aortic stenosis, Coarctation of aorta, Interrupted aortic arch, Shone complex

Ductus dependent pulmonary circulation: TOF with pulmonary atresia, Pulmonary atresia with intact ventricular septum, Critical pulmonic stenosis, Single ventricle with pulmonary atresia, Severe Ebstein's anomaly, Complete TGA with intact ventricular septum.

Answer: 112. A. Double outlet right ventricle with pulmonary stenosis

Because of pulmonic stenosis, there is decreased pulmonary blood flow.

Answer: 113. D. Noonan's syndrome with sever PS due to dysplastic PV

Answer: 114. D. 50% valvular stenosis have dysplastic valves

Answer: 115. B. Aortic ejection click

Aortic ejection click is seen in valvular AS.

Answer: 116. A. Short PR interval

Short PR interval is seen in Ebstein when associated with pre-excitation.

Answer: 117. B. VSD with AR

12 Cardiac Hemodynamics and Interventional Cardiology

Right Heart Catheterization

1. **Normal mean pulmonary capillary wedge pressure is:**
   A. 2-4 mm Hg B. 4-12 mm Hg
   C. 12-18 mm Hg D. 18-24 mm Hg

2. **Higher value of oxygen saturation (out of the given choices) will be observed under normal conditions in:**
   A. Inferior vena cava
   B. Superior vena cava
   C. Coronary sinus
   D. Right atrium

3. **Which of the following is true regarding the 'v wave' in the right atrial pressure trace?**
   A. It occurs just after the tricuspid valve-opening
   B. It is due to filling of right atrium by blood returning from vena cavae and coronary sinus
   C. It occurs during the period of ventricular diastole
   D. It is of higher amplitude than left atrial v wave

4. **Gorlin formula for calculation of stenotic mitral valve area in cm2:**
   A. {[CO(liters/min) × 1000]/(44.3) (HR)(SEP)}
   B. {[CO(liters/min) × 1000]/(37.7) (HR) (DFP)}
   C. {[CO (liters/min) × 1000]/(44.3) (HR) (DFP)}
   D. {[CO (liters/min) × 1000]/(37.7) (HR) (SEP)}

5. **All are useful for computing mitral valve area by cardiac catheterization except:**
   A. Cardiac output
   B. Duration of cardiac cycle
   C. Systolic ejection period
   D. Mean valve gradient

6. **All of the following represent normal values except:**
   A. LV mass-76 gm/m2 in male
   B. PCWP-6-12 mm Hg
   C. PVR- 6-7 wood unit
   D. AV 02 difference : 40

7. **All of the following represent normal values except?**
   A. LVEDP – 18 mmHg
   B. Pulmonary vascular resistance – 70 dyne-sec.cm^{-5}
   C. Cardiac output – 4.9 L/min in females
   D. Mean pulmonary artery pressure – 15 mmHg

8. **Gorlin formula for MV include all except:**
   A. HR
   B. Mean gradient
   C. Systolic ejection period
   D. CO

9. Pulmonary blood flow can be calculated by:

A. VO_2/ pulmonary Venous O_2 saturation- pulmonary arterial O_2 saturation
B. VO_2/ pulmonary Venous O_2 saturation – IVC satuartion
C. VO_2/ pulmonary Venous O_2 saturation – aortic saturation
D. VO_2/ Aortic saturation – Mixec venous saturation

10. Pulmonary congestion with systemic hypoperfusion present with following values of PCWP and cardiac index:

A. PCWP > 18 mmHg and cardiac index > 2.2 L/min
B. PCWP > 18 mmHg and cardiac index < 2.2 L/min
C. PCWP < 18 mmHg and cardiac index > 2.2 L/min
D. PCWP < 18 mmHg and cardiac index < 2.2 L/min

11. On cardiac catheterization of a patient with mitral stenosis, the mean gradient between pulmonary capillary wedge pressure and left ventricular end-diastolic pressure was16 mmHg at a heart rate of 60 bpm. The cardiac output by the Fick method was 4.0 L/min. The calculated mitral valve area is approximately:

A. 0.5 cm2 B. 1.0 cm2
C. 1.5 cm2 D. 2.0 cm2

12. Pressure half time across a stenotic mitral valve is 250ms. What is the mitral valve area?

A. 0.46 cm2 B. 0.88 cm2
C. 1.26 cm2 D. 1.52 cm2

13. Pulmonary capillary wedge mean pressure is not equal to left ventricular end diastolic pressure in:

A. Mitral stenosis
B. Placement of catheter in non-dependent zone of the lung
C. Decreased ventricular compliance
D. All the above

14. The likely management of a 45-year-old female patient having the oximetry and hemodynamic data as shown below should be?

Chamber	O_2 Saturation	Pressure
SVC	65	
IVC	60	
RA	82	a 16, v 16, m 14
RV	80	60, ed 16
PA	80	60/24, m 36
PCW	98	a15, v16, m14
LA	98	a16, v16, m14
LV	98	100, ed 16
FA	98	100/68, m 77

A. Medical treatment with Sildenafil and Bosentan
B. Open heart surgery for ASD
C. Open heart surgery for ASD and mitral valvotomy
D. Open heart surgery for ASD and pulmonary valvotomy

15. Calculate the shunt fraction in left to right shunt with the following information:

SaO2 – 98%
MVO2 – 72%
PAO2 – 85%

A. 2 : 1 B. 3 : 2
C. 5 : 2 D. 3 : 1

16. Which of the following causes elevation of pulmonary capillary wedge pressure?

A. Ebstein's Anomaly
B. Atrial septal defect
C. Constrictive pericarditis
D. Severe tricuspid regurgitation with low cardiac output

17. Pulmonary capillary wedge pressure is lower than pulmonary artery diastolic pressure in all conditions stated below except:

A. Primary pulmonary arterial hypertension
B. Pulmonary artery embolism
C. Pulmonary vein stenosis
D. Tachycardia

Left Heart Catheterization

18. Mach effect in coronary angiography is suggestive of:
A. Lumen lucency due to eccentric lesions
B. Lumen lucency due to tortuosity
C. Lumen lucency due to thrombus
D. Lumen reduction due to passage of stiff wire

19. All of the following are true about myocardial bridging except:
A. Most common artery involved is LAD
B. Seen in 5-10% normal population
C. Seen in 40% of HCM population
D. Causes obligatory ischemia

20. Sellers grading is for:
A. Mitral regurgitation
B. Aortic regurgitation
C. Both of the above
D. None of the above

21. To assesses viability of myocardium following test is not useful:
A. PET imaging
B. MRI imaging
C. Dobutamine stress echo
D. Coronary angiography

22. Coronary Angiography was first done by:
A. Mason Sones B. Andre Cournand
C. Charles Dotter D. Seldinger

23. Type C coronary lesion:
A. Eccentric
B. Total occlusion > 3 months
C. Bifurcation lesion
D. Ostial lesion

24. Which is not a correct match for the characteristics of type A, B and C coronary lesions as per ACC/AHA classification?
A. Type B - Tubular
B. Type C - Ostial
C. Type A - Concentric
D. Type C - Total occlusion more than 3 months old

25. Myocardial bridges are most common in:
A. LAD B. RCA
C. Major OM D. Diagonal

26. "Milking effect" phenomenon on coronary angiography has been described in:
A. Critical left main stenosis
B. Myocardial bridge
C. Coronary aneurysm
D. Coronary arteriovenous fistula

27. Which one of following is not true in classification of TIMI flow grade?
A. TIMI grade 1 B. TIMI grade 2
C. TIMI grade 3 D. TIMI grade 4

28. The commonest benign congenital coronary anomaly is:
A. Left circumflex (LCx) coronary artery arising from right aortic sinus
B. Left main coronary artery (LMCA) arising from right aortic sinus
C. Single coronary artery
D. Right Coronary Artery (RCA) arising from left aortic sinus

29. Most common coronary artery anomaly seen on coronary angiography:
A. Left main arising from right sinus
B. RCA arising from left sinus
C. LAD arising from right sinus
D. LCX arising from right sinus

30. Coronary ischemia not caused by:
A. ALCAPA
B. Myocardial bridging

C. Abnormal RCA from left sinus
D. ALCAOS

Percutaneous Coronary Interventions

31. Which one of the following drug is not used in drug eluting stent?
A. Zotarolimus B. Cyclosporine
C. Sirolimus D. Paclitaxel

32. Rotational atherectomy is not done in:
A. Ostial lesions
B. Calcified lesions
C. Instent restenosis
D. Degenerated vein grafts

33. In the setting of primary percutaneous coronary intervention (Primary PCI), the benefit of drug eluting stent (DES) over bare metal stent (BMS) is:
A. Reduced stroke
B. Reduced death
C. Reduced target vessel revascularization
D. Reduced stent thrombosis

34. A 55 year old male underwent CT coronary angiography in view of a mildly positive treadmill test on routine health checkup. Anomalous left main coronary artery from noncoronary sinus coursing retro aortic between aorta and left atrium was reported. He should be advised:
A. No therapy
B. Restricted physical activity
C. Stenting of the retro aortic portion to prevent systolic compression
D. Surgical implantation of left main coronary artery to left coronary sinus

35. All of the following drugs are useful in coronary 'no flow' phenomenon except:
A. Nitroglycerine
B. Adenosine
C. Nicorandil
D. Sodium nitroprusside

36. What drug is commonly used in drug eluting balloon?
A. Sirolimus B. Zotarolimus
C. Paclitaxel D. Everolimus

37. Which of the following statements is true for intra-aortic balloon counterpulsation (IABP)?
A. Balloon is deflated at beginning of diastole
B. Balloon is positioned just distal to left common carotid artery
C. It augments subendocardial myocardial blood flow
D. Cannot be used in patients having permanent pacemaker implant

38. Which is FALSE about IABP?
A. Useful in cardiogenic shock in relation to acute MI
B. Useful in LV failure in relation to acute AR
C. IABP decreases afterload
D. Useful in hypotension in relation to left main artery disease

Coronary Artery Bypass Grafting

39. Patency rate of left internal mammary artery for LAD artery at 10-years is approximately?
A. 75% B. 86%
C. 90-95% D. 99%

40. Saphenous venous grafts patency rates seen post CABG on long term follow up of 10 years is:
A. 25% B. 35%
C. 50% D. 75%

41. Which of the following was evaluated in SYNTAX trial?
A. Role of ICD vs antiarrhythmics in post-myocardial infarction and left ventricular dysfunction

B. Role of CRT in heart failure
C. Role of renal denervation
D. Role of PCI vs CABG in coronary artery disease

Intravascular Diagnostics

42. On angiography of a patient, there was proximal LAD 60% disease, FFR came out to be 0.70. What should be the next step?
A. Stress thallium
B. Repeat with nicorandil
C. Repeat CAG+FFR after 6 months
D. Stent implantation

43. All of the following are true about FFR except:
A. Adenosine used in dose of 12 mg intravenous bolus during FFR estimation
B. Non-invasive FFR may be estimated during CT angiography
C. FFR may also be useful in estimation of lesion severity in tandem lesions
D. FFR values reduced following acute MI

44. The frequency of intravascular ultrasound catheter:
A. 2-5 MHz B. 7-10 MHz
C. 20-45 MHZ D. 10-15 MHz

45. What is the probe frequency used for IVUS?
A. 1-10 MHz B. 10-20 MHz
C. 20-40 MHz D. 40-60 MHz

46. Left main lumen area as measured by IVUS which correlates with significant stenosis is?
A. < 5 mm^2 B. < 6 mm^2
C. < 7 mm^2 D. < 8 mm^2

47. IVUS is indicated in all except:
A. Left main coronary artery disease
B. In-stent restenosis
C. Primary angioplasty
D. Transplant vasculopathy

48. Which of the following is true about fractional flow reserve (FFR)?
A. Specific index of epicardial coronary artery stenosis
B. Value < 0.9 indicate functionally significant stenosis
C. Dopamine infusion is used to induce hyperaemia
D. Lack reproducibility as it is dependent on BP and heart rate

49. All of the following true about OCT (optical coherence tomography) except:
A. Higher resolution but poor penetration compared to IVUS
B. Flowing blood cells interfere with vessel visualisation
C. Cannot differentiate between red and white thrombus
D. Visualisation of adventitia is suboptimal

50. All of the following are true about OCT except:
A. Has higher resolution but better penetration than IVUS
B. Needs RBC 's devoid field
C. Cannot differentiate between red and white thrombi
D. Adventitial visualization is suboptimal

51. Most common complication of intracoronary use of IVUS during catheterization:
A. Coronary dissection
B. Coronary perforation
C. Coronary vasospasm
D. Coronary thrombosis

52. OCT is better than IVUS to detect lesions of:
A. Intima
B. Media
C. External elastic membrane
D. Adventitia

53. It is reasonable to use IVUS for which of the following coronary intervention procedure?
A. Assessment of angiographically indeterminant left main CAD
B. One year after cardiac transplantation to exclude donor CAD
C. Determine the mechanism of stent restenosis
D. All the above

54. Which of the following is true regarding Intravascular ultrasound (IVUS) and Optical coherence tomography (OCT) imaging of coronary arteries?
A. IVUS has better axial resolution than OCT
B. IVUS detects thrombus better than OCT
C. IVUS is better for detection of far-field signals than OCT
D. IVUS detects vulnerable plaque better than OCT

55. All of the following are true about OCT except;
A. Higher resolution and poorer penetration
B. Differentiate between red and white thrombus
C. Adventitia can be imaged
D. Lipid and calcification is better seen

56. The following coronary imaging modalities conveys the histological tissue characteristics, except:
A. Optical coherence tomography
B. Near-infrared spectroscopy
C. Virtual histology intravascular ultrasound
D. Magnetic resonance imaging

Complications

57. Osmolality of Iodixanol (mosm/kg):
A. 590 B. 490
C. 290 D. 190

58. All of the following are features of cholesterol embolization following cardiac catheterization except?
A. Eosinophilia
B. Renal dysfunction
C. Livedo reticularis of lower limb
D. Absent popliteal artery pulsation

59. Which of the following is incorrect regarding prevention of contrast induced nephropathy?
A. Preprocedure hydration with 0.9% NaCl is better than 0.45% NaCl
B. Low osmolar contrast media is better than iso-osmolar contrast media
C. Preprocedure use of N-acetyl cysteine is not recommended
D. Biplane angiography is useful in reducing the dose of contrast

60. Cardiac chamber air embolises most commonly to which coronary artery:
A. LAD B. LCx
C. RCA D. Ramus

Miscellaneous

61. All of the following are true about coronary AV fistula except?
A. Most commonly involved artery is RCA
B. May lead to myocardial steal
C. CXR shows massive cardiomegaly
D. Coil embolization may be done

62. True match:
A. First ECG – Kouwenhoven
B. First cardiac catheterization – Grube
C. First cardiac angiogram – Sones
D. First percutaneous pulmonary valve replacement – Cribier

63. True all except:
A. Coronary angiography- Sones
B. First cardiac catheterization- Forssmann

C. ICD-Kriklin
D. Coronary Stent- Puel and Sigwart

64. Coronary angiogram in human first done by:
A. Mason Sones B. Werner Forrsmann
C. Charles Dotter D. William Cournand

65. Which of the following is wrongly matched pair?
A. Cardiac MRI – LV function
B. CT - Pericardial calcification
C. Post cardiac transplant atherosclerosis - Fractional flow reserve
D. Echocardiography - Fetal tachycardia

66. Which of the following is wrongly matched?
A. First cardiac catheterisation – Forsmann
B. First coronary angiography – Sones
C. First coronary stent – Gruentzig
D. First ICD – Michel Mirowski

67. Left ventricular pressure tracing differs from right ventricle by shorter duration of:
A. Isovolumetric contraction
B. Ejection period
C. Systole
D. Isovolumetric relaxation

68. Aortic pulse wave velocity is used in estimating:
A. Endothelial dysfunction
B. Arterial stiffness
C. Severity of aortic regurgitation
D. Allograft vasculopathy

ANSWERS

RIGHT HEART CATHETERIZATION:

Answer: 1. B. 4-12 mm Hg

Answer: 2. A. Inferior vena cava. Coronary sinus has the lowest saturation.

Answer: 3. B. It is due to filling of right atrium by blood returning from vena cavae and coronary sinus

Answer: 4. B. {[CO (liters/min) × 1000]/(37.7)(HR)(DFP)}

Answer: 5. C. Systolic ejection period

→ Diastolic filling period is used

Answer: 6. C. PVR-6-7 wood unit

→ Normal PVR: 0.25 to 2 wood units

Answer: 7. LVEDP – 18 mmHg

→ Normal LVEDP: 4 to 12 mmHg

Answer: 8. C. Systolic ejection period

Answer: 9. A.VO2/ pulmonary Venous 02 saturation- pulmonary arterial 02 saturation

Answer: 10. B. PCWP > 18 mmHg and cardiac index < 2.2 L/min

Answer: 11. B. 1.0 cm2

→ Use Hakki's formula

Answer: 12. B. 0.88 cm2

Answer: 13. D. All the above

Answer: 14. B. Open heart surgery for ASD

Answer: 15. A. 2 : 1

Qp/Qs= (SaO2-MVO2)/(PVO2-PAO2)=(98-72)/(98-85) = 26/13 = 2/1

Take Pulmonary venous saturation as systemic saturation.

Answer: 16. C. Constrictive pericarditis

Answer: 17. C. Pulmonary vein stenosis

Atrial pressure:

Three waves

– (a) atrial systole

– (c) closing of AV valve

– (v) RV systole

Two descents

– (x) atrial relaxation with open AV valve

– (x') continued atrial relaxation with closed AV valve

– (y) tricuspid valve opening

Cardiac output measurement:

Cardiac output = Stroke volume × heart rate

Cardiac index = Cardiac output / Body surface area

Normal stroke volume = 35-65 ml/ m_2

Normal Cardiac Output: 4 to 8 L/min

Normal Cardiac Index: between 2.5 and 4.2 L/min/m²

Thermodilution method

Tends to underestimate CO with aortic regurgitation (AR), mitral regurgitation (MR) or tricuspid regurgitation (TR)

Inaccurate in low CO state (CO <2.5 L/min), shunt or irregular rhythm

Fick Method

CO (L/m) = O_2 consumption (ml/min) / A-V O_2 difference × 1.36 × Hb × 10

Fick's method is **not** affected by TR or low output state.

Should not be used with severe MR or AR and high cardiac output states.

Angiographic Method

CO = (end-diastolic volume – end-systolic volume) x heart rate

Shunts:

By measuring saturations at various levels

Left to right shunts: Step up of oxygen in right sided chambers

Right to left shunts: Step down of oxygen in left sided chambers

Shunt fraction (Qp/Qs) calculation

Pulmonary blood flow (Qp) = O_2 consumption / (PV saturation – PA saturation)

Systemic blood flow (Qs) = O_2 consumption / (Systemic artery saturation – Mixed venous saturation)

Qp/Qs= (SAO_2-MVO_2) / (PVO2-PAO_2)

Mixed venous saturation (MVO2) is calculated by **Flamm's formula:**

MVO2= [3(SVC O_2) + (IVC O_2)] / 4

Identification of intracardiac shunts:

Level of shunt	Difference in O_2 saturation	Differential diagnosis
Atrial (SVC/IVC to RA)	>7%	ASD, PAPVC, RSOV, VSD with TR, Coronary to RA fistula
Ventricular (RA to RV)	>5%	VSD, PDA with PR, Primum ASD, Coronary to RV fistula
Great vessel (RV to PA)	>5%	PDA, AP window, Aberrancy coronary a rtery origin
Any level (SVC to PA)	>7%	Any of the above

Vascular resistance:

Systemic vascular resistance (Woods) = (Mean arterial pressure – RA pressure)/ Cardiac output

Pulmonary vascular resistance (Woods) = (Mean PA pressure – PCWP)/Cardiac output

Pulmonary vascular resistance index (PVRI) = (MAP – RA pressure)/ Cardiac index

= PVR × Body surface area

→ 1 Wood = 80 dyn × s/cm^5

RHC NORMAL VALUES

Measure	Pressures (Normal range)
Right atrium	1-6 mmHg
Right ventricle	15-25/ 1-8 mmHg
Pulmonary artery	15-25/4-12 mmHg

PCWP	4-12 mmHg
Left atrium	2-12 mmHg
Left ventricle	100-140/4-12 mmHg
Aorta	100-140/70-90 mmHg
Cardiac output	4-6 L/min
Cardiac index	2.4-4 L/min/m2
Systemic vascular resistance	700-1600 dyn.s/cm^5 (8 – 20 wood units)
Pulmonary vascular resistance	20-130 dyn.s/cm^5 (0.25 – 2 wood units)

Pulmonary capillary wedge pressure:

It is measured by wedging a pulmonary catheter with an inflated balloon into a small pulmonary arterial branch. It estimates the left atrial pressure.

Normal PCWP: 4-12 mmHg

Elevated PCWP is seen in LV failure, Mitral stenosis.

Operability criteria on catheterization in left to right acyanotic congenital heart diseases:

1. Pulmonary vascular resistance index (PVRI) < 6 WU × m^2
2. PVR/SVR < 0.3

Calculation of Stenotic Valve Area (Gorlin Formula):

Based on relationship between flow velocity, pressure gradient and area of stenotic valve

– AV area (AVA) calculated based on flow during systole only (systolic ejection period)

– Mitral valve area (MVA) is calculated based on flow during diastole (diastolic flow period).

AVA= (CO × 1000)/(44.3 × HR × SEP × √Mean systolic gradient)

MVA= (CO × 1000)/(37.7 × HR × DFP × √Mean diastolic gradient)

Simplified Hakki formula:

AVA or MVA= CO/ √Mean pressure gradient across valve

LEFT HEART CATHETERIZATION

Answer: 18. B. Lumen lucency due to tortuosity

Answer: 19. D. Causes obligatory ischemia

Answer: 20. C. Both of the above

Answer: 21. D. Coronary angiography

Answer: 22. A. Mason Sones

Answer: 23. B. Total occlusion >3 months

Answer: 24. B. Type C – Ostial

Answer: 25. A. LAD

Answer: 26. B. Myocardial bridge

Answer: 27. D. TIMI grade 4

Answer: 28. A. Left circumflex (LCx) coronary artery arising from right aortic sinus

Answer: 29. D. LCX arising from right sinus

Answer: 30. C. Abnormal RCA from left sinus

Percutaneous coronary interventions

Answer: 31. B. Cyclosporine

Answer: 32. D. Degenerated vein grafts

Answer: 33. C. Reduced target vessel revascularization

Answer: 34. A. No therapy

Answer: 35. A. Nitroglycerine

Answer: 36. C. Paclitaxel

Answer: 37. C. It augments subendocardial myocardial blood flow

→ Balloon is placed just distal to left subclavian artery (not left common carotid artery).

Answer: 38. B. Useful in LV failure in relation to acute AR

Left ventriculography:

Left ventriculography: Done for LV function, RWMA assessment, to detect presence of VSD or LV aneurysm, to quantify valvular regurgitation.

RAO view: Anterior, anterolateral, apical and inferior/posterior walls

LAO view: Anterior, lateral, inferior and septal walls.

Left ventriculogram contraindicated when LVEDP >25 mmHg or critical LM coronary artery disease

Assessment of valvular regurgitation (AR and MR):

Sellar's grading:

Grade 1: Partial filling of proximal chamber,

Grade 2: Complete filling of proximal chamber but less dense than distal chamber,

Grade 3: Equal opacification of proximal chamber in 4–5 beats,

Grade 4: Equal opacification of proximal chamber in ≤3 beats.

CORONARY ANGIOGRAPHY

Normal Coronary Anatomy

LMCA arises above the left aortic sinus and the **right coronary artery (RCA)** above the right coronary sinus. Best viewed in antero-posterior (AP) projection.

LMCA courses divides in to left anterior descending (LAD) and left circumflex (LCx) (30 % of population have a ramus intermedius branch).

Ramus courses similarly to diagonal or obtuse marginal artery.

LAD gives rise to 1–3 diagonal arteries (supplying anterior wall, anterolateral papillary muscle, and anterior RV wall) and septal arteries (supplying apical and anterior two-thirds of septum). Best viewed with cranially angulated projections.

LCx gives rise to 1–3 obtuse marginal arteries supplying the lateral wall. Best viewed with caudally angulated projections.

RCA gives rise to conus branch, marginal arteries (supply RV free wall), posterior descending artery (PDA) (supply posterior third of septum), and posterolateral branches (PLB) (supply inferior wall).

Sinoatrial artery arises from RCA in 60 % of patients.

Dominance determined by the artery supplying the PDA. Eighty- five percent are right dominant.

Dampening of pressure wave form or **ventricularization** of waveform (decrease in diastolic pressure) due to occlusion of coronary artery, clot in catheter or catheter embedded in arterial well, selective engagement of conus artery when searching for RCA, coronary spasm.

Mach effect:

Lucency is caused by severe eccentric coronary stenotic lesion. However, sometimes similar lucency may appear at normal segment near the area of darker contrast through a perceptual artefact known as Mach effect. It is caused by tortuosity or overlapping of vessels in the absence of true abnormality at the site.

Concertina effect:

Transient angiographic appearance of stenosis during percutaneous coronary intervention in a tortuous vessel induced by a stiff guide wire.

These pseudolesions disappear when stiff guide wire is removed.

Also known as **Accordion effect.**

Syndrome X:

Angina with signs associated with decreased blood flow to heart tissue but with normal epicardial coronary arteries on angiography.

The frequency of angiographically normal coronary arteries in patients with angina is approximately 10% to 30%.

Mechanisms: Microvascular coronary disease, endothelial dysfunction and enhanced pain perception.

MINOCA:

Myocardial infarction with non-obstructive coronary arteries.

Clinically defined by the presence of the universal acute myocardial infarction (AMI) criteria, absence of obstructive coronary artery disease (≥50% stenosis), and no overt cause for the clinical presentation at the time of angiography (e.g., takotsubo cardiomyopathy).

Incidence: Around 6% of Acute MI patients, More common in women.

Poorer prognosis than general population; 12 months all-cause mortality: 4.7%.

TIMI criteria for coronary blood flow assessment on angiography:

TIMI flow grade	Feature
0	Absence of any antegrade flow beyond a coronary occlusion
1	Faint antegrade coronary flow beyond the occlusion, although filling of the distal coronary bed is incomplete
2	Delayed or sluggish antegrade flow with complete filling of the distal territory
3	Normal flow that fills the distal coronary bed completely

Collateral Circulation:

Rentrop classification

– 0 = no filling

– 1 = side branch filled

– 2 = partial filling occluded artery

– 3 = complete filling of occluded artery.

Assessment of Coronary Lesions:

Type A: Discrete (<10 mm), concentric, non-angulated segment, smooth contour, minimal calcium, non-ostial, no thrombus, no significant side branch involvement.

Type B: Tubular (<20 mm), eccentric, moderate angulation (45–90°), irregular, calcified, ostial, bifurcation, thrombus present, total occlusion <3 months.

Type C: Diffuse (> 20 mm), angulated >90°, bifurcation but unable to protect side branch, total occlusion >3 months, degenerated SVG.

Anomalous Coronary Arteries:

Occur in up to 5 % of population.

Majority are discovered incidentally and are of no clinical significance.

Coronary artery anomalies are the second most common cause of SCD among young athletes, first being HCM.

Absence of ischemia	Most anomalies (split RCA, ectopic RCA from right cusp; ectopic RCA from left cusp)
Episodic ischemia	Anomalous origin of a coronary artery from the opposite sinus (ACAOS); coronary artery fistulas; myocardial bridge
Typical ischemia	Anomalous left coronary artery from the pulmonary artery (ALCAPA); coronary ostial atresia or severe stenosis

Anomalous Origin of Coronary Artery:

The LCA arising from the right aortic sinus may follow one of these four courses: prepulmonic, retroaortic, interarterial, or transseptal.

The **interarterial course** of an anomalous LCA from the right sinus is associated with SCD during or shortly after exercise in young individuals.

Similarly, origin of the RCA from the left aortic sinus with an interarterial course is associated with myocardial ischemia and SCD.

Once this anomaly is diagnosed, CABG is recommended.

Most common anomalies:

1st: Separate origins of LAD and LCx

2nd: LCx from Right sinus

Myocardial bridges:

A myocardial bridge is a segment of a coronary artery that travels **into the myocardium** instead of the normal epicardial course.

An estimated prevalence of approximately **25%** in autopsy series.

Most common in middle segment of **LAD artery**.

Considered as **benign "normal variants"** however sometimes may be associated with ischemic symptoms.

In coronary angiography, it produces **"milking effect"** i.e. the vessel is filled in diastole whereas it is squeezed in systole due to myocardial contraction.

Treatment involves **myotomy or coronary artery bypass grafting** if symptoms are recalcitrant to medical therapy.

Stenting is contraindicated as there is high risk of stent fracture and restenosis in the intramyocardial segment of coronary artery.

Percutaneous coronary intervention (PCI)

BMS vs DES

	Advantages	**Disadvantages**
Balloon angioplasty	Dilates stenotic segment	Elastic recoil of artery High early restenosis
Bare metal stent	Less elastic recoil due to stent manifold Lower early restenosis	Metal scars endothelial tissue Leads to neointimal growth response Contributes to late restenosis
Drug eluting stent	Antiproliferative drug mitigates adverse response to metal → reduces in-stent restenosis by reducing neointimal proliferation and reduced need for target vessel revascularization.	Incomplete healing and delayed endothelization Increased risk of stent thrombosis

Drug eluting stents:

1st generation: Sirolimus eluting stents, Paclitaxel eluting stents

2nd generation: Zotarolimus and Everolimus eluting stents

3rd generation: Biodegradable stents or bioresorbable vascular scaffolds

Bioresorbable vascular scaffolds (BVS):

Mainly useful for the restoration of functional endothelial coverage, enables prevention of acute recoil or occlusion, provide inhibition of in segment restenosis through efficient drug elusion and no foreign material left behind.

Disadvantage:

Increased risk of stent thrombosis

Higher target lesion revascularization rates compared with Drug Eluting Stents (DES).

Eluting drug: Everolimus (most common), Sirolimus, Paclitaxel

Composition:

Currently there are four materials used in BVS

Lactide polymers particularly Poly-L-lactic acid (PLLA) form the basis of most devices

other materials include magnesium poly anhydrates (salicylic acid and adipic acid) and amino acids.

→ The most frequently used polymer in the current generation of BVS is **PLLA.**

Drug eluting balloons (DEB):

Conventional semi-compliant angioplasty balloons are covered with an anti-proliferative drug which is released into the vessel during inflation of the balloon.

DEBs are used and evaluated in **re-stenotic lesions** where previously stented segments have developed neointimal hyperplasia and luminal obstruction.

Also being evaluated in **peripheral arterial diseases** where stents have not been much useful.

Advantage: This local drug delivery method does not require foreign material implantation.

Drugs used in DEB: Paclitaxel (Most common), Preclinical status: Everolimus, zotarolimus and sirolimus.

No- flow phenomenon:

Less than TIMI 3 flow in a coronary artery after PCI in the absence of dissection, spasm, stenosis or thrombus of epicardial vessel.

Four pathologic components:

1. Distal atherothrombotic embolization
2. Ischemic injury
3. Reperfusion injury
4. Individual susceptibility of coronary microcirculation to injury

→ Drugs used for treatment of No-reflow phenomenon:

- Adenosine
- Sodium nitroprusside
- Nicorandil
- Verapamil
- Adrenaline

Stent thrombosis:

Mechanisms and causes:

1. Endothelial denudation
2. Medial dissection
3. Exposure of sub-intimal components
4. Thrombogenicity of metal

Increased rates of late stent thrombosis with drug eluting stents as compared to bare metal stents because endothelization is delayed with DES.

Appropriate dual antiplatelet therapy is must to prevent stent thrombosis. Period of DAPT is longer with DES.

Presentation: As STEMI or ACS

Types: 4 types according to the duration from stent implantation

Acute: <24 hours

Subacute: 24 hours to 30 days

Late: 30 days to 1 year

Very late: >1 year

In-stent restenosis:

Stent restenosis is secondary to tissue ingrowth (neointimal hyperplasia) within the stent.

Mechanism: Reaction to stent struts → Production of cytokines, mitogens, chemotaxic factors by macrophages → Activation of vascular smooth muscle cells → Proliferation and migration of vascular smooth muscle cells → Restenosis.

Drug eluting stent decrease neointimal hyperplasia and hence in stent restenosis as compared to bare metal stents.

Presentation: Chronic stable angina

Types:

I: Focal (≤10 mm)

II: Diffuse intrastent (>10 mm)

III: Diffuse proliferative (>10 mm, exceeding the boundaries of the stent)

IV: Total in-stent occlusion

Management:

Focal: Balloon angioplasty or short DES

Diffuse: DES placement (Treatment of choice), Brachytherapy, Drug eluting balloon (DEB)

Rotational atherectomy:

Atherectomy device removes atheromatous plaque by abrasion of the inelastic calcified plaque.

Microscopic (20 to 50 μm) **diamond chips** embedded on the surface of a rapidly rotating (160,000 rpm) olive-shaped **atherectomy burr**.

Generates 2- to 5-μm microparticles that pass through the coronary microcirculation for removal by the reticuloendothelial system.

Burr diameters range from 1.25 to 2.50 mm (0.25 mm increments).

Once adequate lumen in created, further balloon dilation and stent placement is performed.

Principle: Differential cutting

Normal vascular tissue has elastic properties that allow it to deflect away from advancing diamonds on the rotating burr.

It selectively ablates inelastic tissue (i.e. plaque) which is composed of calcium and fibrotic tissue.

Indications:

Used for **ostial and heavily calcified lesions** that cannot be dilated with balloon angioplasty or those that prevent the delivery of coronary stents.

Calcified and undilatable lesions

In-stent restenosis

Ostial lesions

Chronic total occlusions

Contraindications:

Thrombotic lesions (Usually in the setting of STEMI and ACS)

Saphenous venous grafts (Usually have high thrombotic burden)

Dissection in the lesion

Heavily tortuous vessel

Intra-Aortic Balloon Pump (IABP)

IABP consists of a balloon catheter which is positioned distal to left subclavian artery and a pump console to control the timing of balloon inflation and deflation.

Helium is used because its low viscosity facilitates rapid transfer in and out of the balloon, and because it absorbs very rapidly in blood if the balloon ruptures.

The balloon inflates with the **onset of diastole**, which roughly corresponds with electrophysiologic repolarization or the middle of the T wave on the surface ECG, or just after the dicrotic notch on the aortic pressure tracing.

Following diastole, the balloon rapidly deflates at the **onset of LV systole**, which is timed electrocardiographically to the peak of the R wave on the surface ECG.

The IABP increases diastolic blood pressure, decreases afterload, decreases myocardial oxygen consumption, increases coronary artery perfusion, and modestly enhances cardiac output.

SHOCK II trial: Compared IABP therapy with best available medical therapy for treatment of AMI complicated by cardiogenic shock

The use of IABP counter pulsation did not significantly reduce 30-day mortality in patients with AMI complicated by cardiogenic shock for whom an early revascularization strategy was planned

Contraindications of IABP:

Aortic regurgitation

Severe peripheral vascular disease

Aortic dissection

Aortic aneurysm

Severe sepsis

Severe coagulopathy

Coronary artery bypass grafting (CABG)

Answer: 39. C. 90-95%

Answer: 40. C. 50%

Answer: 41. D. Role of PCI vs CABG in coronary artery disease

CABG:

In 1964, Garrett, Dennis, and DeBakey first used CABG as a "bailout" procedure

Use of an internal mammary artery (IMA) graft was pioneered by Kolessov in 1967

Grafts:

Arterial grafts are better and more durable than veins

Arterial grafts:

1. Internal mammary artery (Internal thoracic artery)- Most common bypass graft.

   It is left intact at its origin; and distal end is cut and sewn to the coronary artery below the site of the blockage.

   It has best long-term results

   LIMA to left anterior descending artery (LAD) gives best results as compared to other graft.

Use of both ITAs as bypass grafts is more complex and is not appropriate for some patients specially in diabetics and obese patients as this can make wound healing more difficult due to reduced blood flow to the sternum.

2. Radial artery:

   Radial artery is a muscular artery, hence higher tendency for spasm.

   Patients usually kept on calcium channel blockers post bypass.

   Before radial artery is used, Allen's test performed to check the integrity of palmer arch and patency of ulnar artery.

3. Gastroepiploic artery

4. Inferior epigastric artery

Venous grafts:

Saphenous veins:

Long term results poorer than arterial grafts

Reasons for elevated failure rates include variable quality and size of the veins, the presence of valves within the veins and the potential for areas of dilatation (varicosities) within the veins. These and other factors can lead to flow pattern disturbances within the veins that can lead to early failure. The 10-year patency of vein grafts is approximately 60 percent,

Graft patency rates:

	LIMA	**SVG**
1 year	98%	87%
5 years	98%	78%
10 years	95%	60%
15 years	>90%	46%
20 years	>90%	35%

Techniques for CABG:

1. On-pump CABG:

Conventional technique

Arrested heart with cardioplegia and using cardiopulmonary bypass.

2. Off-pump CABG (OPCAB):

With a beating heart and without the use of cardiopulmonary bypass.

Epicardial stabilizers used to stabilize beating heart during surgery. E.g.: Octopus.

Advantages of OPCAB:

Low morbidity with faster recovery and reduced procedural cost.

Less strokes at 30 days, Less post-operative AF and respiratory failure.

Less procedure time and ventilation time.

Advantages of On-pump CABG:

Less graft occlusion at 30 days and 1 year

Less mortality beyond 1 year

Less need for coronary intervention at 1 year

ROOBY trial:

In comparison with on-pump revascularization, off-pump coronary artery bypass (CABG) led to lower 5-year survival (84.8% vs 88.1%; P = .02)

Bypass graft patency is inferior compared with on-pump CABG.

Usual grafted vessels include:

Anterior wall: LAD

Inferior wall: RCA, PDA

Lateral wall: Obtuse marginal

Important points:

Bilateral IMA grafts: Higher rate of postoperative complications, including bleeding, wound infection, and prolonged ventilatory support.

Early occlusion (before hospital discharge) occurs in 8% to 12% of venous grafts, and by 1 year, 15% to 30% have become occluded. After the first year the annual occlusion rate is 2% and rises to approximately 4% annually between years 6 and 10. Patency rates with IMA grafts are superior.

Arterial grafts are more susceptible to failure because of competitive flow from native blood vessels than saphenous vein grafts (SVGs); thus, arterial grafts should not be used to revascularize borderline stenoses without clear evidence of flow limitation.

Operative mortality: 2%

Other complications: 1.3% for stroke, 2.0% for renal failure, 0.3% for mediastinitis, and 23.4% for AF, 3% for Perioperative MI

Post-operative AF:

AF occurs in up to 40% of patients, primarily within 2 to 3 days.

Up to 80% of patients spontaneously revert to sinus rhythm within 24 hours without treatment other than agents used for controlling the ventricular rate

AF causes twofold to threefold increase in postoperative stroke.

Older age, hypertension, previous AF, and HF are associated with a higher risk for AF after cardiac surgery.

Statin therapy and off-pump techniques may be associated with less frequent postoperative AF.

Prophylactic use of beta-blocking agents reduces the frequency of postoperative AF.

Amiodarone is also effective in prophylaxis against postoperative AF and may be considered in patients at high risk for its development

INTRAVASCULAR DIAGNOSTICS

Answer: 42. D. Stent implantation

Answer: 43. Adenosine used in dose of 12 mg intravenous bolus during FFR estimation

Answer: 44. C. 20-45 MHZ

Answer: 45. C. 20-40 MHz

Answer: 46. B. < 6 mm2

Answer: 47. C. Primary angioplasty

Answer: 48. A. Specific index of epicardial coronary artery stenosis

Answer: 49. C. Cannot differentiate between red and white thrombus

Answer: 50. C. Cannot differentiate between red and white thrombi

Answer: 51. C. Coronary vasospasm

Answer: 52. A. Intima

Answer: 53. D. All the above

Answer: 54. C. IVUS is better for detection of far-field signals than OCT

Answer: 55. C. Adventitia can be imaged

Answer: 56. D. Magnetic resonance imaging

Functional assessment of coronary artery disease

Coronary Flow Reserve (CFR):

CFR is defined as the ratio of the maximally augmented coronary flow velocity to the resting flow velocity.

Limitations:

1. Influenced by changes in resting myocardial flow, as occurs with post-PCI reactive hyperemia and changes in heart rate, preload, and contractility.
2. Abnormal in case of microvascular dysfunction, which is present in patients with coronary atherosclerosis.

To address this limitation, relative CFR can be measured but with additional measurements and instrumentation of a normal vessel. Relative CFR is the ratio of the CFR in the culprit vessel divided by the CFR in a normal reference vessel.

A ratio of 0.65 or less is indicative of a physiologically significant epicardial stenosis.

Fractional flow reserve (FFR):

→ Myocardial FFR is defined as the ratio of the hyperemic flow in a diseased target artery to the hyperemic flow in the same target artery if no lesion is present.

→ In normal coronary arteries, the distal pressure equals the aortic pressure during hyperemia and the myocardial FFR equals 1.

→ Values of 0.80 or less indicate physiologically significant lesions and are predictive of abnormal findings on non-invasive function tests.

Method:

Pressure gradient measured across lesion using a 0.014-in. angioplasty guidewire equipped with pressure sensor.

Pressure gradient is measured after coronary vasodilation by administration of adenosine for fractional flow reserve (FFR).

Coronary hyperemia can be achieved by **intracoronary or intravenous adenosine.**

FFR = Distal coronary artery pressure (Pd)/ Central aortic pressure (Pa)

The normal value of FFR is 1 for every coronary artery regardless of size.

FFR recordings ≤0.80 correlate with ischemia and warrant intervention.

Advantages:

Myocardial FFR is much less dependent on microcirculatory function and it does not vary appreciably with changing heart rate, blood pressure, or contractility.

Indications for Intracoronary Pressure Measurements

1. Indeterminate Coronary Stenoses

Determines the physiological significance of coronary artery stenotic lesion

Stenoses of intermediate severity (40%–70% diameter stenoses) myocardial FFR cut-off value of 0.80 or less may be used to identify lesions (left main and other locations) that merit revascularization.

For patients with multivessel disease, the FAME trial demonstrated that angiography plus a myocardial FFR-guided (≤0.80) strategy for lesion selection during PCI leads to superior outcomes compared with a strategy based on angiography alone

2. Coronary Interventions

After PTCA, patients with a low myocardial FFR (0.75–0.90) and adequate angiographic results (<30% residual stenosis by quantitative coronary angiography) have an increased rate of restenosis compared with patients with higher myocardial FFR values (>0.90).

In the absence of serial lesions or diffuse disease, optimal stent deployment should result in a myocardial FFR greater than 0.90

Uses of FFR:

1. Intermediate severity of lesion in coronary artery (50 to 70% disease)
2. Multivessel PCI
3. Left main disease
4. Ostial and side branch stenosis
5. Postprocedural measurement of FFR

Instantaneous Wave-Free Ratio (iFR):

iFR is a new physiologic index for assessment of the hemodynamic **severity of a coronary stenosis**.

It **does not** require vasodilators, so safer than measurement of FFR which requires coronary vasodilation with adenosine.

Measurement of iFR is based on a specific period in diastole called the wave-free period, during which resistance at rest is stable.

This resting state occurs spontaneously in each cardiac cycle during **diastole**.

It is calculated as the mean pressure distal to the stenotic segment divided by the mean aortic pressure during the diastolic wave-free period.

Best iFR cut-off for hemodynamically significant disease in coronary artery seems to be **less than 0.90**.

Intravascular Ultrasound (IVUS):

High ultrasound frequencies (20 to 40 MHz) are used which result in higher resolution (150 μm).

But resolution is less than OCT (10-15 μm).

Provides cross-sectional image of vessel lumen and wall.

Minimal luminal area by IVUS: **LM > 6 to 7.5 mm^2 and for other native vessels > 3 to 4 mm^2.**

Most common complication: Coronary vasospasm (1 to 3%).

Indications:

- Assess lesion severity when unclear by angiography
- Ostial LMCA disease (significant if minimum lumen area <6.0 mm2)
- Bifurcation lesion
- Borderline lesions
- Measure plaque burden and characterize plaque content
- Guide PCI
- Determine stent size and extent of stent expansion.
- Re-evaluate stent in patients with in-stent thrombosis or restenosis.
- Evaluation of transplant vasculopathy (IVUS is gold standard for detection of silent vasculopathy at present)

Optical Coherence Tomography (OCT):

- Analogous to IVUS, OCT uses backscattered infrared light ("optical echoes").
- It is similar in principle to IVUS but uses light rather than acoustic waves.
- Unlike IVUS, requires blood free vessel (flushed with contrast or saline or ringer's lactate continuously) during image acquisition.
- Significantly higher resolution (~10-15 μm) than IVUS (150 μm) but with less tissue penetration, allowing for detailed visualization of superficial coronary plaque morphology; can differentiate between red and white thrombus.

- Due to lesser penetration, adventitia is poorly imaged.
- Experimental use to identify presence of vulnerable plaques with thin fibrous caps
- Indications (similar to IVUS): assess severity of lesion if unclear by angiography, guide PCI, evaluate etiology of post-PCI complications.

Complications of catheterization:

Answer: 57. C. 290

Answer: 58. D. Absent popliteal artery pulsation

Answer: 59. B. Low osmolar contrast media is better than iso-osmolar contrast media

Answer: 60. C. RCA

Radiation side effects:

Stochastic effects:

1. These effects occur by chance and are not dependent on the radiation dose.
2. No lower threshold of radiation dose where it is certain that an adverse effect cannot occur.

E.g.: Cancer, genetic defects

Deterministic effects:

Effects are directly related to dose of radiation received.

There is a clear relationship between radiation dose and effect.

E.g.: Skin burns, hair loss, cataract, sterility, gastrointestinal ulcers, bone marrow suppression.

Contrast side effects:

Iodinated contrast agents are used which are divided based on osmolality (high, low, isosmolar)

Class	Trade name	Generic name	Osmolality
Ionic			
High osmolar	Angiovist	Sodium diatrizoate	2076
Low osmolar	Hexabrix	Ioxaglate	600
Nonionic			
Low osmolar	Omnipaque	Iohexol	844
Isosmolar	Visipaque	Iodixanol	290

The majority of contrast agents used in current practice are non-ionic low osmolar or isosmolar because high-osmolar agents have been found to have more hypotension, myocardial depression, heart failure, and electrical abnormalities.

Allergic reaction to contrast

Result in skin reactions (itch, rash) or anaphylaxis. Prevalence: 1%.

Prior history of contrast induced nephropathy- Give steroid and antihistaminic prophylactically.

Contrast induced nephropathy (CIN)

Transient increase in creatinine by 0.5 mg/dl or 25% increase from baseline.

Occurs in **<2%** of patients following cardiac angiography.

It is non-oliguric, peak within 1 to 2 days and then return to baseline by 7 days but may rarely require chronic dialysis.

Risk factors:

DM

Pre-existing renal dysfunction

Multiple myeloma

Volume depletion

Other nephrotoxic drug therapy

The recommended maximum dose of contrast to limit CIN is **3 ml/kg (or 5 ml/kg divided by S. creatinine in patients with elevated baseline creatinine).**

Strategies to minimize risk of CIN-

Smaller catheter is associated with lower amount of contrast per case.

Use of biplane angiography helps in minimizing the amount of contrast used for angiography.

Hydration protocol:

Isotonic saline 0.9%) is better than 0.45% saline.

0.9% NS 1 ml/kg/h starting 12 h before the procedure and continued for 12 h after the procedure.

2 ml/kg bolus infusion of NS 1 h before contrast administration, followed by an infusion of 1.5 ml/kg/h during the procedure and for 4 h thereafter.

Safety of contrast media used:

Iso-osmolar (Visipaque) > Low osmolar (Omnipaque) > High osmolar

The use Soda bicarbonate and NAC is not recommended.

Preprocedure statin use has been found to be associated with lower incidence of CIN and other complications of PCI.

Air embolism: Rare.

Most common artery involved: Right coronary artery.

Complications following cardiac catheterization

Local vascular complications	Hematoma	Most common complication
	Retroperitoneal bleeding	0.2%
	Pseudoaneurysm	
	Arteriovenous fistula	
	Thrombosis and embolism	

Other major complications	Death	0.05%
	Myocardial infarction	0.1%
	Stroke	0.05 to 1% Diagnostic0.18 to 0.4% Intervention
	Dissection and perforation of great vessel	
	Athero-embolism	
	Allergic reaction	1%
	Acute renal failure	3.3 to 16.5% (Average 7%)
	Infection	
	Radiation injury	
	Arrhythmias	

Miscellaneous:

Answer: 61. C. CXR shows massive cardiomegaly

Answer: 62. C. First cardiac angiogram – Sones

Answer: 63. C. ICD-Kriklin

Answer: 64. A. Mason Sones

Answer: 65. C. Post cardiac transplant atherosclerosis - Fractional flow reserve

Answer: 66. First coronary stent – Gruentzig

Answer: 67. D. Isovolumetric relaxation.

Aortic valve has shorter hangout interval than pulmonary valve due to higher systemic vascular pressure which leads to shorter isovolumic relaxation period of left ventricle.

Answer: 68. B. Arterial stiffness

Inventions and 1st use:

ECG: Einthoven

Cardiac catheterization: Werner Forssmann

Coronary angiography: Sones

Balloon angioplasty (Peripheral artery): Charles Dotter and Judkins

Coronary balloon angioplasty (POBA): Andreas Gruentzig

Coronary stent (Bare metal stent- Self expanding): Puel and Sigwart

Coronary stent (BMS- Balloon expandable): Palmaz and Schatz

Coronary stent (Drug eluting stent): Sousa

ICD: Dr. Michel Mirowski

13 Infectious Diseases

Infective Endocarditis

1. Streptococcus gallolyticus endocarditis is commonly associated with:
A. Cirrhosis of liver
B. Gastrointestinal lesion
C. Skin lesions
D. Uremia

2. All of the following are true about endocarditis in intravenous drug abusers, except:
A. More common in HIV seropositive individuals
B. Left side valves are not affected/usually spared
C. Usually are culture negative
D. Not seen in structurally normal valve

3. Which of the following has highest IE risk?
A. RHD
B. Prosthetic valve
C. I/V drug user
D. MVP with MR

4. According to modified Duke's criteria, following is not true for diagnosis of infective endocarditis?
A. 2 major criteria
B. 5 minor criteria
C. 1 major & 2 minor criteria
D. 1 major & 3 minor criteria

5. Following is not true for janeway lesions:
A. It is painless hemorrhagic macules
B. Common over soles & palms
C. Commonly associated with staphylococcal endocarditis
D. It results from immune complex deposition & focal vasculitis

6. Which one of following is not an indication for surgery in patients with infective endocarditis?
A. Persistence of vegetation after antimicrobial therapy
B. Highly mobile vegetation of > 10 mm size over anterior mitral leaflet
C. Embolic episodes during first 2 week of therapy.
D. Valve perforation

7. Prophylaxis of infective endocarditis in highest risk patients is indicated for which of the following procedures?
A. Bronchoscopy or laryngoscopy
B. Placement or adjustment of removable prosthodontic or orthodontic appliances or braces
C. Colonoscopy or transesophageal echo-cardiography
D. None of the above

8. IE Relapse most commonly seen with:
A. Candida albicans
B. Staphylococcus aureus

C. Streptococcus viridans
D. Enterobacteriaceae

9. Maximum relapse after IE is seen with:
A. Enterococcus
B. Fungal
C. Streptococcus viridans
D. Staphylococcus aureus

10. As per the new guidelines, IE prophylaxis is not indicated in:
A. Post-transplant
B. Prior IE
C. Ischemic MR
D. Prosthetic valve

11. Which one of following organism is associated with culture negative endocarditis?
A. Salmonella
B. Coxiella burnetii
C. Pseudomonas species
D. Enterococcus faecalis

Human Immunodeficiency Virus

12. In AIDS patients with infective endocarditis following organism is uncommon as a causative organism for endocarditis?
A. Salmonella species
B. Streptococcus pneumoniae
C. Streptococcus aureus
D. Clostridium septicum

13. Which of the following complication of HIV has not been reduced by anti-retroviral therapy?
A. Pericardial effusion
B. Heart failure
C. Pulmonary hypertension
D. Opportunistic infections

Acute rheumatic fever

14. Which of the following is not a major Jones criterion for the diagnosis of acute rheumatic fever?
A. Carditis
B. Chorea
C. Erythema nodosum
D. Subcutaneous nodules

15. Which of the following is true about WHO criteria for recurrence of RF in patient with RHD?
A. One minor + evidence of recent GAS infection is enough for diagnosis in patients with established RHD
B. 1 major is needed to diagnose recurrence in patients with established RHD
C. Recent streptococcal infection is mandatory to diagnose recurrence
D. Recent scarlet fever is not considered as essential criterion

16. Which of the following is true of arthritis associated with acute rheumatic fever?
A. Spine and axial joints are frequently affected
B. Usually painless
C. Resolves in most patients within 3-4 weeks
D. Joint aspirates are usually acellular

17. Which one of following is not true for sydenham chorea in rheumatic fever?
A. It may persist for 2 years
B. It is never unilateral
C. It does not occur simultaneously with arthritis
D. Emotional lability is common

18. Which one of following is not true for subcutaneous nodules in rheumatic fever?
A. Usually firm & painful
B. Freely movable over the subcutaneous tissue
C. Usual size is 0.5 cm to 2 cm
D. Occurs in crops

19. Which one of following is not true for erythema marginatum in rheumatic fever?
A. The rash is evanescent, pink & non pruritic

B. It has irregular serpiginous border
C. It becomes less prominent after taking hot bath
D. It extends centrifugally, whereas skin at centre returns to normal

20. Which of the following is not an acceptable prophylactic antibiotic regimen for rheumatic fever?
A. Benzathine penicillin 1.2 million units once a month
B. Penicillin V 250 mg BID
C. Sulfadiazine 1 g once a week
D. Erythromycin 250 mg BID

21. Which of the following is true regarding duration of secondary prevention of rheumatic fever?
A. For carditis with residual valvular disease, at least 10 years from last episode and till the age of 40 years
B. For carditis with no residual valvular disease, at least 10 years from last episode and till the age of about 21 years
C. For those with no carditis, at least 10 years from last episode and till the age of about 21 years
D. All of the above

22. Which one of following is not true for Jaccoud arthritis?
A. It occurs after repeated attacks of rheumatic fever
B. It is painless without signs of inflammation
C. Ulnar deviation of 4th & 5th fingers are common
D. Hyperextension of metacarpophalangeal joints are common

Miscellaneous

23. Features of acute streptococcal pharyngitis in children all except:
A. Fever
B. Coryza
C. Tonsillar enlargement
D. Tender cervical lymphadenopathy

24. Risk of anaphylaxis with benzathine penicillin is:
A. 1%
B. 3.2%
C. 5%
D. 0.2%

25. Which of the following is not a major criteria for ARF in low risk population according revised Jones criteria (2015)?
A. Subclinical carditis
B. Chorea
C. Erythema marginatum
D. Monoarthritis

ANSWERS

INFECTIVE ENDOCARDITIS

Answer: 1. B. Gastrointestinal lesion

Answer: 2. D. Not seen in structurally normal valve

Answer: 3. C. I/V drug user

Answer: 4. C. 1 major & 2 minor criteria

Answer: 5. D. It results from immune complex deposition & focal vasculitis

Answer: 6. A. Persistence of vegetation after antimicrobial therapy

Answer: 7. D. None of the above

Answer: 8. A. Candida albicans

Answer: 9. B. Fungal

Answer: 10. C. Ischemic MR

Infective endocarditis:

Most common symptom is fever.

Streptococcus gallolyticus endocarditis is associated with **gastrointestinal lesions.**

Diagnosis

	Sensitivity	Specificity
Transthoracic echo	60%	90%
Transesophageal echo	90%	95%

Intravenous drug users:

Most common pathogen is Staphylococcus aureus.

Right sided valves (TV and PV) are particularly affected and patients present with pulmonary septic embolic symptoms.

Affects structurally normal valves

Modified Duke's criteria:

Major criteria

1. Blood culture positive for IE:

   Typical microorganisms consistent with IE from 2 separate blood cultures: Viridans streptococci, Streptococcus bovis, HACEK group, Staphylococcus aureus; or community acquired enterococci in the absence of a primary focus.

   or

   Microorganisms consistent with IE from persistently positive blood cultures, defined as follows:

   At least two positive cultures of blood samples drawn > 12 h apart or single positive blood culture for Coxiella burnetii or IgG antibody titre > 1:800

2. Evidence of endocardial involvement:

   Echocardiogram positive for IE, defined as follows:

   Oscillating intracardiac mass on valve or supporting structures, in the path of regurgitant jets,

   or Abscess

   or New partial dehiscence of prosthetic valve

   New valvular regurgitation (worsening or changing of pre-existing murmur not sufficient)

Minor criteria

1. Predisposition, predisposing heart condition, or IDU

2. Fever (temperature >38 °C)
3. Vascular phenomena:

   Major arterial emboli, septic pulmonary infarcts, mycotic aneurysm, intracranial hemorrhage, conjunctival hemorrhages, and Janeway lesions
4. Immunologic phenomena

   Glomerulonephritis, Osler's nodes, Roth spots, and rheumatoid factor
5. Microbiological evidence: positive blood culture but does not meet a major criterion as noted above or serologic evidence

Definite infective endocarditis

1. Two major criteria; or
2. One major criterion and three minor criteria; or
3. Five minor criteria

Possible infective endocarditis

1. One major criterion and one minor criterion; or
2. Three minor criteria

Janeway lesions:

Painless and non-tender hemorrhagic macules seen of soles and palms, caused by septic emboli which have deposits of bacteria and microabscesses.

More common with staphylococcus aureus infection.

Osler nodes:

Painful, red, raised lesions found on the hands and feet; caused by immune complex deposition.

Osler's nodes present with tenderness and are of immunologic origin.

Commonly indicative of subacute bacterial endocarditis.

Roth spots:

Roth's spots are retinal hemorrhages with white or pale centers.

Caused by immune complex mediated vasculitis seen in bacterial endocarditis.

Other causes of Roth spots are leukemia, diabetes, subacute bacterial endocarditis, pernicious anemia, ischemic events, and hypertensive retinopathy.

Complications of infective endocarditis:

Heart failure

Most common and feared complication of IE.

Heart failure is most commonly associated with IE of **aortic valve**. Frequency of acute HF depends on location of IE: 29 % (aortic), 20 % (mitral), versus 8 % (tricuspid).

Embolization:

Most common site of embolization is **CNS** followed by kidney and spleen.

65 % of emboli involve the central nervous system (CNS), especially in the middle cerebral artery distribution.

Most common valve leading to embolization is **mitral valve**.

Risk factors for embolization may include: vegetation size, mitral valve involvement, staphylococcal species, prior emboli

Indications of surgery in infective endocarditis:

Class I:

Heart failure

Valvular dehiscence, rupture or perforation

Perivalvular abscess or periannular extension

Fungal IE or multidrug-resistant aggressive pathogens

Persistently positive blood cultures after >1 week of targeted antimicrobials

≥1 embolic event during the initial 2 weeks of antimicrobials

Class IIa:

Anterior mitral leaflet, specially if >10mm

Class IIb:

Increased vegetation size despite antibiotics

Fungal endocarditis:

Rare (<10%)

Most common cause is candida.

Risk factors: Prosthetic valves, nosocomial exposures, catheter, immunocompromise, antibiotic use, IDU, TPN.

Complication: Most common is embolization due to large size of vegetations.

Heart failure is less common.

Recurrence rates are **very high**.

Prosthetic valve endocarditis:

Early prosthetic valve endocarditis: ≤ 1 year post valve surgery

Late prosthetic valve endocarditis: >1 year post-valve surgery

S. aureus and coagulase-negative staphylococcus are the most common organisms in the early prosthetic valve endocarditis.

High morbidity and mortality, and more often require surgical intervention.

Endocarditis prophylaxis:

Cardiac conditions with indications for prophylaxis:

1. Prosthetic cardiac valve or prosthetic material in valve repair
2. History of prior IE
3. Specific forms of congenital heart disease (CHD)
   - Completely repaired CHD if prosthetic material or device was placed within past 6 months
   - Repaired CHD with residual defects at or adjacent to site of prosthetic material or device
   - Unrepaired cyanotic CHD
4. Cardiac transplant with valvulopathy

Surgical procedures which require prophylaxis:

Dental procedures:

Any procedure that involves manipulation of gingival tissue or the periapical region of teeth or perforation of the oral mucosa.

Respiratory procedures:

If procedure is invasive with incision or biopsy. Not indicated in bronchoscopy.

GI/GU procedures:

No prophylaxis indicated

Recommended prophylactic antibiotic regimen:

All regimens are single doses to be given 30–60 min prior to procedure.

REGIMEN	ANTIBIOTICS
Preferred	Amoxicillin 2 g PO
PCN allergy	Clindamycin 600 mg PO OR Azithromycin 500 mg PO
Unable to take oral medication	Ampicillin 2 g IV OR Cefazolin 1 g IM or IV
Unable to take oral and PCN allergy	Cefazolin 1 g IM or IV OR Clindamycin 600 mg IM or IV

Answer: 11. B. Coxiella burnetii

Causes of culture negative endocarditis:

1. Starting antibiotics prior to collection of blood for cultures
2. Right sided endocarditis
3. Non bacterial pathogen (fungi, mycobacteria)
4. Fastidious organisms that require different diagnostic tools
   - Coxiella burnetiid (Q fever)
   - Bartonella

- Brucella
- Mycoplasma
- Tropheryma whipelii
- HACEK organisms (Haemophilus, Actinobacillus, Cardiobacterium, Eikenella, Kingella)

Human immunodeficiency virus

Answer: 12. D. Clostridium septicum

Answer: 13. C. Pulmonary hypertension

HUMAN IMMUNODEFICIENCY VIRUS (HIV) AND CARDIOVASCULAR COMPLICATIONS

1. Pericarditis:

Most common cardiac involvement in HIV is pericarditis and pericardial effusion.

Pericardial effusion is common in HIV not on antiretroviral therapy. Patients on ART have reduced prevalence of pericardial effusion.

Cause- Infections (TB), bacterial, viral, fungal, parasitic and malignancy.

2. Myocarditis:

Cause: Opportunistic infections or direct invasion of myocardium

3. Atherosclerosis:

HIV infection is associated with premature atherosclerosis and increased incidence of cardiovascular events.

Cause: Dyslipidemia (related to HIV and antiretroviral treatment), increased visceral adiposity, chronic inflammation due to HIV infection, increased prevalence of traditional risk factors (smoking).

4. Cardiomyopathy and heart failure:

Both HFrEF and diastolic dysfunction may occur.

Prevalence decreased in ART era as compared to pre-ART era.

Cause: Chronic inflammation, nutritional deficiency, ART

5. Pulmonary artery hypertension (PAH):

Rare complication (0.5%) but with high mortality.

Risk not related to immunosuppression.

ART does not reduce incidence of PAH.

6. Infective endocarditis:

It is usually due to Staphylococcus aureus and is more commonly localized to the right side of the heart. Other common organisms include Salmonella sps and streptococcus pneumoniae.

Cardiovascular drug interactions in HIV patients:

Ritonavir and other protease inhibitors are strong CYP 3A4 inhibitors.

HIV patients may have QT prolongation, so QT prolonging drugs should be carefully administered.

ACUTE RHEUMATIC FEVER

Answer: 14. C. Erythema nodosum.

Answer: 15. C. Recent streptococcal infection is mandatory to diagnose recurrence

Answer: 16. C. Sulfadiazine 1 g once a week.

Answer: 17. B. It is never unilateral (hemichorea)

Answer: 18. A. Usually firm & painful

Answer: 19. C. It becomes less prominent after taking hot bath

Answer: 20. C. Sulfadiazine 1 g once a week

Answer: 21. D. All of the above.

Answer: 22. D. Hyperextension of metacarpophalangeal joints are common

Epidemiology of ARF

Acute rheumatic fever and rheumatic heart disease are rare in more affluent populations, however still common in developing countries.

Overcrowding, close person-to-person contact, and poor health care facilities seem to be consistent predisposing condition.

ARF is a disease of the young, occurs most commonly between 5 to 14 years of age.

Both acute rheumatic fever and rheumatic heart disease are more common in females.

Pathogenesis:

Acute rheumatic fever results from an exaggerated immune response to group A streptococci.

Pharyngeal streptococcal infection is necessary for acute rheumatic fever to develop.

Clinical features:

Incubation period: 2 to 4 weeks after an episode of pharyngitis.

Diagnosis is based on Jones criteria.

Jones Criteria for Diagnosis of Acute Rheumatic Fever

Major manifestations

1. Carditis
2. Polyarthritis
3. Chorea
4. Erythema marginatum
5. Subcutaneous nodules

Minor manifestations

1. Fever
2. Arthralgias
3. Previous rheumatic fever or rheumatic heart disease
4. Elevated C-reactive protein concentration or erythrocyte sedimentation rate
5. Prolonged PR interval on electrocardiogram

Evidence of antecedent group A streptococcal infection (Essential criteria)

1. Positive throat culture or rapid antigen test positive for group A streptococci
2. Increased or increasing streptococcal antibody titre
3. Recent scarlet fever

For diagnosis:

1) 2 major manifestations or 1 major and 2 minor manifestations and
2) Evidence of a recent streptococcal infection

When chorea or carditis is clearly present, evidence of antecedent group A streptococcal infection is not necessary.

World Health Organization Criteria for Diagnosis of Acute Rheumatic Fever

1. First episode—same as the Jones criteria
2. Recurrent episode in a patient without established RHD—same as for first episode
3. Recurrent episode in a patient with established RHD—requires 2 minor manifestations from the Jones criteria and evidence of an antecedent group A streptococcal infection

Major manifestations of ARF:

Carditis:

Carditis is most common major manifestation and develops in 90% of patients with rheumatic fever.

It is pancarditis i.e. involves pericardium, myocardium and endocardium.

Endocardial involvement with valve leaflet thickening occurs as a rule.

In young patients, mitral valve regurgitation is the predominant cardiac lesion.

Mitral stenosis becomes progressively more common in early to mid adulthood.

Myocarditis: Myocardium is infiltrated by mononuclear cells, interstitial connective tissue shows degenerative changes. 30-40% biopsy samples show **Aschoff bodies**, which are pathognomonic of rheumatic fever.

Subclinical carditis, is thought to occur in approximately 12% to 21% of persons with acute rheumatic fever which can be detected by echocardiography.

Rheumatic myocarditis is rare without rheumatic valvular disease.

Arthritis:

Beyond fever, arthritis is typically the earliest manifestation of acute rheumatic fever.

Arthritis is classically migrating from joint to joint.

Large joints are affected and knees and ankles are often first affected.

Duration of joint inflammation is typically short (≤1 week). Resolve in all patients by 3-4 weeks. If arthritis persists more than 4 weeks, then alternative diagnosis should be considered.

Pain is very responsive to salicylates and NSAIDs.

Synovial fluid is acellular and sterile on examination.

Sydenham chorea or St Vitus dance:

Neurologic movement disorder characterized by abrupt, purposeless involuntary movements of the muscles of the face, neck, trunk, and limbs. It can be both unilateral or bilateral.

Muscular weakness (hypotonia), behavioural disturbances such as obsessive-compulsive behaviors and emotional lability may be seen.

Symptoms progressively worsen over 1 to 2 months and spontaneously resolve gradually after 3 to 6 months. In some patients, may persist for years.

20% of patients may have recurrences.

It does not occur simultaneously with arthritis.

Subcutaneous nodules:

Diameter up to 2 cms occur over bony surfaces or near tendons; are freely movable under the skin.

They are firm and **painless**, overlying skin is not inflamed.

They are smaller and short lived as compared to rheumatoid arthritis.

Erythema marginatum:

Rash is evanescent, pinkish red and non-pruritic with irregular serpiginous borders.

It extends centrifugally, and skin at centre returns to normal.

Typically occurs on truck and proximal limbs; becomes more prominent after hot bath.

Erythema marginatum and subcutaneous nodules usually occur only in patients with carditis.

Jaccoud's arthritis:

Chronic painless non-erosive reversible joint disorder, may occur after repeated bouts of arthritis.

In Jaccoud's arthropathy, the deformities result from soft-tissue abnormalities, such as laxity of ligaments, fibrosis of the capsule, and muscular imbalance, rather than from destruction of the bone of joints, as occurs in rheumatoid arthritis.

Classically described in rheumatic fever, Jaccoud's arthropathy has also been described in SLE and other diffuse connective-tissue diseases.

These deformities are reducible and are characteristic of Jaccoud's arthropathy. Magnetic resonance imaging of the hands shows no erosions.

Treatment of acute rheumatic fever:

Fever and arthritis resolve quickly with salicylates.

Conventional therapy for congestive heart failure.

Steroids: For severe carditis, dose is 2 mg/kg per day for 1 to 2 weeks, followed by tapering of dose.

Antibiotic therapy: Penicillin to eradicate group A streptococcal infection from upper respiratory tract to all individuals. Injection benzathine penicillin 1.2 MU for adults or 600,000 U when weight is less than 27 kg can be given.

Antibiotic prophylaxis:

For all patients who have acute rheumatic fever or rheumatic heart disease.

Best drug for prophylaxis is benzathine penicillin G IM every 3 weeks. Recommended dose is same as for treatment.

Oral drugs include 1. Penicillin V 250 mg BD 2. Sulfadiazine 1 gm OD 3. Erythromycin 250 mg BD 4. Azithromycin 250 mg OD

Patients allergic to penicillin can take sulfadiazine or erythromycin.

Duration of prophylaxis:

Indication	Duration
1. Rheumatic fever with carditis and persistent valvular disease	10 y or at least until age 40, whichever is longer.
2. Rheumatic fever with mild or healed carditis but without valve disease	10 y or until age 21, whichever is longer.
3. Rheumatic fever without carditis or valve disease	5 y or until age 21, whichever is longer.

Miscellaneous

Answer: 23. B. Coryza

Acute streptococcal pharyngitis	Viral infection
Fever	Conjunctivitis
Headache	Coryza
Tonsillopharyngeal inflammation (Tonsillar enlargement)	Rhinorrhoea
Patchy tonsillopharyngeal exudates	Cough
Anterior cervical adenitis (tender nodes)	Hoarseness
History of exposure to streptococcal pharyngitis	Viral exanthem
Scarlatiniform rash	

Answer: 24. D. 0.2%

Penicillin allergy:

Estimated frequency of anaphylaxis is at 1-5 per 10,000 cases of penicillin therapy, however with injectable penicillin such as benzathine penicillin anaphylaxis occurs at the rate of 0.2%.

Answer: 25. D. Monoarthritis

Revised Jones criteria (2015) for acute rheumatic fever:

Low-risk population: ARF incidence ≤2 per 100 000 school-aged children or all-age RHD prevalence of ≤1 per 1000 population year

Moderate/high-risk population: Children not clearly from a low-risk population

Major criteria

Low risk population	Moderate/high risk population
Clinical or subclinical carditis	Clinical or subclinical carditis
Polyarthritis	Monoarthritis, Polyarthritis or polyarthralgia
Chorea	Chorea
Erythema marginatum	Erythema marginatum
Subcutaneous nodules	Subcutaneous nodules

Minor criteria

Low risk population	Moderate/high risk population
Prolonged PR interval	Prolonged PR interval
Polyarthralgia	Monoarthralgia
Fever: ≥38.5°C	Fever: ≥38°C
Inflammatory markers: Peak ESR ≥60 mm in 1 h and/or CRP ≥3.0 mg/dL	Inflammatory markers: Peak ESR ≥30 mm in 1 h and/or CRP ≥3.0 mg/dL

Subclinical carditis: Findings seen only on echocardiography without ausculatory findings

The echocardiographic criteria suggestive of rheumatic heart disease:

I. Echocardiographic (Doppler) criteria:

Pathological mitral regurgitation – 4 criteria (all must be met)	**Pathological aortic regurgitation** – 4 criteria (all must be met)
Visible at least in 2 projections.	Visible at least in 2 projections.
Regurgitation jet length ≥2 cm at least in 1 projection.	Regurgitation jet length ≥1 cm at least in 1 projection.
Regurgitation peak velocity > 3 m/s.	Regurgitation peak velocity > 3 m/s.
Regurgitation pansystolic.	Regurgitation pandiastolic.

II. Echocardiographic (morphological) criteria:

Acute mitral valve involvement	Chronic mitral valve involvement (invisible in acute involvement)	Lesions in acute and chronic aortic valve involvement
Dilatation of mitral annulus.	Thickening of leaflets.	Symmetrical or focal thickening of leaflets.
Elongation of chordae tendineae.	Thickening of chordae tendineae, with their fusion.	Disturbed leaflet coaptation leaflet closing during systole).
Rupture of chorda tendinea with acute mitral regurgitation.	Limited mobility of leaflets.	Limited mobility of leaflets.
Prolapse of anterior (less often posterior) leaflet.	Calcifications.	Prolapse of leaflets.

14 Cardiac Masses, Systemic Disorders and Pregnancy

Cardiac Masses and Tumors

1. Papillary fibroelastoma occurs on:
A. Heart valves
B. Inter atrial septum
C. Atrium
D. Ventricle

2. Most common primary sarcoma of heart in children is:
A. Angiosarcoma
B. Leiomyosarcoma
C. Rhabdomyosarcoma
D. Fibrosarcoma

3. All of the following are true regarding Rhabdomyoma except:
A. Have tendency to regress spontaneously
B. Commonly arise from ventricular wall
C. Usually present as solitary tumor causing obstruction
D. Originate from cardiac myocytes

4. Identify the wrong statement in rhabdomyoma of the heart:
A. Probably hamartomas
B. Can mimic restrictive cardiomyopathy
C. Most often require resection
D. 90% are multiple

5. Most common site of origin of cardiac metastasis?
A. Lung
B. Stomach
C. Breast
D. Esophagus

Systemic Disorders

6. False statement about cardiovascular effects of hypothyroidism:
A. Systemic vascular resistance decreases
B. Heart rate decreases
C. Cardiac output decreases
D. Blood volume decreases

7. All of the following are true about hypothyroidism except:
A. Diastolic hypertension more common
B. Decreased pulse pressure
C. Increased serum renin levels
D. Increased systemic vascular resistance

8. Subclinical hypothyroidism all except:
A. Elderly M:F-1:1
B. Associated with increased cholesterol
C. Odds ratio for MI risk is twice
D. Decrease lsovolumic relaxation time

9. Cardiovascular manifestations of Acromegaly include all except:
A. Accelerated atherosclerosis
B. Secondary hypertension with dramatic response to ARBs
C. Four fold increase in ventricular arrythmias
D. Late potentials in SAECG

10. What is the incidence of dilated cardiomyopathy in Duchenne muscular dystrophy, after age of 18 years?
A. Up to 20%
B. Up to 50%
C. Up to 70%
D. Up to 90%

11. All of the following are true about Becker's muscular dystrophy except:
A. Heart failure can be the only initial symptom
B. Marked improvement is seen with glucocorticoids in early period
C. Size of gene deletion does NOT predict severity
D. Facial weakness is uncommon

12. Following cardiomyopathy is common in Friedreich ataxia:
A. Asymmetrical septal hypertrophy
B. Concentric hypertrophic cardiomyopathy
C. Dilated cardiomyopathy
D. Restrictive cardiomyopathy

13. Cardiovascular effects of acromegaly include?
A. Left ventricular hypertrophy
B. Hypertension
C. Insulin resistance and diabetes mellitus
D. All of the above

14. Cushing's syndrome is not associated with?
A. Hypertension
B. Diabetes mellitus
C. Atrial myxomas
D. Mitral regurgitation

15. Cardiac effects of hyperthyroidism include?
A. Atrial fibrillation
B. High-output heart failure
C. Higher blood volume
D. All of the above

16. Which of the following are cardiac effects of hypothyroidism?
A. Pericardial effusion
B. Elevated serum cholesterol level
C. Low cardiac output and elevated peripheral vascular resistance
D. All of the above

17. All of the following are true for hypothyroid except?
A. Increase SVR
B. Increase renin level
C. Pulse pressure -decreases
D. Diastolic HTN

18. All of the following are true about hypothyroidism except:
A. Reduced myocardial contractility
B. Increased systemic vascular resistance
C. Decreased pulmonary artery pressure
D. Increased peripheral oxygen consumption

19. Which of the following may occur with acute subarachnoid hemorrhage?
A. Giant T wave inversion
B. Takotsubo-like syndrome with cardiac dysfunction and troponin release
C. QT prolongation and torsades
D. All of the above

Chemotherapeutic Agents

20. At what level of doxorubicin therapy do cardiotoxic effects increase exponentially:
A. 300 mg/m2
B. 450 mg/m2
C. 600 mg/m2
D. No threshold

21. What factors increase the toxic effects of doxorubicin on the heart?
A. Radiation to chest
B. CAD
C. Age >65 years
D. All of the above

22. In addition to Adriamycin, which other cancer chemotherapeutic agents are potentially cardiotoxic?
A. Herceptin
B. Cyclophosphamide
C. Mitoxantrone
D. All of the above

23. 5-fluorouracil can potentially cause:
A. Coronary vasospasm, especially in those with CAD
B. Myocarditis
C. Pericarditis
D. None of the above

24. Anticancer drug associated with arterial or venous thromboembolism is:
A. Cisplatin
B. Cyclophosphamide
C. Adriamycin
D. None of the above

Perioperative Evaluation

25. Which of the following is not included in the risk calculation using RCRI?
A. Age
B. Creatinine >2 mg/dL
C. CAD
D. Type of surgery

26. What is an elevated risk according to RCRI:
A. RCRI ≥2
B. RCRI ≥3
C. RCRI ≥4
D. RCRI ≥5

27. High cardiac risk for non cardiac surgery all except:
A. DM on insulin
B. Pancreaticoduodenectomy
C. Ejection fraction =40%
D. History of TIA

28. High risk of cardiac events during non-cardiac surgery all except:
A. BP 180/104
B. Creatinine- 2.5mg%
C. History of TIA
D. Insulin for NIDDM

29. High risk of adverse cardiovascular events during non-cardiac surgery associated with all except:
A. Prior transient ischemic attack
B. Whipple surgery
C. Serum creatinine > 2.1 mg/dL
D. History of syncope

30. Which of the following are class I indications for beta blockade perioperatively?
A. Those on chronic beta blockade
B. Those with moderate or high risk myocardial ischemia on preoperative stress testing
C. Those with three or more revised clinical risk index (RCRI) risk factors; for example, diabetes mellitus, heart failure, coronary artery disease (CAD), renal insufficiency, cerebrovascular accident
D. All of the above

31. POISE trial addressing perioperative beta blockade yielded which of the following results?
A. Use of beta blocker reduced risk of atrial fibrillation
B. Use of beta blocker reduced risk of myocardial ischemia
C. Beta blocker use resulted in higher risk of stroke and noncardiac death
D. All of the above

32. What is the prevalence with regard to atrial fibrillation after cardiac surgery?
A. 10%
B. 20%
C. 30–50%
D. 80%

33. Which of the following drugs does not reduce the risk of post-operative atrial fibrillation?
A. Beta blocker
B. Sotalol
C. Amiodarone
D. Digoxin

Pregnancy

34. Hemodynamic changes during pregnancy:
A. Heart rate increases
B. Blood volume increases

C. Pulmonary vascular resistance decreases
D. All of the above

35. All the following statements about hemodynamic changes during pregnancy are true except?
A. Heart rate increases by 10-20%
B. Blood volume increases by 30-40%
C. Arterial blood pressure increases by 10-20%
D. Cardiac output increases by 30%

36. All of the following are true regarding pregnancy except:
A. Stroke volume is increased
B. Decreased plasma colloid oncotic pressure
C. Low pulmonary vascular resistance
D. Elevated pulmonary capillary wedge pressure

37. Identify the wrong statement regarding hemodynamic changes during pregnancy:
A. Plasma volume increases by about 40-50% above baseline
B. Heart rate increase by 10-20%
C. Pulmonary vascular resistance increases by 10-15%
D. Venous pressure in lower limbs increases

38. Normal physiologic changes during pregnancy include?
A. Fall in systemic blood pressure occurs predominantly during the last trimester
B. Increase in cardiac output predominantly occurs due to increase in stroke volume which occurs during last trimester
C. Pulmonary artery systolic and diastolic pressures remain normal
D. Physiological anaemia during pregnancy reduces the placental perfusion

39. All of the following can be seen in normal pregnancy except?
A. Elevated ESR
B. Elevated serum creatinine
C. Decreased systemic vascular resistance
D. Increased chance of coronary dissection

40. All of the following drugs are unsafe in pregnancy except:
A. Spironolactone
B. Propylthiouracil
C. Olmesartan
D. Telmisartan

41. Mismatch in drugs during pregnancy:
A. B blockers- Teratogenic
B. Aspirin- Premature ducal closure
C. Amiodarone- Neonatal goitre
D. ACE inhibitor- Oligohydramnios

42. Pregnancy is contraindicated in which of the following cardiovascular conditions?
A. Hypertrophic cardiomyopathy
B. Repaired tetralogy of Fallot
C. Fontan circulation
D. Native severe coarctation

43. All are risk factors for peripartum cardiomyopathy except?
A. Primipara
B. Older maternal age
C. Preeclampsia
D. Twin pregnancy

44. 27 years old lady with history of peripartum cardiomyopathy during previous pregnancy comes for expert opinion regarding second pregnancy. Evaluation reveals LV function of 40% which has improved considerable from 20%. She is asymptomatic on low dose diuretic, beta blocker and ACE inhibitor. What do you recommend?
A. To go ahead with pregnancy
B. Recommend reassessing LV function in 6 months and if normal, then proceed
C. Counsel against pregnancy
D. Stop ACE inhibitor and then proceed with pregnancy

45. Which of the following is rare finding in preeclampsia?
A. Left ventricular hypertrophy
B. Proteinuria
C. Elevated plasma uric acid
D. Sudden weight gain

46. Which of the following is associated with highest maternal mortality during pregnancy?
A. Marfan syndrome with aortic root measurement of 4.5 cm
B. Family history of cardiomyopathy
C. Severe mitral regurgitation
D. Ventricular septal defect (VSD) with a right-to-left shunt

47. Which of the following disorders are associated with the highest risk with pregnancy?
A. Primary pulmonary hypertension with a PA systolic pressure of 110 mmHg
B. Surgically corrected tetralogy of Fallot
C. Severe pulmonary stenosis
D. Large atrial septal defect with a shunt ratio of 3:1 and PA systolic pressure of 50 mmHg

48. Maternal risk of pregnancy is very high in all except:
A. VSD with severe PAH
B. Marfan syndrome with aortic root > 40 mm
C. Dilated cardiomyopathy with EF < 40%
D. Pulmonary stenosis with gradient of 50 mmHg

49. Spontaneous coronary artery dissection (SCAD) is most commonly seen in which of the following groups?
A. Young women
B. Young men
C. Elderly women
D. Elderly men

Miscellaneous

50. All of the following are true regarding 'Fetal echocardiography' except?
A. Should be done in the last trimester of pregnancy as the fetal heart is well developed
B. Fetal arrhythmias can be diagnosed on echocardiography
C. Hypoplastic left heart syndrome can be easily diagnosed
D. Imaging of coarctation of aorta is difficult

51. Cardiac hypertrophy is seen all except:
A. Acromegaly
B. Pheochromocytoma
C. Hyperparathyroidism
D. After space flight

52. All are age related cardiovascular changes except:
A. Increase in LA size
B. Decrease â receptor sensitivity
C. Increased heart rate variability
D. Endothelium dependent vasodilation impaired

53. What is not true about cardiovascular disease in women?
A. Women with MI have less comorbid conditions
B. With PCI, women have more vascular complications than men
C. With CABG, women have more postoperative depression
D. Women have more atypical features

54. Cardiac surgery during pregnancy is associated with about what fetal loss:
A. 5% B. 30%
C. 70% D. 100%

55. Kissing vegetations on mitral valve may be seen in?
A. Takayasu arteritis

B. APLA
C. Rheumatoid arthritis
D. Rheumatic fever

56. Ankylosing spondylitis true except:
A. Only 20% of HLA B-27 patients have AS
B. Coronary arteritis is common
C. AR in children may precede joint manifestations
D. Ophthalmic involvement includes anterior uveitis

57. What is the investigation of choice to diagnose hepatopulmonary syndrome?
A. Saline contrast echocardiography
B. Pulmonary CT angiography
C. Contrast pulmonary angiography (invasive)
D. Magnetic resonance angiography

ANSWERS

Cardiac tumors

Answer: 1. A. Heart valve

Answer: 2. C. Rhabdomyosarcoma

Answer: 3. C. Usually present as solitary tumor causing obstruction

Answer: 4. C. Most often require resection

Answer: 5. A. Lung

Cardiac tumors

Most common cardiac mass: Thrombus

Most common cardiac tumor: Secondary

Secondary tumors are 20–40 times more common than primary cardiac tumors.

The most common primary cardiac tumors in adults are myxomas

Secondary Tumors (Metastatic):

Pericardium most commonly affected (69.4 %), followed by epicardium (34.2 %) and myocardium (41.8 %) then endocardium (5 %)

Most common cancer to metastasize to heart: **Lung cancer**

Cancer having most propensity for heart metastasis: **Melanoma**

Cardiac Myxomas

Most common location is **left atrium (75%)** followed by right atrium (15%), RV (5%), LV (5%).

May result in systemic symptoms, largely due to embolic phenomena or to secretion of interleukin 6.

Constitutional symptoms include fever and weight loss

Presenting symptoms of left-sided cardiac myxomas: Dyspnea on exertion, paroxysmal nocturnal dyspnea, and fever, but sudden death and hemoptysis also may occur.

The most common physical finding with a left atrial myxoma is a **mitral diastolic murmur** (similar to mitral stenosis but without the opening snap) or a **mitral systolic murmur** due to mitral incompetence. Other features tumor plop, raynaud's phenomenon, and clubbing.

Familial myxoma:

Approximately **10%** of myxomas and have an autosomal dominant inheritance.

In contrast to sporadic myxoma, they occur in younger patients, have less of a female preponderance, are frequently multiple, recur more frequently postoperatively.

Carney syndrome: Cardiac myxoma, pigmentation of skin (pigmented nevi), endocrine tumors (pituitary adenoma), adrenocortical disease or testicular tumors.

NAME syndrome: Nevi, Atrial myxoma, Myxoid neurofibromas, and Ephelides.

LAMB syndrome: Lentigines, Atrial myxoma, and Blue nevi.

Cardiac rhabdomyomas

Associated with the tuberous sclerosis syndrome, which is characterized by **hamartomas** in multiple organs, epilepsy, mental deficiency, and adenoma sebaceum.

Rhabdomyomas develop almost exclusively in children, mostly before the age of one year, and arise from ventricular wall; most of them are multiple.

About 80 to 90 percent are associated with tuberous sclerosis.

Most rhabdomyomas regress spontaneously, and resection is usually not required unless a child is symptomatic.

Symptoms are rare and are caused by obstruction of blood flow through the heart or consist of rhythm disturbances, such as heart block of ventricular tachycardia.

Cardiac fibromas

Benign connective tissue tumors that occur predominantly in children

Lipomatous Hypertrophy of the Atrial Septum

Accumulation of adipose tissue within atrial septum.
More common in elderly, obese women

Cardiac Sarcomas

Cardiac sarcomas are the most common primary malignant tumor of the heart.

Prognosis is poor, with median survival of less than 1 year.

Papillary Fibroelastoma

Benign tumors that arise from the cardiac valves

May cause thromboembolic complications
Surgical resection is curative.

Carcinoid Heart Disease

Characterized by plaque-like deposits of fibrous tissue on the endocardial surface of valve cusps and leaflets, usually on the right heart valves (90% of cases) but less commonly on the left heart valves (10% of cases) if there is a patent foramen ovale or the carcinoid tumor is a bronchial carcinoid.

Although carcinoid tumor cells not found in the heart, but remote secretion of serotonin is considered the mechanism of carcinoid heart disease

Systemic disorders

Answer: 6 A. Systemic vascular resistance decreases

Answer: 7. C. Increased serum renin levels

Answer: 8. D. Decrease Isovolumic relaxation time

Answer: 9. B. Secondary hypertension with dramatic response to ARBs

Answer: 10. D. Up to 90%

Answer: 11. B. Marked improvement is seen with glucocorticoids in early period

Answer: 12. B. Concentric hypertrophic cardiomyopathy

Answer: 13. D. All of the above.

Answer: 14. D. Mitral regurgitation.

→ Association with myxoma is seen in Carney complex.

Answer: 15. D. All of the above.

Answer: 16. D. All of the above.

Answer: 17. B. Increase renin level

Answer: 18. D. Increased peripheral oxygen consumption

Answer: 19. D. All of the above.

Friedreich Ataxia

Autosomal recessive neuromuscular disorder characterized by ataxia, muscle weakness, and sensory loss

Hypertrophic cardiomyopathy is present which differs from classical one (Myofibrillary disarray is absent and concentric LVH is more common than asymmetric septal hypertrophy).

Duchenne Muscular Dystrophy

X-linked recessive disorder characterized by the absence of the protein dystrophin

Causes dilated cardiomyopathy.

Heart blocks and atrial/ventricular arrhythmias are also common.

ECG: Tall R waves and increased R/S amplitude in V1 and deep narrow Q waves in the left precordial leads possibly related to the posterolateral left ventricular involvement

Steroids decrease progression to dilated cardiomyopathy.

Cerebral Hemorrhage

Marked ECG changes, including QT prolongation, prominent U waves, ST-segment elevation or depression, and deep symmetrical T-wave inversion in the precordial leads.

Takotsubo like syndrome with apical LV dysfunction and ballooning

Acromegaly

Cardiomegaly, hypertension, diabetes mellitus, focal myocardial fibrosis, and premature atherosclerosis.

ACE inhibitors and ARBs can cause a paradoxical **increase** in blood pressure in patients with acromegaly.

Thyroid Disease

Hyperthyroidism:

Heart is hyperdynamic, with an increase in heart rate, systolic blood pressure, cardiac output, and stroke volume and a decrease in systemic vascular resistance.

Atrial fibrillation occurs in 25% of patients.

Thyroid hormone increases renin secretion from kidneys.

Hypothyroidism:

Decrease in heart rate, ventricular contractility, and cardiac output but an **increase** in systemic vascular resistance and diastolic blood pressure.

Decrease in pulmonary vascular resistance.

Pericardial effusion (1/3rd patients) and an abnormal lipid profile (an increase in low-density lipoprotein cholesterol and triglyceride levels)

Cancer chemotherapeutic agents:

Answer: 20. A. 300 mg/m2.

Answer: 21. D. All of the above.

Answer: 22. D. All of the above.

Answer: 23. A. Coronary vasospasm, especially in those with CAD.

Answer: 24. A. Cisplatinum.

Chemotherapeutic agents

Agents	**Cardiac side effects**
Anthracyclines	
Doxorubicin, daunorubicin, mitoxantrone	Cardiac dysfunction and heart failure
Taxanes	
Paclitaxel	Arrhythmia, myocardial ischemia
Alkylating and Alkylating-Like Agents	
Cyclophosphamide	Myopericarditis
Cisplatin, carboplatin,	Arterial vasospasm, HTN, Arterial and venous thrombosis

Antimetabolites	
5-Fluorouracil, capecitabine	Coronary vasospasm, myocardial ischemia,
Monoclonal Antibody Tyrosine Kinase Inhibitors	
Bevacizumab	HTN, CM, HF, arterial and venous thrombosis
Trastuzumab (Herceptin)	Cardiac dysfunction and heart failure
Proteasome Inhibitors	
Bortezomib	Cardiac dysfunction, heart failure
Small-Molecule Tyrosine Kinase Inhibitors	
Sunitinib, Sorafenib	HTN, CM, HF, thrombosis
Nilotinib, Ponatinib	Peripheral vascular disease, ischemic heartdisease
Dasatinib	Pulmonary HTN, pericardial effusion
Immune-Modulating Agents	
Thalidomide, Lenalidomide	Edema, thrombosis, arrhythmia
Androgen-Deprivation Therapy	
Leuprolide, goserelin, triptorelin, flutamide, bicalutamide	Metabolic syndrome, ischemia, coronaryartery disease
Estrogen-Receptor Modulators	
Tamoxifen	Thrombosis
Aromatase inhibitors (anastrozole, letrozole, exemestane)	Hypercholesterolemia, HTN, valvular disease, and pericarditis
Radiation Therapy	Valvular disease, pericardial disease, coronary artery disease, cardiac dysfunction

Anthracyclines:

Incidence of cardiotoxicity: 9%, mostly reversible.

Mechanism: Formation of reactive oxygen species, formation of anthracycline-iron complexes, and topoisomerase-2β inhibition

Risk factors for doxorubicin induced cardiotoxicity:

Cumulative dose, conventional CV risk factors (Old age, smoking, dyslipidemia, DM, HTN); young age, additional cardiotoxic therapies, including radiotherapy or trastuzumab.

Cumulative dose of doxorubicin: 300 mg/m^2 or more increase the risk of cardiac dysfunction.

Incidence of HF: 1.7% at a cumulative dose of 300 mg/m2, 4.7% at 400 mg/m2, 15.7% at 500 mg/m2, and 48% at 650 mg/m2.

Cardioprotective agent: Dexrazoxane

It is a derivative of EDTA, may provide cardioprotection against anthracyclines.

Perioperative evaluation

Answer: 25. A. Age

Answer: 26. A. RCRI ≥2

Answer: 27. C. Ejection fraction =40%

Answer: 28. A. BP 180/104

Answer: 29. D. History of syncope

Answer: 30. A. Those on chronic beta blockade.

Answer: 31. D. All of the above.

Answer: 32. C. 30–50%

Answer: 33. D. Digoxin

Risk stratification	Cardiac risk	Procedure
High	>5%	- Aortic or other major vascular surgery - Peripheral or infrainguinal vascular surgery
Intermediate	1 %-5%	- Intraperitoneal and intrathoracic surgery - Carotid endarterectomy - Head and neck surgery - Orthopedic surgery - Prostate surgery
Low	<1%	- Endoscopic procedures - Superficial procedures - Cataract surgery - Breast surgery

Revised Goldman cardiac risk index (RCRI)

Six independent predictors of major cardiac complications:

1. High risk surgery (e.g. Vascular surgery and any open intraperitoneal or intrathoracic procedures)
2. History of ischemic heart disease (H/o of MI or a positive exercise test, present complaint of chest pain considered to be secondary to myocardial ischemia, use of nitrate therapy, or ECG with pathological Q waves; do not count prior coronary revascularization procedure unless one to the other criteria for ischemic heart disease is present.

3. History of heart failure
4. History of cerebrovascular disease
5. Diabetes mellitus requiring treatment with insulin
6. Preoperative creatinine >2.0 mg/dl

→ Elevated cardiac risk when RCRI is two or more. Score of 0 or 1 is considered low risk.

→ Rate of cardiac death, nonfatal MI, and nonfatal cardiac arrest:

- No risk factors: 0.4%
- One risk factor: 1.0%
- Two risk factors: 2.4%
- Three or more risk factors: 5.4%

Peri-operative beta blockers:

Indication	Recommendation
Patients who have been on beta blockers chronically	I
Intermediate or high risk myocardial ischemia noted in pre-operative risk stratification tests	IIb
Patients with 3 or more RCRI risk factors	IIb
Beta blocker therapy should not be started on day of surgery	III

Peri-operative atrial fibrillation after cardiac surgery:

AF occurs in up to 40% of patients, primarily within 2 to 3 days.

Up to 80% of patients spontaneously revert to sinus rhythm within 24 hours without treatment other than agents used for controlling the ventricular rate

AF causes twofold to threefold increase in postoperative stroke.

Older age, hypertension, previous AF, and HF are associated with a higher risk for AF after cardiac surgery.

Statin therapy and off-pump techniques may be associated with less frequent postoperative AF.

Prophylactic use of beta-blocking agents reduces the frequency of postoperative AF.

Amiodarone is also effective in prophylaxis against postoperative AF and may be considered in patients at high risk for its development.

Pregnancy

Answer: 34. D. All

Answer: 35. C. Arterial blood pressure increases by 10-20%

Answer: 36. D. Elevated pulmonary capillary wedge pressure

Answer: 37. C. Pulmonary vascular resistance increases by 10-15%

Answer: 38. C. Pulmonary artery systolic and diastolic pressures remain normal

Answer: 39. B. Elevated serum creatinine

Answer: 40. B. Propylthiouracil

Answer: 41. A. B blockers-teratogenic

Answer: 42. D. Native severe coarctation

Answer: 43. A. Primipara

Answer: 44. C. Counsel against pregnancy.

Pregnancy is not recommended when LVEF is <25% at initial presentation or there is persistent decrease in LVEF

Answer: 45. A. LVH

Answer: 46. D. Ventricular septal defect (VSD)with a right-to-left shunt.

Answer: 47. A. Primary pulmonary hypertension with a PA systolic pressure of 110 mmHg.

Eisenmenger's complex is also associated with one of the highest risks.

Answer: 48. D. Pulmonary stenosis with gradient of 50 mmHg

Answer: 49. A. Young women

Hemodynamic Changes During Normal Pregnancy

- There is a 20% to 30% increase in red blood cell mass and a 30% to 50% increase in plasma volume which results in increased blood volume with relative anemia.
- HR increases about 10 bpm (by 10-20%).
- SVR and PVR decrease.
- BP generally decreases slightly during pregnancy.
- Cardiac output increases by 30 to 50%.
- Oxygen consumption increases by 30%.
- Venous pressure in lower limbs increases.

Cardiac findings in pregnancy

Normal Cardiac Findings	Abnormal findings
JVP increases slightly with prominent a and v waves. S1 is louder than normal. P2 is prominent with persistent splitting of S2. Audible S3 Pulmonary ejection systolic murmur Venous hum and mammary continuous murmur Peripheral edema	Fourth heart sound (4) Loud systolic murmur (grade 3/6 or louder) Diastolic murmur Fixed splitting of the second heart sound

Cardiac indications of caesarean delivery:

Anticoagulation with warfarin (Risk of fetal intracranial haemorrhage)

Critical or symptomatic fixed cardiac obstructive lesions

Markedly enlarged or enlarging aorta during pregnancy

Pulmonary hypertension

Obstructive cardiac lesions are poorly tolerated than regurgitant lesions

Cardiac Contraindications to Pregnancy:

Severe pulmonary hypertension

Eisenmenger syndrome

Cardiomyopathy with NYHA class III or IV congestive heart failure

Systemic ejection fraction <40%

Severe obstructive cardiac lesions (Severe MS, Severe AS, Severe Coarctation of aorta)

Marfan syndrome with aortic root e"40 mm

Severe cyanosis

History of peripartum cardiomyopathy

Peripartum Cardiomyopathy

Congestive heart failure that occurs in the **last trimester or up to 6 months** post-partum (most commonly within 1st month post-partum) in the absence of other recognized cause of heart failure.

Incidence: 1:3000 to 1:15000 live births, and is higher in some parts of world such as Africa and Haiti.

Risk Factors:

Multifetal pregnancies

Multiparous women

Women older than 30 years

Black women

Women with gestational hypertension or preeclampsia

Women treated with tocolytic therapy

Prognosis:

Maternal mortality: 10 to 15%, mortality increased if LV dysfunction persists.

Improvement in LV function is expected in 50% within 6 months after delivery.

Recurrence in subsequent pregnancies is common, hence subsequent pregnancies should be avoided. And, pregnancy is contraindicated with persistent LV dysfunction.

Treatment:

Management of CHF. Specific therapy: Bromocriptine, Pentoxifylline, IVIG.

Teratogenic drugs:

ACE inhibitors

ARBs

Aldosterone antagonists (Spironolactone and Eplerenone)

Warfarin

Statins.

Nonteratogenic drugs:

Loop and thiazide diuretics, Digoxin, beta blocker, calcium channel blockers, Adenosine, Heparin, Aspirin.

Aspirin is non-teratogenic but can cause premature ductus arteriosus closure like other NSAIDs.

Warfarin Embryopathy

Incidence of warfarin embryopathy is less than 10%

Risk lesser with a warfarin dose less than 5 mg daily

Bone and cartilaginous abnormalities with chondrodysplasia, nasal hypoplasia, optic atrophy, microphthalmia, blindness and seizures.

Important points

DC cardioversion may be used safely in pregnancy.

Atenolol should be avoided during pregnancy and breastfeeding.

When cardiac surgery is necessary during pregnancy, the optimal time is between weeks 24 and 28 of pregnancy, and the duration of cardiopulmonary bypass should be as short as possible.

Pregnancy and hypertension:

Gestational hypertension refers to mild blood pressure elevations that occur in the second half of pregnancy and are unaccompanied by proteinuria. Blood pressures usually return to normal within 12 weeks after delivery.

Pre-eclampsia is a disorder of pregnancy in which there is hypertension associated with proteinuria.

Eclampsia, which is considered a complication of severe preeclampsia, is commonly defined as new onset of grand mal seizure activity and/or unexplained coma during pregnancy or postpartum in a woman with signs or symptoms of preeclampsia.

Most cases of eclampsia occur in third trimester or within 48 hours of delivery.

Delivery is the definitive treatment for preeclampsia. Pending delivery, magnesium sulfate is the pharmacologic treatment of choice.

Spontaneous coronary artery dissection:

Rare non-atherosclerotic cause of acute coronary syndromes (ACS).

Usually young females are affected during pregnancy or just after delivery who are without any cardiovascular risk factors.

This is not atherosclerotic, but may be associated with fibromuscular dysplasia. There could be genetic and hormonal factors.

Presentation with chest pressure and ST elevations in the anterior leads points to pathology in the left anterior descending artery.

Avoid heavy exertion. The artery may remodel, and about 80% of the lesions disappear with conservative management. Intravascular ultrasound and CT are very useful in making a diagnosis.

Conservative management is the preferred option with spontaneous healing of the dissection in the majority of uncomplicated cases.

Sometimes require PCI or CABG.

Miscellaneous

Answer: 50. A. Should be done in the last trimester of pregnancy as the fetal heart is well developed

→ It's typically done in the second trimester, between weeks 18 to 24.

Answer: 51. D. After space flight

Cardiac atrophy may be seen after space flight.

Answer: 52. C. Increased heart rate variability

Answer: 53. A. Women with MI have less comorbid conditions

Answer: 54. B. 30%

Answer: 55. B. APLA

Answer: 56. A. Only 20% of HLA B-27 patients have AS

Answer: 57. A. Saline contrast echocardiography.

In hepatopulmonary syndrome there is formation of pulmonary AV fistulas, and shunting of blood can be detected with saline contrast echocardiography.

Saline contrast echocardiography: By late appearance of bubbles on the left side (after four beats) and without Valsalva maneuver. The shunt can be qualitatively graded depending upon degree of left-sided opacification. This gets better after liver transplant.

Cardiovascular changes after long duration space flight:

- Decreased cardiac muscle mass
- Decrease HR and BP
- Decrease in cardiac output
- Increased arteriosclerosis and calcification of vessels.
- Decreased sympathetic nervous system activity
- Decreased baroreceptor reflex
- Decreased plasma volume
- Increased antidiuretic hormone

Age related cardiovascular changes:

- Decreased heart rate variability
- Decreased beta-adrenergic response
- Reduced baroreceptor sensitivity
- Reduced SA node automaticity
- Sclerosis of aortic and mitral valve
- Impaired diastolic function due to LV thickening and fibrosis
- Increase in LA size
- Impaired endothelium dependent vasodilation
- Thickening of arteries due to atherosclerosis and arteriosclerosis leading to increased afterload.
- Ejection fraction is preserved

15 Cardiac Anatomy and Physiology

Cardiac Anatomy

1. **Acute marginal artery is a branch of:**
   A. Right coronary artery
   B. LM
   C. LCx
   D. Ramus intermedius
2. **Oblique vein of Marshall drains into:**
   A. Right atrium B. Coronary sinus
   C. Left atrium D. Right ventricle
3. **The venous drainage of right ventricle is through:**
   A. Small cardiac vein
   B. Great cardiac vein
   C. Middle cardiac vein
   D. Vein of Marshall.
4. **The boundaries of the triangle of Koch do not include:**
   A. Coronary sinus
   B. Tricuspid annulus
   C. Tendon of Todaro
   D. Crista terminalis
5. **Which of the following is not an anatomic part of interatrial septum?**
   A. PFO
   B. Torus aorticus
   C. Limbus fossa ovalis
   D. Noduli of Arantius
6. **Following is an extra pericardial structure:**
   A. Ascending aorta
   B. 4 pulmonary veins
   C. Right and left pulmonary arteries
   D. Main pulmonary artery
7. **Which of the following statement is true about mitral valve?**
   A. Anterior mitral leaflet is rectangular and is divided into 3 scallops
   B. Posteromedial papillary muscle usually has multiple heads and is supplied by right coronary artery
   C. Dilatation of MV annulus primarily affects the anterior leaflet
   D. Anterolateral papillary muscle bas single blood supply
8. **All are true regarding conduction system of the heart except:**
   A. SA nodal artery arises from RCA in 55-60% of persons
   B. His bundle and bundle branches have a single blood supply from 1st septal perforator of Left anterior descending artery
   C. Both SA and AV nodes are richly innervated by sympathetic and parasympathetic fibers
   D. SA node is situated on the epicardial surface of the heart
9. **Torus aorticus is caused by:**
   A. Right aortic sinus
   B. Left aortic sinus

C. Non-coronary aortic sinus
D. Transverse sinus of pericardium

10. Most of the blood from right ventricular muscle returns through:
A. Thebasian veins
B. Oblique vein of Marshall
C. Anterior cardiac veins
D. Coronary sinus

Cardiac Physiology

11. At constant pressure if radius is doubled, the flow increases by:
A. 2 times B. 4 times
C. 8 times D. 16 times

12. LV afterload increased in all except:
A. Systolic HTN B. Aortic stiffness
C. Moderate AS D. VSD

13. LV afterload determined by:
A. Vascular distensibility
B. Ventricular wall tension
C. Vascular resistance
D. Ejection fraction

14. All are determinants of myocardial oxygen demand except:
A. Heart rate
B. Oxygen carrying capacity of blood
C. Myocardial wall tension
D. Inotropic state of heart

15. All of the following are true except?
A. Increased heart rate is associated with decreased LV contractility in normal hearts
B. Normal heart works on the steep curve part of starling forces with < 12 mmHg
C. In systolic dysfunction, stroke volume depends on preload
D. Stroke volume is dependent on afterload

16. The longest phase of the cardiac action potential is:
A. Phase 0 B. Phase 1
C. Phase 2 D. Phase 3

17. All of the following are true about Calcium channel except?
A. Membrane influx with L type channel
B. Membrane efflux with T type channel
C. SERCA for flux Ca into SR
D. Ryanodine for Ca mediated Ca release

18. Which of the following is molecular unit of gap junction?
A. Connexin
B. Desmosome
C. Phospholamban
D. Thin actin filaments

19. Which of the following statements is true regarding the cardiac cycle?
A. Cardiologic systole extends from A_2 to M_1.
B. Physiologic systole extends from the start of isovolumic contraction phase to the end of the ejection phase
C. Cardiologic systole starts and ends later than the physiologic systole
D. Cardiologic diastole includes filling phases and reduced ejection

20. Following statements are true about 'hang out' interval except:
A. Duration is related to the impedance of the vascular bed into which blood is being received
B. Normal intervals is 15 to 30 ms in systemic circulation
C. Normal interval in pulmonary circulation is 43 to 86 ms
D. Decrease in impedance in systemic vascular bed alters hang out interval and causes wide splitting of 2nd heart sound

21. Resting normal coronary blood flow in ml/minute/100 gm of myocardium:
A. 30-60 B. < 30
C. 60~90 D. 90-120

22. True about coronary flow:
A. Arterial flow is phasic and venous is continuous
B. Intramyocardial vascular volume is highest in diastole
C. Myocardial compressive force higher on epicardial vessels than on subendocardial vessels
D. Subendocardial/subepicardial ratio < 0.6

23. All of the following constrict atherosclerotic coronaries except?
A. Serotonin
B. Thromboxane
C. Endothelin
D. Papaverine

24. Which of the following is a false statement?
A. Acetylcholine requires intact endothelium to cause vasoconstriction
B. Decreased CO_2 causes cerebral vasoconstriction and syncope
C. Hypoxia causes pulmonary vasoconstriction and systemic vasodilation
D. Adenosine causes coronary vasodilation independent of endothelial function

25. All of the following are true about Nitric oxide except?
A. Selectively acts on pulmonary vessels and decreases pulmonary vascular resistance
B. Metabolized in RBCs
C. Sudden withdrawal leads to rebound increases PA pressure
D. Prolonged usage leads to methemoglobinemia

26. Excessive production of the following substance by the endothelial cells can inactivate Nitric oxide:
A. Hydrogen peroxide
B. Endothelium derived hyperpolarizing factor
C. Endothelin
D. Superoxide anion (02)

Miscellaneous

27. Contribution of cardiac myocytes to the ventricular mass is about:
A. 90%
B. 50%
C. 75%
D. 60%

28. Which of the following is not a physiological response to hypoxia?
A. Erythrocytosis
B. Hyperventilation
C. Systemic arterial vasoconstriction
D. Increased cardiac output

29. Who discovered SA node?
A. Shamroth
B. Flack and Keith
C. E Braunwald
D. Joseph Perloff

30. Tracer used to assess cardiac sympathetic denervation is:
A. 11C-meta-hydroxyephedrine
B. Technetium (99mTc) sestamibi
C. Fluorodeoxyglucose (18F)
D. None of the above

31. All of the following are true about exercise physiology except:
A. In sedentary persons, cardiac output can increase 4 times on maximal exercise
B. Pulmonary stretch receptors contribute to increased heart rate
C. Stroke volume increases with isometric exercise
D. LV enlargement reverses after few months of stopping the exercise

ANSWERS

Cardiac anatomy

Answer: 1. A. Right coronary artery

Answer: 2. B. Coronary sinus

Answer: 3. A. Small cardiac vein

Answer: 4. D. Crista terminalis

Answer: 5. D. Noduli of Arantius

Answer: 6. C. Right and left pulmonary arteries

Answer: 7. B. Posteromedial papillary muscle usually has multiple heads and is supplied by right coronary artery

Answer: 8. B. His bundle and bundle branches have a single blood supply from 1st septal perforator of Left anterior descending artery

Answer: 9. C. Non-coronary aortic sinus

Answer: 10. C. Anterior cardiac veins

The pericardium encloses the heart, portions of the vena cavae, most of the ascending aorta, the main pulmonary artery and the four pulmonary veins.

The ligament of Marshall is a pericardial fold containing the remnant of the embryonic left superior vena cava.

The right heart forms the largest part of the anterior surface, whereas the left heart is largely posterior

Posteriorly the crux ("cross") is the intersection of the AV interatrial, and interventricular grooves.

Cardiac Chambers

Right Atrium

Muscular anterior portion of RA contains pectinate muscles.

Eustachian valve: At the opening of IVC, directs blood towards foramen ovale.

Thebesian valve: Valve of coronary sinus

When the eustachian or thebesian valves are large and fenestrated, it is described as a Chiari net

Crista terminalis is a C-shaped muscular ridge on the right atrial fee wall which separates the smooth posterior portion of RA from the muscular anterior portion

The **right atrial appendage** is a large triangular structure that overlies the right coronary artery and contains pectinate muscles

In the lower medial portion of the RA, **Koch triangle** is present. The **tendon of Todaro** is a fibrous band located between the valves of the inferior vena cava and the coronary sinus.

Boundaries of Kock triangle:

1. Coronary sinus orifice
2. Tendon of Todaro
3. Septal leaflet of the right atrioventricular valve

Anatomical significance: **Atrioventricular node** is located at the apex of the triangle.

Right Ventricle

The right ventricle is the most anterior chamber of the heart

Conus (infundibulum) is present in RV while it is absent in LV.

Right ventricular apex is heavily **trabeculated**

Right ventricle contains three papillary muscles,

Crista supraventricularis (supraventricular crest) separates the inûow and outflow portions of the right ventricle

Moderator band is an intracavity muscular bridge that connects the distal septum with the right ventricular free wall at the anterior papillary muscle

Left Atrium

LA does not contain pectinate muscles except in LA appendage.

The left atrial appendage, overlying the left circumûex coronary artery is **smaller, longer, more tortuous**, and less triangular than the right atrial appendage, often containing two or more lobes

Left Ventricle

High-pressure, muscular chamber, 2.5 to 3 times thicker than the right ventricle

Two papillary muscles, the larger anterolateral and the smaller posteromedial, arise from LV free wall

True chordae attach papillary muscle to mitral leaflet.

False chordae occur in half of normal hearts, and may connect walls, papillary muscles, and the septum, but are not attached to the mitral leaflets.

Cardiac valves

Tricuspid Valve

Largest of the heart valves

Three leaflets: anterior, posterior, and septal.

The anterior leaflet is the largest and the most mobile.

Posterior leaûet is the smallest, and septal leaflet is the least mobile.

Pulmonic Valve

Most anterior and smallest valve of the heart.

Mitral valve

Two mitral leaflets, the anterior and the posterior.

The anterior leaflet is semicircular or oval shaped, broader but narrow transversely

The posterior leaflet is crescent shaped, longer and narrower, half the height but twice the length of the anterior leaflet. Both of leaflets have approximately same cross sectional area.

Unlike the tricuspid chordae, mitral chordae do not have insertions into the septum.

Aortic valve

The **nodules of Arantius** are small fibrous mounds at the center of the free edge of each cusp.

Torus aorticus: **Torus aorticus** (aortic mound) is the prominent region of the right atrial septum, which marks the projection of the non-coronary aortic sinus into the right atrial wall. The bulge is superior to the coronary sinus and anterior to the fossa ovalis.

It is superior to the coronary sinus and anterior to the fossa ovalis

→ Largest cardiac valve: Tricuspid valve

→ Smallest cardiac valve: Pulmonary valve

Coronary Arteries

Proximal aorta (aortic root) is dilated and contains the aortic valve and the sinuses of Valsalva

Coronary arteries, the first two branches of the aorta, arise from the left and the right sinus of Valsalva, respectively

Branches of right coronary artery (RCA)

Conal artery: 1st branch of RCA, supplies RVOT. In 50% people, it directly arises from right sinus of Valsalva.

SA nodal artery

Acute marginal artery

AV nodal artery

Posterior descending artery (PDA)

Posterolateral ventricular branches (PLV)

Dominant RCA (70-80%) gives PDA and PLV branches. **Codominant RCA (10-15%)** gives PDA, PLV comes from LCx; and **non-dominant RCA (10-15%)** does not give rise to PDA and PLV as both these comes from LCx.

Left main trunk varies from 3 to 10 mm in diameter and from 1 to 4 cm in length.

Bifurcates into left anterior descending (LAD) and left circumflex (LCx). In 30% people trifurcates with additional branch being ramus intermedius.

LAD travels into anterior interventricular septum and gives septal and diagonal branches.

LCx travels into left atrioventricular grove and supplies lateral and posterior wall of heart through obtuse marginal branches.

The size of LCx is inversely proportional to the RCA.

In 60% people SA nodal artery is a branch of RCA and in rest 40% it comes from LCx.

Heart gets its blood supply **during diastole** because during diastole the aortic valve will close and opens the pathway for blood to enter coronary vessels.

Increase in heart rate (tachycardia) will have shorter diastolic period and thus decreased filling time or decrease in cardiac output.

Coronary artery occlusion in myocardial infarction

Left anterior descending artery **in 50% cases**, Right coronary artery **in 30% cases** and Left circumflex artery **in 20% Cases.**

Cardiac Veins

Venous system of the heart consists of the coronary sinus, cardiac veins, and the thebesian venous system. Coronary sinus is largest cardiac vein, measuring 2-5 cm in length. It is located in posterior AV groove and drains into RA.

Tributaries of coronary sinus:

Great cardiac vein- Situated in anterior interventricular groove (with LAD)

Small cardiac vein- In posterior part of coronary sulcus (with right marginal artery)

Middle cardiac vein- In posterior interventricular groove (with PDA)

Posterior vein of left ventricle- In diaphragmatic surface of LV

Oblique vein of left atrium (Vein of Marshall)- In posterior surface of LA

Veins directly draining into RA:

Multiple small thebesian veins

Anterior cardiac veins

Coronary sinus valves:

Thebesian valve is a semi-circular fold of membrane at the orifice of coronary sinus.

Prevents regurgitation of blood into sinus during atrial contraction; might pose difficulty during cannulation of coronary sinus.

Vieussens valve is located between the coronary sinus and the great cardiac vein.

Often a flimsy valve composed of one to three leaflets found in 80% to 90% of people.

It is clinically important because it can cause an obstruction to catheters in 20% of patients.

Cardiac physiology

Answer: 11. D. 16 times

Answer: 12. D. VSD

Answer: 13. C. Vascular resistance

Answer: 14. B. Oxygen carrying capacity of blood

Answer: 15. A. Increased heart rate is associated with decreased LV contractility in normal hearts

Answer: 16. C. Phase 2

Answer: 17. B. Membrane efflux with T type channel

Answer: 18. A. Connexin

Answer: 19. C. Cardiologic systole starts and ends later than the physiologic systole

Answer: 20. D. Decrease in impedance in systemic vascular bed alters hang out interval and causes wide splitting of 2nd heart sound

Answer: 21. C. 60~90

Answer: 22. B. Intramyocardial vascular volume is highest in diastole

Answer: 23. D. Papaverine

Answer: 24. A. Acetylcholine requires intact endothelium to cause vasoconstriction

→ Acetylcholine causes vasoconstriction by endothelium independent mechanism.

→ Hypoxia causes pulmonary vasoconstriction and systemic vasodilation.

Answer: 25. A. Selectively acts on pulmonary vessels and decreases pulmonary vascular resistance

Answer: 26. D. Superoxide anion (02)

Determinants of myocardial performance

Preload

Preload is the hemodynamic load on ventricular muscles (or the degree of stretch on the myocardial fibre) at the end of diastole. It is determined mainly by left ventricular **end diastolic** volume & left ventricular end diastolic pressure, in other words - by venous return.

Measures of left ventricular (LV) preload include (a) end-diastolic volume (EDV), (b) end-diastolic pressure (EDP), (c) wall stress at end diastole, and (d) end-diastolic sarcomere length.

Increase venous return such as volume resuscitation, supine body position, atrial contraction, skeletal muscle contraction, and decreased intrathoracic pressure will increase preload, whereas conditions that **decrease venous return** such as decreased intravascular volume (severe anemia, dehydration, diuresis), venodilators (nitrates), upright posture, loss of atrial contraction (atrial fibrillation), increased intrathoracic pressure (Valsalva maneuver, positive pressure ventilation), and increased intrapericardial pressure (pericardial tamponade or constriction) will decrease preload.

Increase in preload results in increase in **contractility** that in turn increases stroke volume **&** thus increase in **ejection fraction**.

A rise in pulmonary capillary wedge pressure is evidence of increased preload on the left ventricle. In some cases, like mitral stenosis or mitral valve prolapse it is **not** a good index of left ventricular preload.

Chronic increase in preload is responsible for **dilated cardiomyopathy**

Afterload

Afterload is the resistance that the ventricle must overcome during contraction in systole.

It is **determined by peripheral arterial resistance**

Chronic increase in afterload (e.g. hypertension, increasing age) will lead to left ventricular hypertrophy.

Several surrogate measures of afterload, the most commonly used are (a) central aortic pressure, (b) systemic arterial pressure, (c) systemic vascular resistance (SVR), (d) arterial impedance, (e) myocardial peak wall stress (affected by LV geometry).

Conceptually, myocardial wall stress is the most applicable measure of afterload.

Afterload is increased by increased blood pressure (hypertension, vasoconstricting drugs), increased LV radius (LV dilatation), reduced arterial elastance (atherosclerotic "stiû" arteries), and decreased wall thickness (eccentric hypertrophy, advanced cardiomyopathy).

Afterload is decreased by decreased blood pressure (vasodilator therapy), increased arterial elastance, and thicker, smaller LV cavities.

Peripheral resistance is calculated as:

Blood flow = Pressure / Resistance (F=ΔP/R), therefore **R = ΔP/F**

$$R \alpha \frac{\eta L}{r^4} \quad and \; F \alpha \frac{r^4 \Delta P}{\eta L}$$

R: Resistance, L: length of vessel, r: Radius of vessel, F: Flow.

Hence, flow is **directly** and resistance is **inversely** proportional **to the 4th power of radius** of vessel.

If the resistance will increase, then the blood flow will decrease and the heart will have to pump more amount of blood against more resistance.

Chronically it will lead to systolic dysfunction (impaired contractility) & diastolic dysfunction (impaired ventricular relaxation).

Myocardial Performance

Myocardial performance reûects the ability of the heart to meet the metabolic demands of the body. The principal determinants of ventricular myocardial performance are

1. Preload
2. Afterload
3. Contractility
4. Lusitropy (diastolic function)
5. Heart rate

Clinically reflected in the form of stroke volume or cardiac output.

Stroke volume

Stroke volume is the **amount of blood** that heart pump out with each beat. It is affected by contractility, afterload & preload.

Stroke volume is calculated as:

SV = EDV (End Diastolic Volume) – ESV (End Systolic Volume)

Ejection fraction

Is the **fraction of blood** that heart pump out during **1 contraction** which is usually 60- 70% in healthy normal adult

Ejection fraction is calculated as – **Ejection Fraction** = Stroke volume/End diastolic volume

Now as SV = EDV – ESV, therefore, **EF** = EDV – ESV/EDV

Cardiac output

Is the **amount of blood** that heart pump out during **1 minute**

Cardiac output is calculated as: **CO** = Heart rate * Stroke volume.

So if the heart rate is 72/min, and stroke volume is 70 ml, then cardiac output in 1 minute = 5000ml or 5 L/min.

According to the Fick's principle,

CO = Rate of oxygen consumption / Arterial oxygen content – Venous oxygen content

Starling's Law

Starling's law dictates that cardiac performance (defined by SV) increases as preload is increased. However, there is a nonlinear relationship between EDP (a measure of preload) and SV.

Anrep effect

An increase in afterload will increase contractility of heart.

Bowditch effect

An increase in heart rate will increase contractility of heart.

Also known as the Treppe phenomenon, Treppe effect or staircase effect.

Action Potential in Fast Response Fibres (Cardiac Muscles, His-Purkinje System)

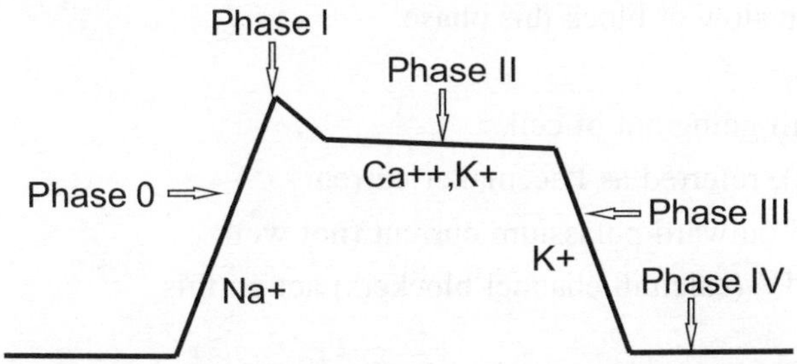

Cardiac Action Potentials in Fast Response Fibres

Phase 0 is phase of depolarization - Depends on number of sodium channels (Na+ coming into the cell) which in turn depends on resting membrane potential of cell.

Contractions occur during this phase (atrial depolarisation – P wave, ventricular depolarization – first half of QRS complex).

Class I antiarrhythmic (procainamide, quinidine) blocks phase 0 in fast response fibres.

Phase I is overshoot - Na+ channels are inactivated. **Overshoot** develops because of potassium going out of cell & inward chloride current.

Phase II is plateau phase - Balanced by slow calcium current going into the cell and slow potassium current going out of cell. It is the longest phase of cardiac action potential.

Phase III is repolarisation phase - Delayed potassium rectifier current rapidly increases and calcium channels get inactivated.

Class III antiarrhythmic (amiodarone, sotalol) slow down this phase.

Atrial repolarization is not seen on ECG, usually hidden behind QRS complex, T wave indicates ventricular repolarization.

Phase IV is return of membrane to resting potential.

Maintained by Na^+/K^+ ATPase pump, which send 2 sodium ions out of the cell in exchange of 3 potassium ions. Phase IV is flat in fast fibres.

Action Potentials in Slow Response Fibres (SA & AV Nodes)

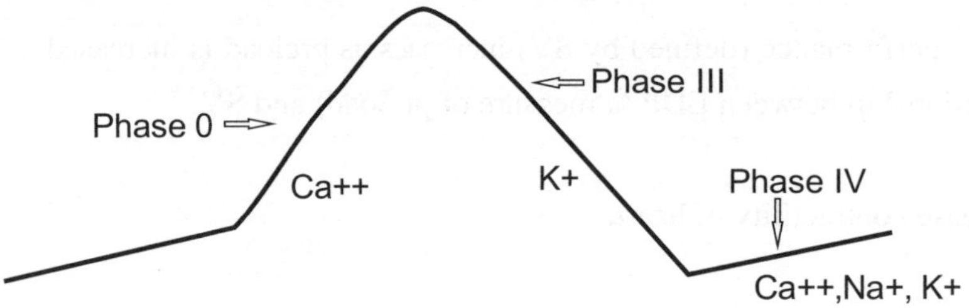

Cardiac Action Potentials in Slow Response Fibres

Phase 0: Dependent on **calcium channels** (not on sodium channels).

With each depolarization SA node sends signal to contract the heart.

Class IV antiarrhythmic (verapamil, diltiazem) can slow or block this phase.

Phase I & II is not present in SA & AV node.

Phase III is repolarisation phase, due to potassium going out of cell.

Phase IV is rising slope (not flat as in fast fibres), referred as Pacemaker current.

It is due to inward sodium & calcium current and outward potassium current (not well understood yet). Class II (beta blockers) & class IV (calcium channel blockers) act on this phase and decreases heart rate.

Gap junctions

GAP junction channels are the functional units that produce direct ionic communication between cardiac cells

Play a major role in the propagation of the AP from one myocardial cell to the next.

The molecular unit of the GAP junction is a protein called connexin.

The oligomerization of six connexins forms a connexon, and two connexons form the final channel called the GAP junction

Connexin 43 is the **most abundant** in myocardial cells.

They are almost absent in the sinus node, are found in low concentration in various areas of the atrioventricular node.

Conduction system

The sinus node is located beneath the **epicardial surface** of the crista terminalis, at its junction with the high right atrium.

Spindle-shaped structure and measures an average 10 to 20 mm in the long axis and 2 to 3 mm in the transverse axis.

Composed of a cumulus of small cells called **P cells;** the main component of the natural pacemaker.

Transitional cells called **T cells** surround the P cells and transmit the impulse generated by the P cells to the surrounding atrium.

Cells within the sinus node demonstrate spontaneous diastolic depolarization, initiating APs in a repetitive fashion.

Sinus node cells **do not** possess the GAP junction protein connexin 43. Therefore, electrical coupling at the node center is poor, reflected as a **low conduction velocity**.

The impulse generated at the sinoatrial node is next transmitted to the AVN through atrial myocytes.

There is anatomic evidence for the presence of **three atrionodal pathways** traversing the right atrium. A fourth pathway called Bachmann bundle, derived from the anterior atrionodal pathway, directs impulse propagation to the left atrium via the interatrial septum.

The **AVN** is a fusiform structure located **subendocardially** along the annular regions of the interatrial septum, with its distal end, the compact node, at the superior corner of the triangle of Koch

The **triangle of Koch** is defined by the insertion of the septal leaflet of the tricuspid valve, the tendon of Todaro, and the line that connect the ostium of the coronary sinus and the tricuspid annulus.

Circulation to the AVN is provided in nearly 90% of individuals by branches of the right coronary artery.

The His bundle is the anatomic structure that connects the compact AVN to the bundle branches.

Speed of conduction - Purkinje > Atria > Ventricles > AV node > SA node

Pacemakers rhythm generation - SA (60-100/min) > AV (40-60/min) > bundle of His/Purkinje (20-40/min).

SA node (Pacemaker) - Uses calcium to generate action potential. Atrial and ventricular **muscle** depolarization is **sodium** dependent

Cardiac contractility

- Each myofibril comprises sarcomeres made up of thick myosin filaments and thin actin filaments that form the basic contractile unit of the cardiac myocyte.
- The active sites of the actin filaments are covered in the resting state by two regulatory proteins, tropomyosin and troponin.

- Both T type (transient) and L type (long lasting) calcium channels cause **influx of calcium into cells** after a depolarizing signal. Intracellular calcium is the most important determinant of myocardial contractility and relaxation.
- Once contraction ensues, calcium entry through L-type calcium channels triggers an exponential release of calcium from the sarcoplasmic reticulum (SR) through **ryanodine receptors.**
- Calcium then binds troponin, leading to a conformational alteration of tropomyosin, exposing the actin active site, facilitating a "sliding" interaction between the actin filaments and the myosin heads as well as the hydrolysis of ATP, thus providing energy for contraction.
- Following a cycle of excitation-contraction coupling, diastolic relaxation is initiated by cytosolic calcium sequestration in the SR by the SR-Ca2• ATPase **(SERCA2a) pump (-75%)** and exportation extracellularly by the Na•/Ca2• exchanger (-25%) located on the sarcolemmal membrane.
- Phospholamban is a regulatory protein that exerts an **inhibitory effect on SERCA2a**, limiting its ability to remove cytosolic Ca2• following contraction.
- In failing hearts, phospholamban expression is altered and SERCA activity is decreased, resulting in diastolic and systolic dysfunction.

Beta adrenergic signalling

- Catecholamines acting on beta 1-adrenergic receptor stimulation leading to G protein-mediated adenyl cyclase activation and cAMP generation.
- It triggers protein kinase A (PKA)¬ dependent phosphorylation of voltage-gated L-type Ca• channels, ryanodine receptors, and phospholamban, which derepresses SERCA2a, leading to excitation-contraction coupling and positive inotropy.
- Beta 2-Adrenergic receptors as well as muscarinic cholinergic receptors, through an inhibitory G protein, provide negative control of adrenergic stimulation by inactivating adenyl cyclase, thereby limiting the generation of cAMP.

Effects of inotropic agents:

Agent	Receptor	Action
Phenylephrine	Only alpha agonist	Increase afterload
Isoproterenol	Beta 1 and 2 agonist	Increase contractility, heart rate and decrease afterload
Nor-epinephrine	Alpha > Beta 1 agonist, No Beta 2 action	Marked increase in afterload, modest increase in cardiac output
Dobutamine	Beta 1 > beta 2 and alpha agonist	Increase CO, decrease SVR, Increase in HR with or without small reduction in BP
Dopamine	Dopamine receptor (<4 μ/kg/min) Beta 1 receptor (4-10 μ/kg/min) Alpha 1 receptor (>10 μ/kg/min)	Moderate dose- Increase contractility, HR and CO. High dose- Vasoconstriction and increase SVR.

Cardiac cycle:

Described by Wiggers and Lewis.

Left Ventricular Contraction
Isovolumic contraction Maximal ejection
Left Ventricular Relaxation
Start of relaxation and reduced ejection
Isovolumic relaxation
LV filling: rapid phase
Slow LV filling (diastasis)
Atrial systole

Physiologic systole lasts from the start of isovolumic contraction to the peak of the ejection phase.

Includes:

- Isovolumic contraction
- Maximal ejection

Physiologic diastole commences as Ca2+ is taken back into the SR, so that myocyte relaxation dominates over contraction, and as the LV pressure starts to fall till the start of isovolumic contraction.

Includes:

- Reduced ejection
- Isovolumic relaxation
- Filling phases

Cardiologic systole is longer than physiologic systole and is demarcated by the interval between the first heart sound (M1) to the closure of the aortic valve (A2).

Includes:

- Major part of isovolumic contraction
- Maximal ejection
- Reduced ejection

The remainder of the cardiac cycle (A2 to M1) automatically becomes cardiologic diastole.

Protodiastole is the early phase of rapid filling, the time when S3 can be heard.

Hangout interval:

Time interval from cross over of pressures to actual occurence of semilunar valve sound (A2 and P2) is called hangout interval.

Hangout interval is lesser on aortic (15-30 ms) than pulmonary side (50-80 ms).

This difference produces normal split of S2.

Systemic circulation: Higher pressure, high resistance and less distensibility (low compliance) in systemic vessels → Recoil from the ejection of blood is brisk → Earlier aortic valve closure; A2 comes immediately after LV ejection → Smaller hangout interval

Pulmonary circulation: Low resistance and high compliance (distensibility) → Recoil is delayed → Delayed PV closure; P2 comes delated after RV ejection → Longer hangout interval

Decrease in the impedance in systemic vascular bed will cause increase in hangout interval of aortic valve and hence, lead to **narrow** split of second heart sound.

Coronary blood flow:

Minimum during systole and maximum during diastole.

Determinants of myocardial consumption:

Myocardial oxygen extraction is **near-maximal at rest**, in contrast to most other vascular beds.

Therefore, increases in myocardial oxygen consumption are primarily met by proportional increases in coronary flow and oxygen delivery.

The **major determinants** of myocardial oxygen consumption:

1. Heart rate
2. Systolic pressure (or myocardial wall tension)
3. Left ventricular (LV) contractility

Coronary autoregulation:

Resting coronary blood flow under normal hemodynamic conditions: **70 to 100 mL/min/100g.**

Can increase between **four and fivefold** during vasodilation.

The ability to increase flow above resting values in response to pharmacologic vasodilation is termed coronary flow reserve.

Subendocardium is more prone for myocardial ischemia as compared to epicardial area.

Subendocardial flow occurs primarily in diastole and begins to decrease below a mean coronary pressure of 40 mm Hg.

In contrast, subepicardial flow occurs throughout the cardiac cycle and is maintained until coronary pressure falls below 25 mm Hg.

Coronary artery resistance

R1 is epicardial conduit artery resistance, which normally is insignificant; R2 is resistance secondary to metabolic and autoregulatory adjustments in flow and occurs in arterioles and small arteries; and R3 is the time-varying epicardial compressive resistance that is higher in subendocardial than subepicardial layers.

In the normal heart: **R2 > R3 > R1.**

The development of a proximal stenosis or pharmacologic vasodilation reduces arteriolar resistance (R2).

In the presence of a severe epicardial stenosis: **R1 > R3 > R2**

Endothelium dependent modulation of coronary tone:

Acetylcholinc normally dilates arteries through an endothelium-dependent relaxing factor which is nitric oxide (NO).

NO binds to guanylyl cyclase and increases cyclic guanosine monophosphate (cGMP),

resulting in vascular smooth muscle relaxation.

When the endothelium is removed or is diseased, the dilation to acetylcholine is converted to vasoconstriction, reflecting the effect of muscarinic vascular smooth muscle contraction.

SUBSTANCE	ENDOTHELIUM DEPENDENT	NORMAL RESPONSE	ATHEROSCLEROSIS
Acetylcholine			
Conduit	Nitric oxide	Net dilation	Constriction
Resistance	Nitric oxide, EDHF	Dilation	Attenuated dilation
Norepinephrine			
Conduit			
Alpha1	—	Constriction	Constriction
Beta1 and Beta2	Nitric oxide	Dilation	Attenuated dilation
Resistance			
Alpha1	—	Constriction	Constriction
Alpha2	Nitric oxide	No effect	Constriction
Beta2		Dilation	Dilation
Platelets			
Thrombin	Nitric oxide	Dilation	Constriction
Serotonin			
Conduit	Nitric oxide	Constriction	Constriction
Resistance	Nitric oxide	Dilation	Constriction
Adenosine Diphosphate (ADP)			
	Nitric oxide	Dilation	Attenuated dilation
Thromboxane			
	Endothelin	Constriction	Constriction
Paracrine Agonists			
Bradykinin	Nitric oxide, EDHF	Dilation	Attenuated dilation
Histamine	Nitric oxide	Dilation	Attenuated dilation
Substance P	Nitric oxide	Dilation	Attenuated dilation
Endothelin (ET)			
ET-1	Nitric oxide	Net constriction	Increased constriction

Nitric oxide:

Nitric oxide is produced in endothelial cells by the enzymatic conversion of **L-arginine** to citrulline via type III nitric oxide synthase (NOS).

Metabolized in RBCs and excreted by kidneys in urine as nitrates and nitrites.

Binds to guanylyl cyclase, increasing cGMP production and causing relaxation through a reduction in intracellular calcium.

NO causes vasodilation in systemic as well as pulmonary vessels, decreases platelet aggregation and leukocyte adhesion to endothelium.

NO-mediated vasodilation is impaired in many disease states such as atherosclerosis, hypertension and diabetes.

This occurs via inactivation of NO by **superoxide anion** generated in response to oxidative stress.

Endothelin:

The endothelins—ET-1, ET-2, and ET-3—are peptide endothelium-dependent constricting factors.

The effects of endothelin are mediated by binding to both ETA and ETB receptors.

ETA-mediated constriction is caused by the activation of protein kinase C in vascular smooth muscle.

ETB predominantly causes **vasodilation** by **ETB-mediated endothelium-dependent NO production**.

Pharmacologic coronary vasodilators:

1. Nitroglycerine
2. Calcium channel blockers
3. Adenosine and A_2 receptor agonists
4. Dipyridamole
5. Papaverine

Miscellaneous

Answer: 27. C. 75%

Answer: 28. C. Systemic arterial vasoconstriction

Answer: 29. B. Flack and Keith

Answer: 30. A. 11C-meta-hydroxyephedrine

Answer: 31. C. Stroke volume increases with isometric exercise

16 Image Based Questions in Cardiology

Electrocardiography

1. **A 45-year-old patient presents to the emergency with severe chest pain. The 12-lead ECG done at the time of presentation is shown below. The likely diagnosis is:**

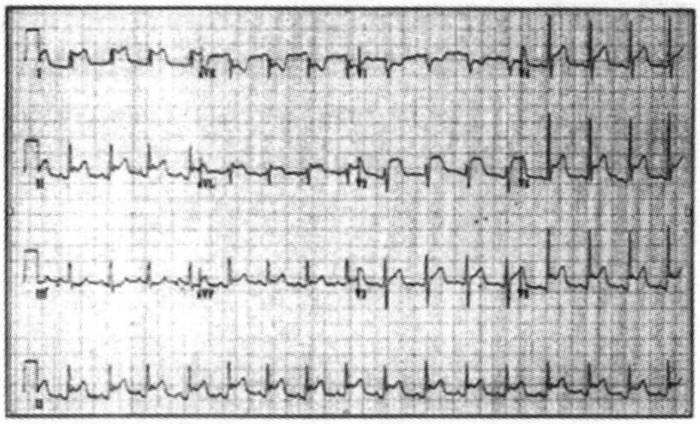

   A. Acute pulmonary embolism
   B. Acute pericarditis
   C. STEMI (left main coronary artery occlusion)
   D. STEMI (distal LAD occlusion)

2. **A 10-year-old child has history of palpitation. The ECG at the time of symptoms is shown below. The likely anatomical site of origin of ventricular premature contraction is:**

   A. Right ventricle outflow tract
   B. Right ventricle apex

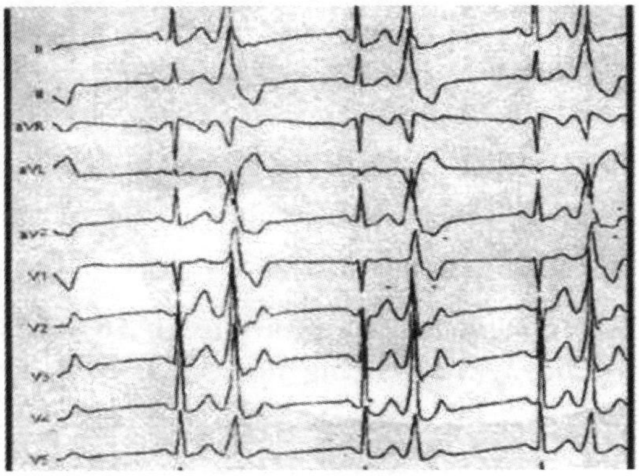

   C. Left ventricular outflow tract
   D. Interventricular septum

3. **20 years old boy with history of witnessed aborted sudden cardiac arrest when he awoke suddenly to answer a telephone call. In hospital he had an episode of ventricular fibrillation for which he was cardioverted. His elder sister had sudden cardiac death at the age of 18 years. What is most probable diagnosis?**

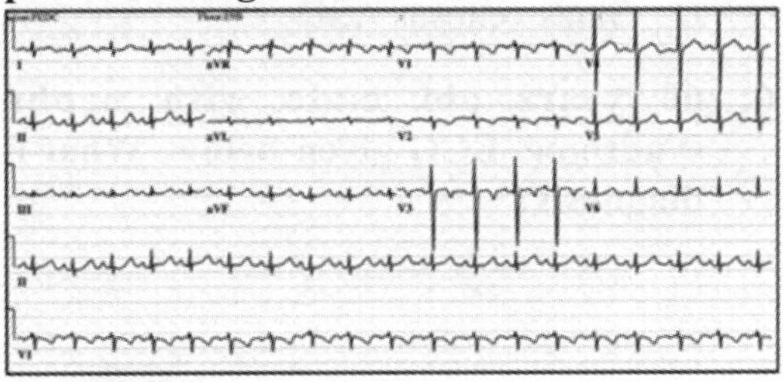

   A. HOCM
   B. Long QT syndrome

C. RVOT tachycardia
D. Idiopathic VF

4. Most likely site of accessory pathway:

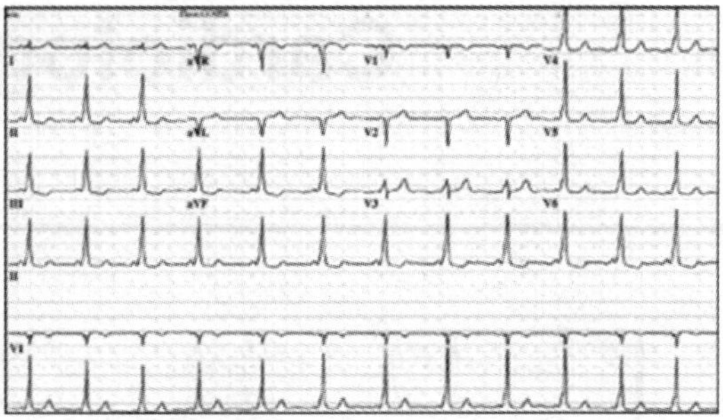

A. Left lateral
B. Left posterior
C. Right posteroseptal
D. Right anterolateral

5. Intermittent palpitations in 16 years old boy. ASD is being suspected:

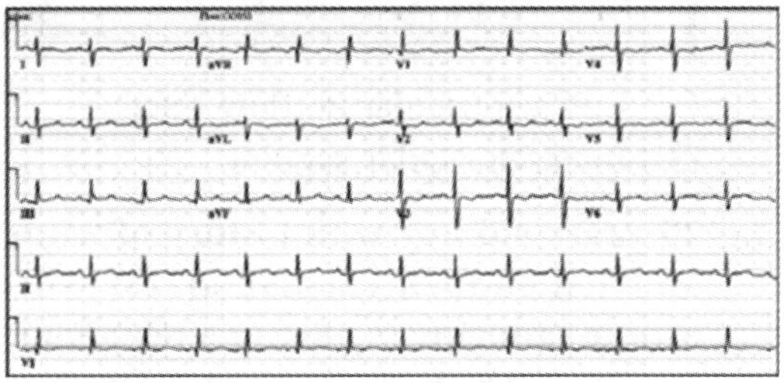

A. OS-ASD
B. OP-ASD
C. Coronary sinus ASD
D. Sinus venosus ASD

6. 60 years old male with nephrotic syndrome. ECG given below. What is the diagnosis?

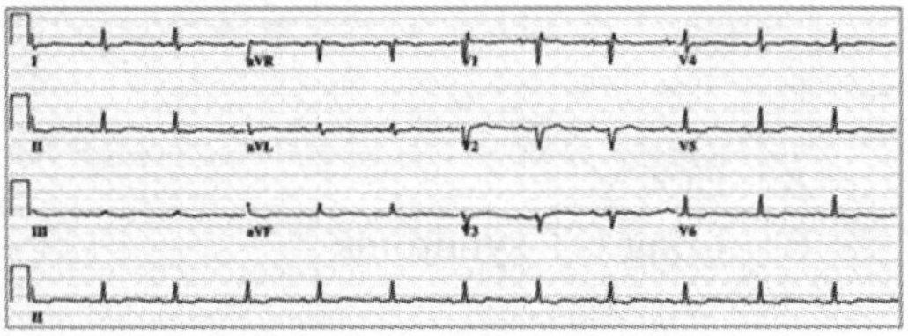

A. Amyloid heart disease
B. HCM
C. Hypertensive heart disease
D. Severe mitral valve regurgitation

7. Which of the following is true about this patient?

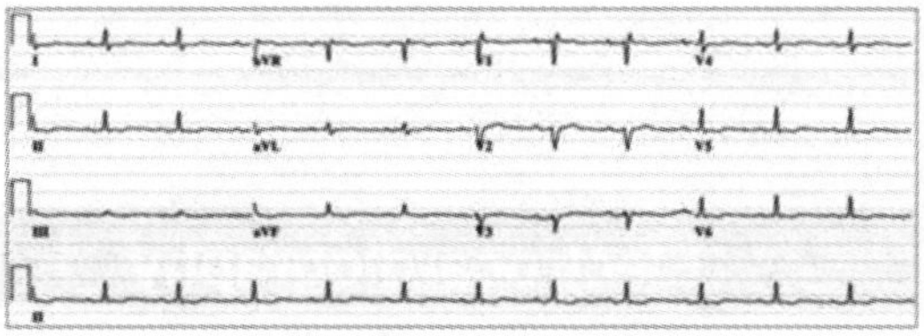

A. Asymmetric septal hypertrophy
B. Hypertrophied interatrial septum
C. Normal BNP
D. Isolated circumflex artery occlusion

8. 60 years old male patient underwent routine ECG (shown below). He does not have any history of heart disease and is presently asymptomatic. What should be the next investigation?

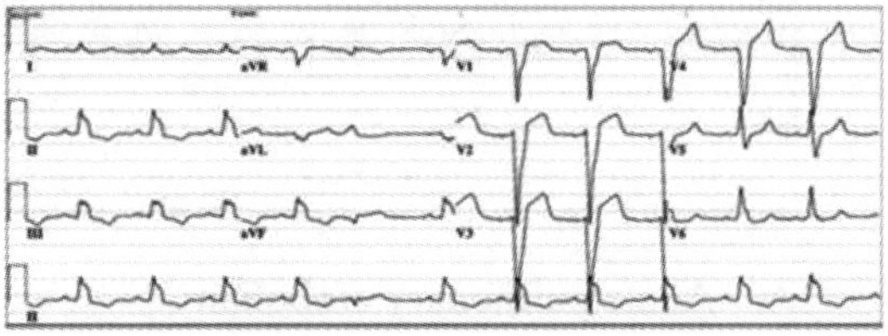

A. Stress thallium
B. Echocardiography
C. Coronary angiography
D. None of the above

9. Patient presents to emergency with chest pain and hypotension. Which of the following is correct diagnosis?

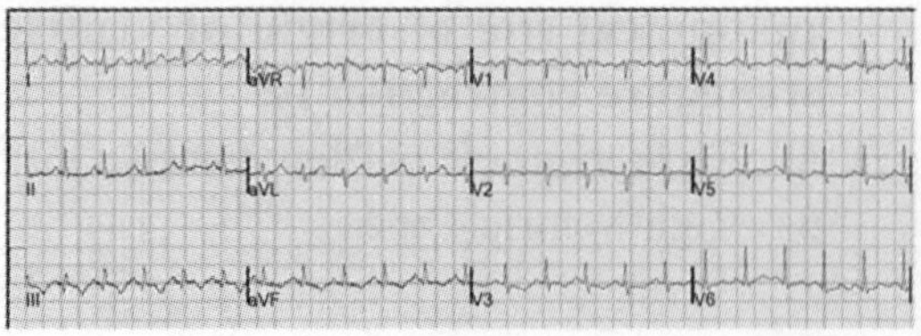

A. Acute pulmonary embolism
B. RCA occlusion
C. Acute stroke
D. ARVC

10. 30-year-old male patient presented with palpitations. What is the diagnosis?

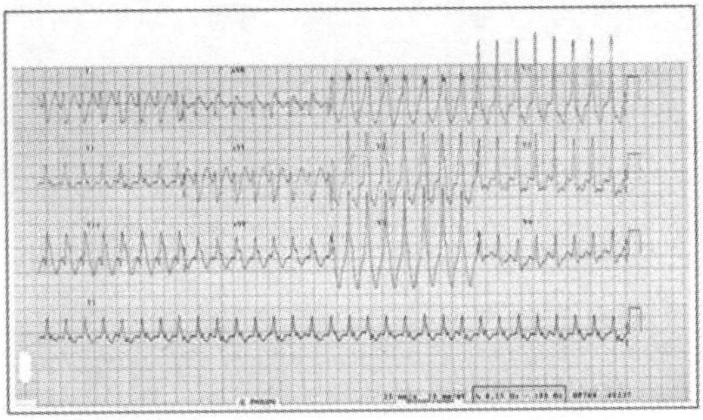

A. Belhassen tachycardia
B. Left accessory pathway tachycardia
C. Atrial tachycardia
D. Anteroseptal MI

11. Patient presents to emergency with palpitations, shortness of breath and shock. Immediate treatment:

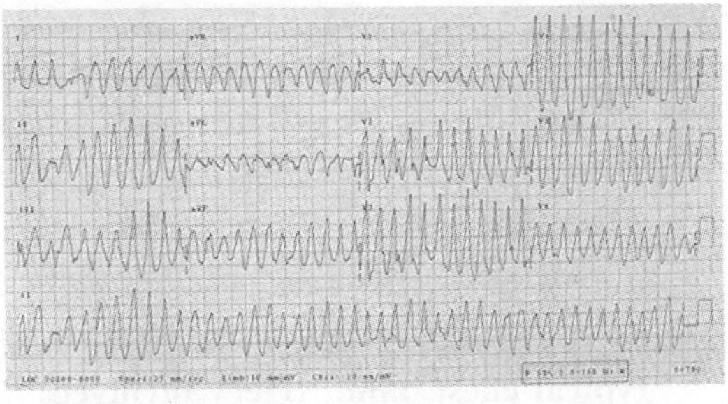

A. DC cardioversion
B. IV Magnesium
C. IV Calcium
D. IV Amiodarone

12. Based on the following ECG, all of the following are correct except:

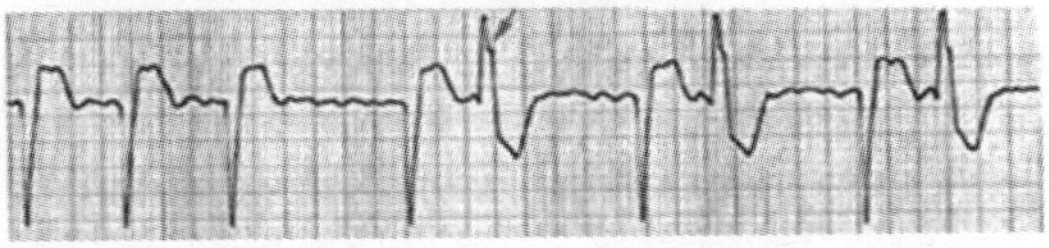

A. Tracing shows RBBB morphology usually
B. Origin of broad QRS below AV node
C. Short coupling predisposed to ventricular fibrillation
D. Baseline rhythm is atrial fibrillation

13. A 16-year-old boy presented with episode of syncope. ECG showed the following. Which of the following tests needs to be done?

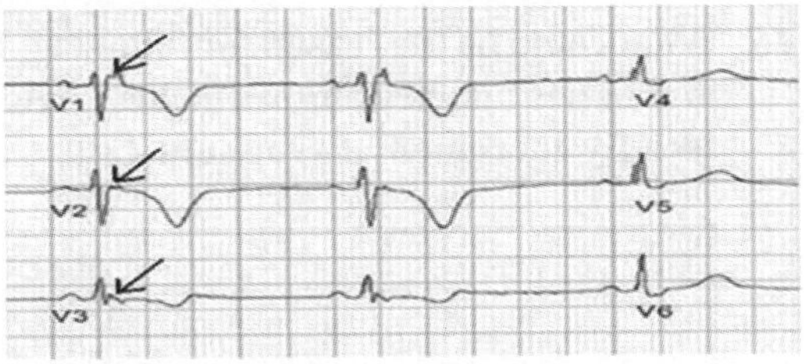

A. MRI
B. Electrophysiologic studies
C. Endomyocardial biopsy
D. Metabolic study

14. All of the following can cause following pattern of ECG except:

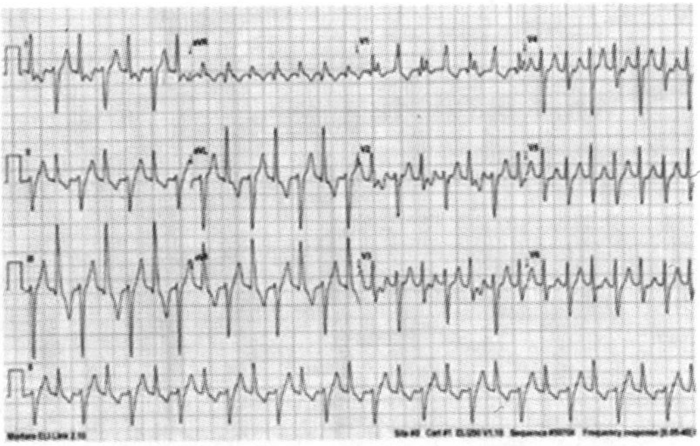

A. Digoxin toxicity
B. Anderson syndrome
C. Aconite poisoning
D. LQTS

15. What is the correct diagnosis?

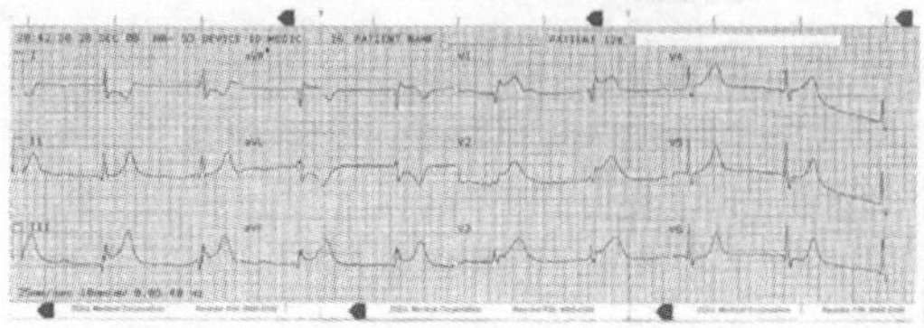

A. Inferior wall MI with AV block
B. Posterior wall MI
C. Anterior wall MI
D. Acute coronary dissection

16. What could be the reason for following ECG in a patient presenting with chest pain and serially incremental troponin I?

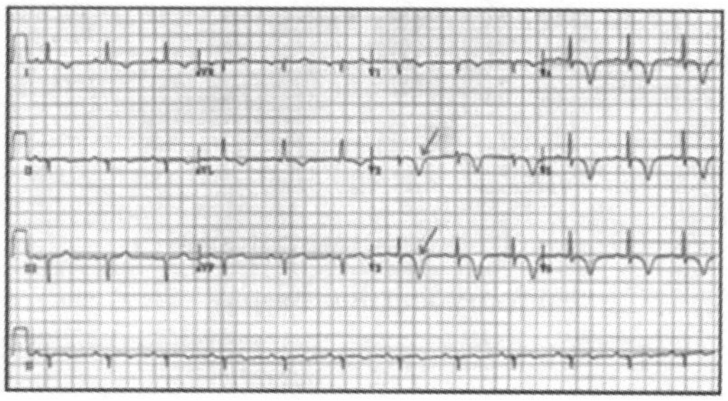

A. Critical LAD stenosis
B. LMCA
C. SAH
D. Electrolyte

17. What is the diagnosis?

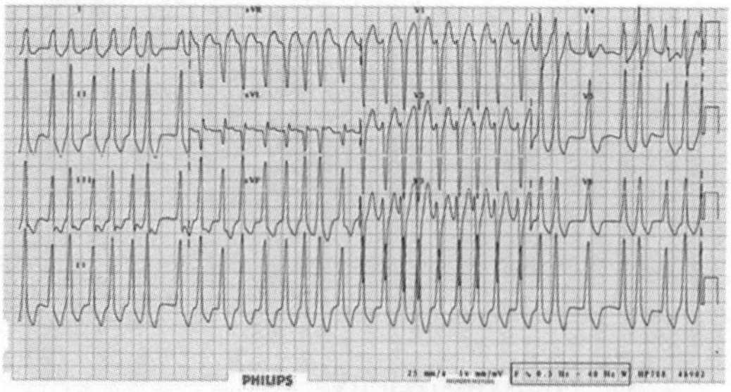

A. AF with antidromic conduction over fast pathway
B. Supraventricular tachycardia with aberrancy
C. Atrial tachycardia with fast ventricular rate
D. Ventricular tachycardia

18. In a 25-year-old male, following ECG is suggestive of:

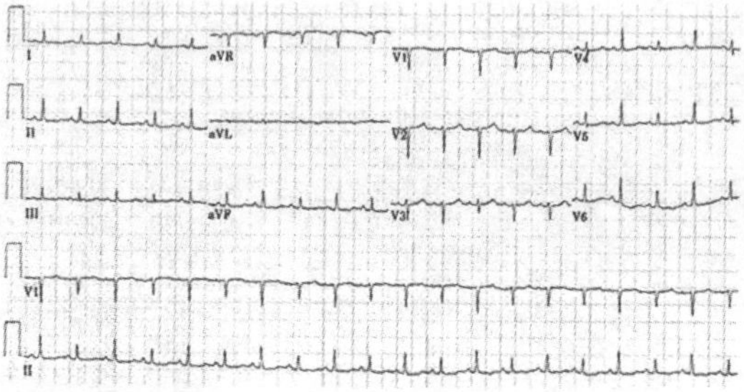

A. Seizure
B. Stroke
C. Metabolic abnormalities
D. Hypotension

19. Which of the following will be seen in this patient?

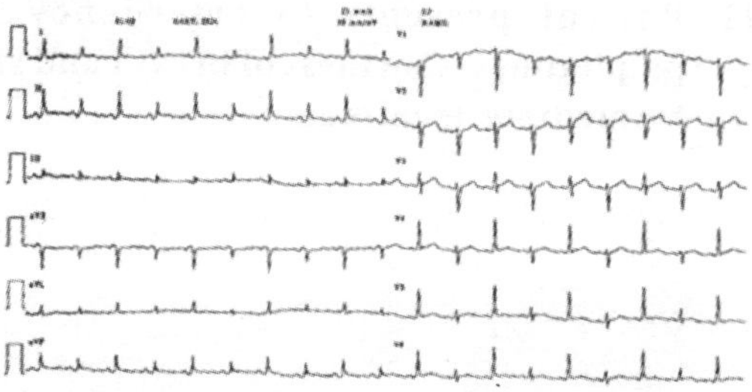

A. Hypotension
B. Cyanosis
C. Hypothyroidism
D. Digoxin toxicity

20. ECG of patient is given who presented with typical chest pain. Artery involved:

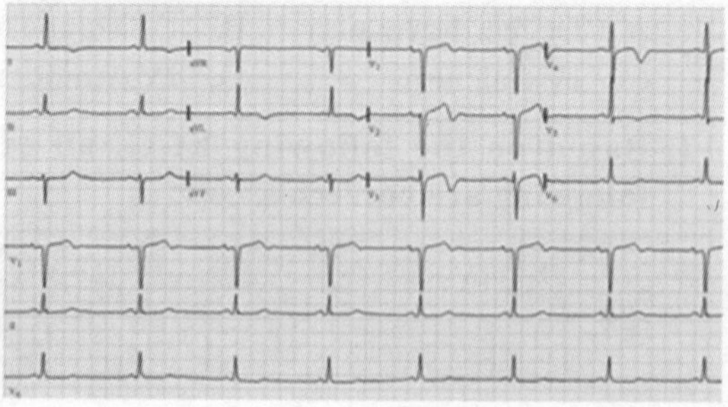

A. Proximal LAD
B. Distal LAD
C. Prominent dominant circumflex
D. Normal coronaries

21. Which of the following is correct diagnosis?

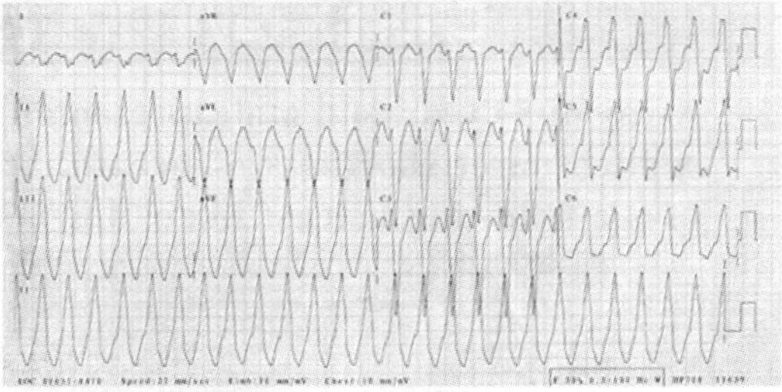

A. RV inflow VT
B. RV outflow VT
C. Mahaim tachycardia
D. LVOT VT

22. Patient is given tenecteplase 30 mins back for acute MI. Chest pain resolved. ECG was done:

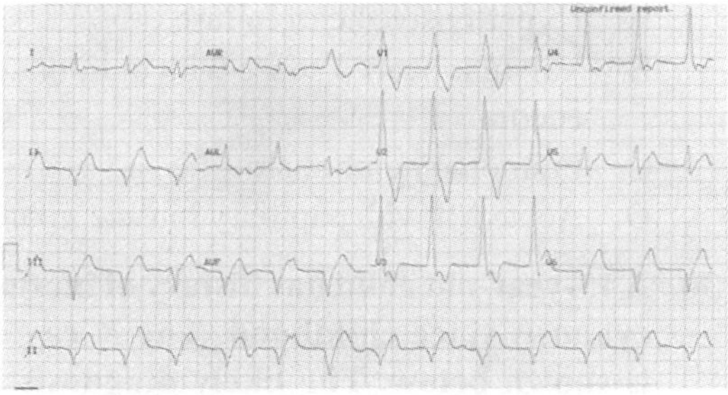

A. Rescue PCI
B. It is highly specific for reperfusion
C. Nothing is to be done
D. Atrial pacing or atropine may help control it

23. A patient present with palpitations and sweating. What should be given?
A. Verapamil
B. Amiodarone

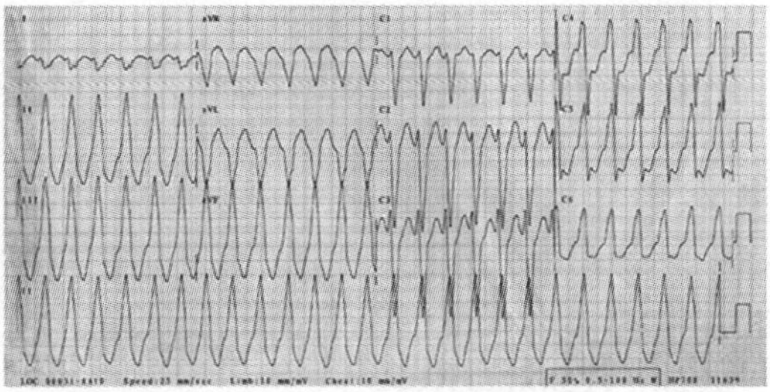

C. Sotalol
D. Flecanide

24. ECG shows:

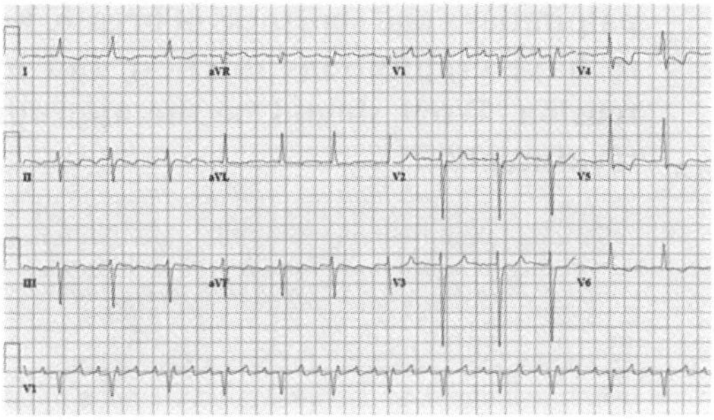

A. Atrial flutter
B. AVNRT with 2:1 block
C. EAT
D. PJRT

25. All of the following can be given for provocation except:

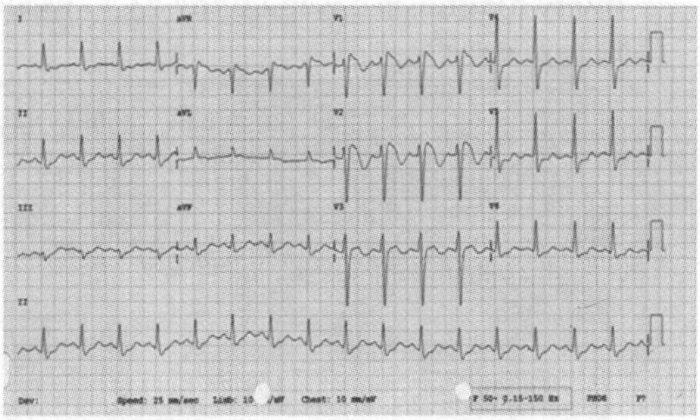

A. Quinidine
B. Ajmaline
C. Procainamide
D. Flecainide

26. A patient presented with history of chest pain. ECG given. What is the site of block?

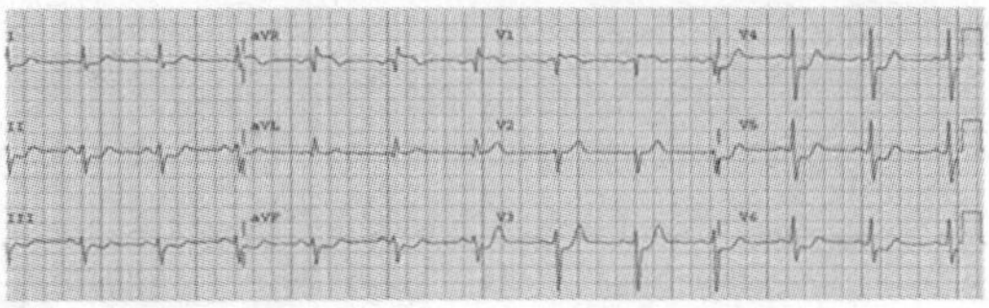

A. Proximal RCA
B. Proximal LAD
C. LMCA
D. Left circumflex

27. 50 years old male patient presented with palpitations and shortness of breath. Found to have crepitations in chest and hypotension. What should be the appropriate treatment?

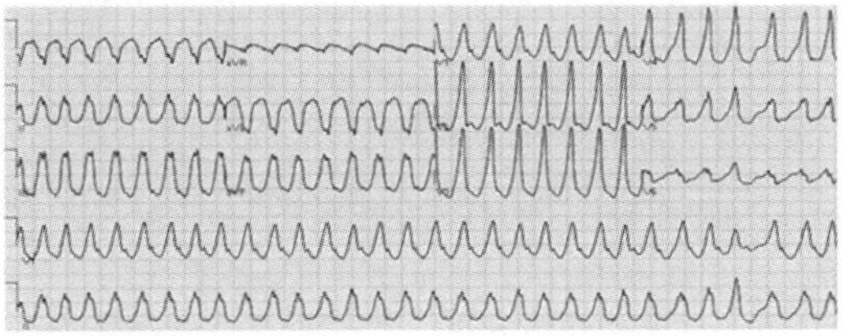

A. DC shock
B. Anticoagulant
C. Thrombolysis
D. CT angiography

28. A 43-year-old patient presents with sudden onset palpitation and hypotension. The likely diagnosis based on the ECG as shown below is:

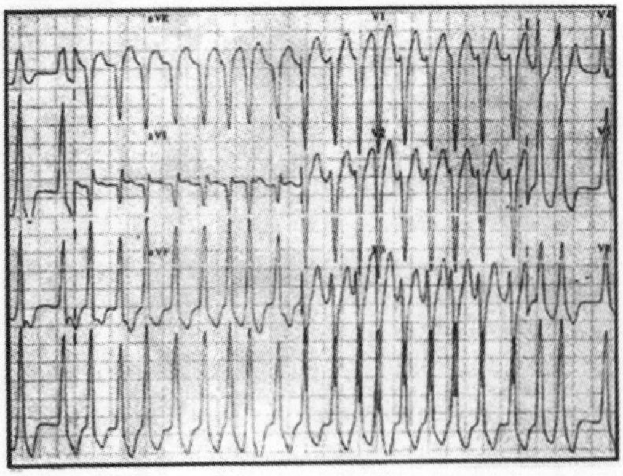

A. Polymorphic ventricular tachycardia
B. Atrial fibrillation with antidromic AVRT
C. Persistent junctional reciprocating tachycardia (MT)
D. PSVT with aberrant conduction

Chest X-ray

29. X-ray of 50 years old male, presented with sudden onset shortness of breath. Which of the following is least likely diagnosis?

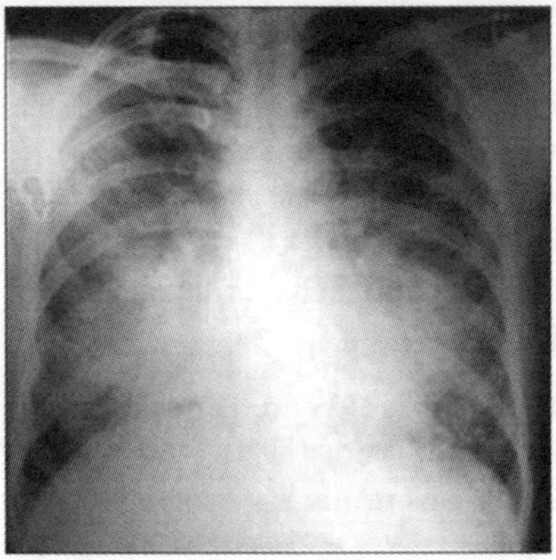

A. Hypertensive heart failure
B. Valvular heart disease with pulmonary edema
C. Pulmonary embolism
D. Acute MI with papillary muscle infarction

30. A 15-year-old child has history of increasing cyanosis since childhood. The X-ray chest is shown below. The likely diagnosis is:

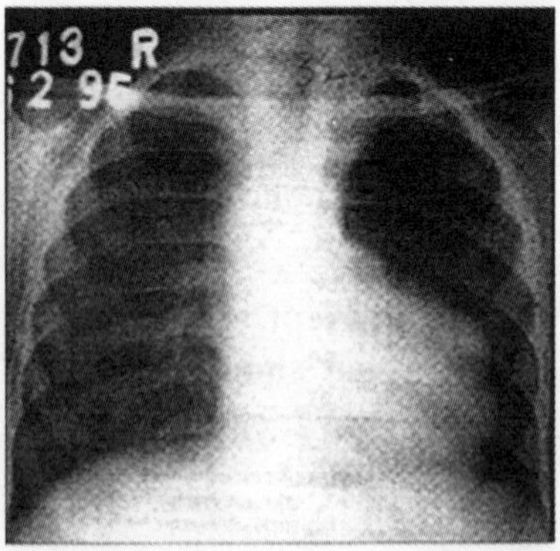

A. ASD with Eisenmenger Syndrome
B. d-transposition of great arteries (d-TGA)
C. Ebstein's anomaly
D. Tricuspid atresia

31. 60 years old male patient with history of CABG, ten years back. Now admitted with drug refractory generalized edema. CXR is shown below. What should be the optimum strategy for the management of this patient?

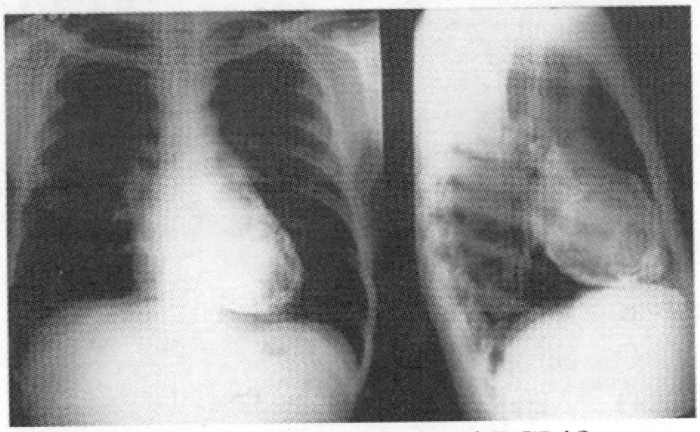

A. Coronary angiography and PCI if required
B. Stress testing
C. CT chest and surgery consultation
D. Discharge and follow up in liver clinic

32. A boy presented for evaluation of shortness of breath. Which of the following is likely diagnosis?

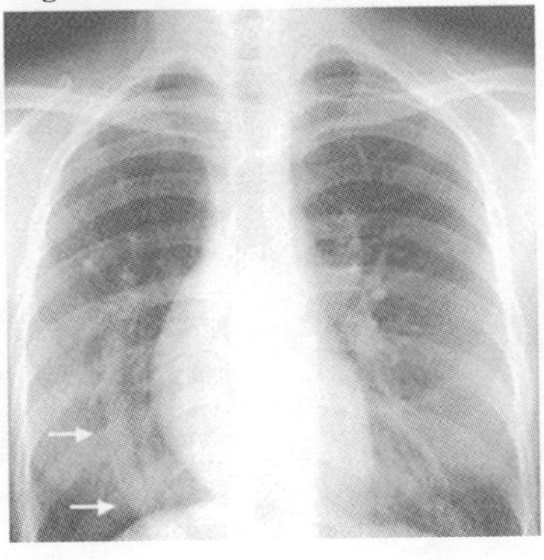

A. Primary pulmonary hypertension
B. Atrial septal defect
C. Ebstein anomaly
D. Scimitar syndrome

33. Which of the following is true about this patient?

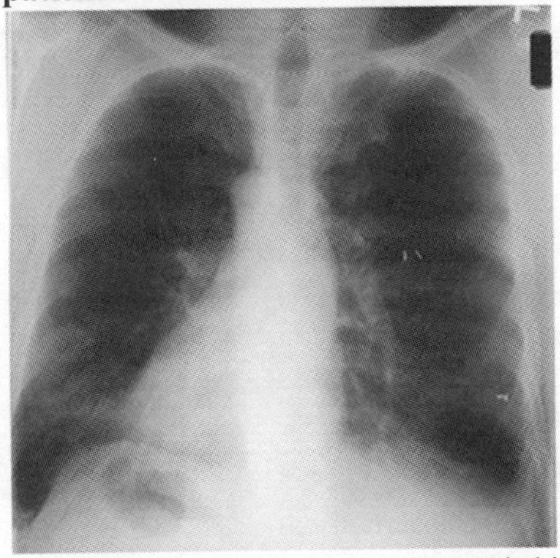

A. Risk of congenital heart disease is high
B. Inheritance is autosomal dominant
C. Chest X-ray shows situs solitus with dextrocardia
D. He is likely to have recurrent otitis media/sinusitis

34. Patient underwent permanent pacemaker implantation. In the evening, the condition of patient worsened. This patient is likely to present with:

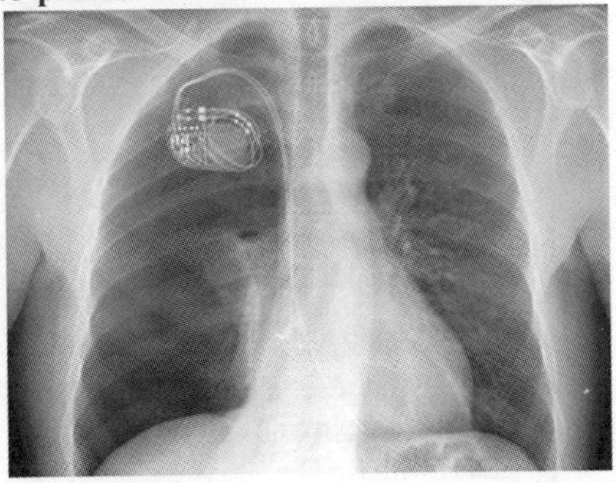

A. Dyspnea B. Dysphagia
C. Syncope D. Anuria

35. Patient underwent permanent pacemaker implantation. In the evening, the patient developed shortness of breath. What should be appropriate management?

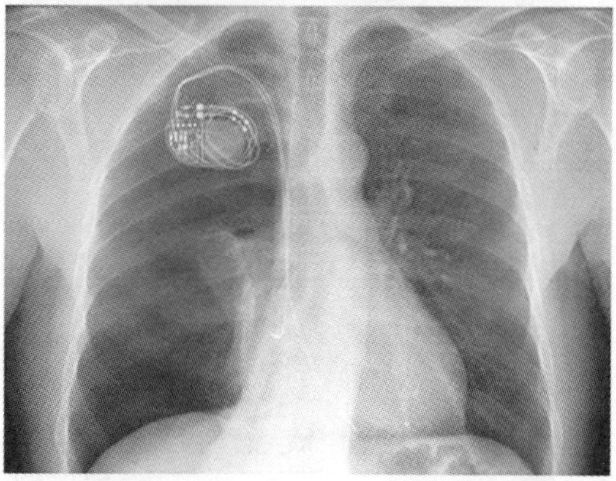

A. ICD insertion
B. Open heart surgery
C. Re-implantation
D. Conservative

36. CXR of a 14-year-old boy with cyanosis is given. ECG will show:

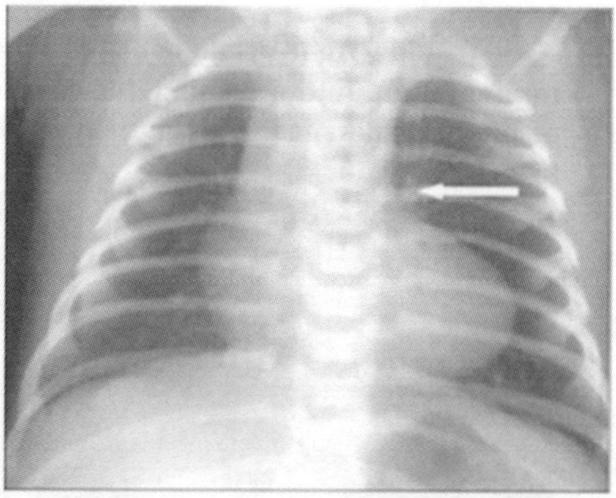

A. RVH with RAD
B. LVH with LAD
C. RVH with extreme axis deviation
D. LVH with RAD

37. A post-operative CXR of a child with congenital heart disease is given. Identify the structure:

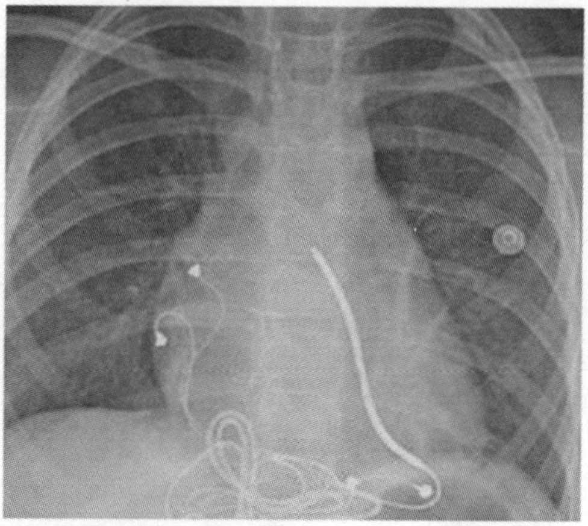

A. Pacemaker lead
B. Displaced Ryle's tube
C. Slipped CV line
D. Artefact

38. Patient is having A.F. on chronic rate controlling drug. Patient developed progressive shortness of breath, presumably due to side effect of the drug. What is false regarding it?

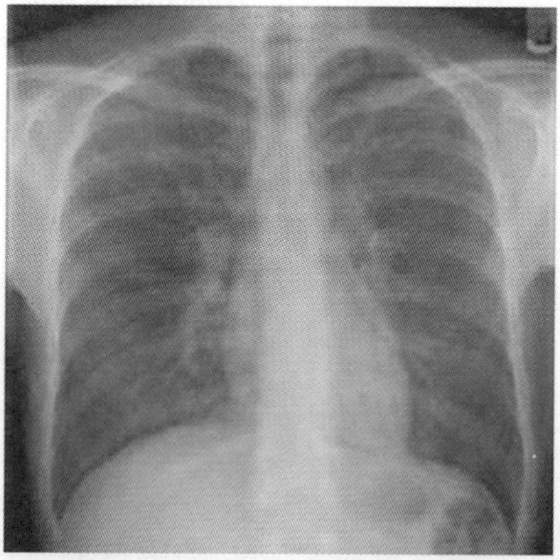

A. DLCO decreases very late in disease

B. Deposition of drug in lung parenchyma
C. BAL S/O cytotoxic T cell
D. Reticular opacities are present

39. All are true except:

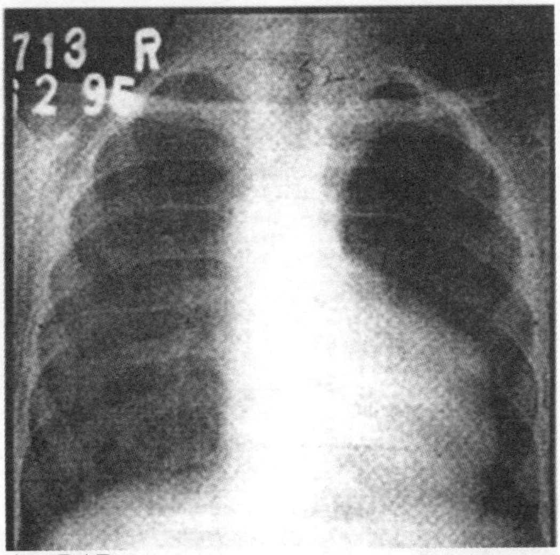

A. RAD
B. Hypoplastic RV
C. Cyanosis
D. Restrictive VSD

40. Two-day-old neonate with respiratory distress. What is the diagnosis?

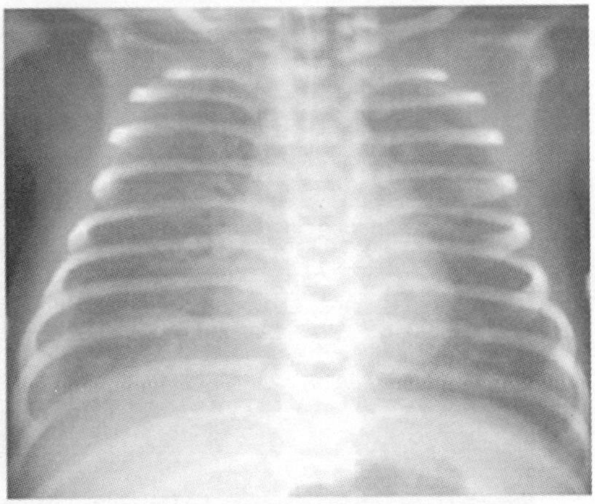

A. Obstructive TAPVC
B. TGA with VSD
C. Coarctation of aorta
D. PDA

41. All of these can present as this, except:

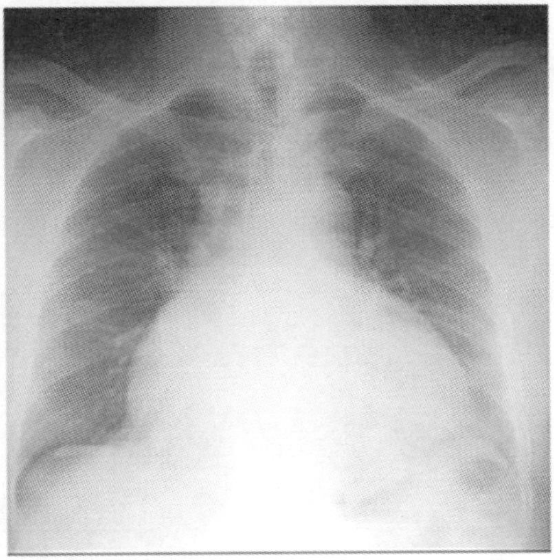

A. Tetralogy of Fallot
B. Cardiac tamponade
C. AR with heart failure
D. Ebstein's anomaly

42. CXR of 8-year-old child with CVP line in situ. What may be the cause of shortness of breath?

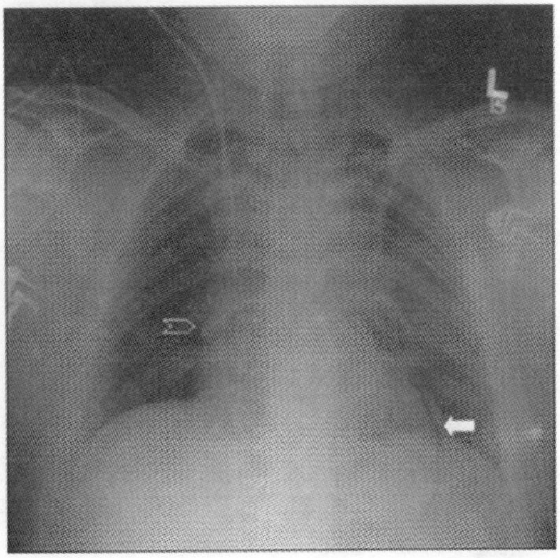

A. Malignancy B. TB
C. Iatrogenic D. Radiation

43. Based on the following chest X-ray, all of the following present in patient except:

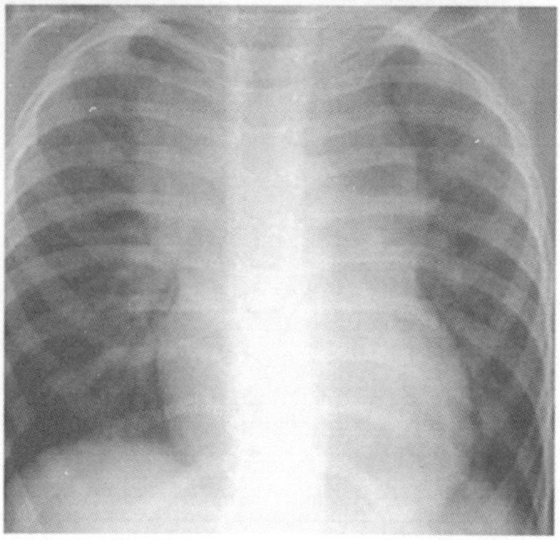

A. Decreased pulmonary blood flow
B. Cyanosis
C. Pulmonary hypertension
D. Right to left shunt

44. What is the diagnosis?

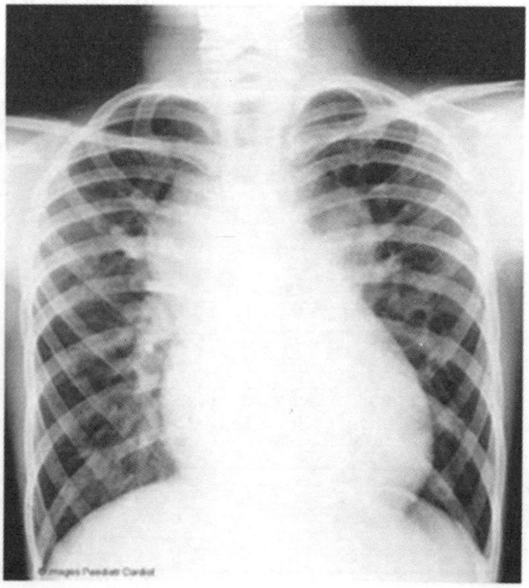

A. Supracardiac TAPVC
B. Aortic Aneurysm
C. Idiopathic pulmonary artery dilatation
D. Thymic mass

45. Young female, presenting with dyspnea and syncope on exertion. Based on the following chest X-ray, what is the diagsosis?

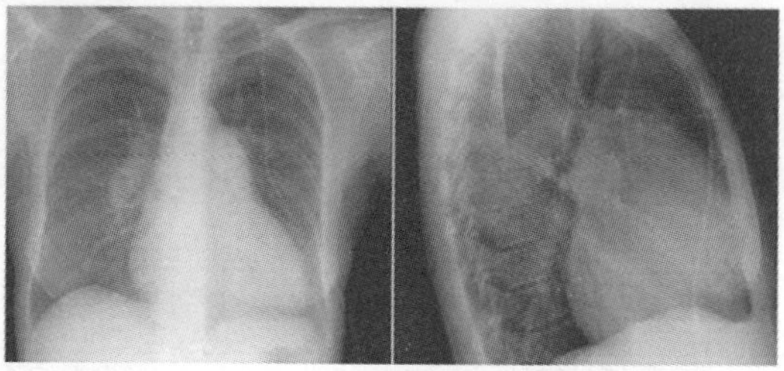

A. IPAH B. Valvular PS
C. Scimitar D. Sarcoid

Echocardiography

46. A 34-year-old male presents with complaints of malaise and shortness of breath on exertion. Physical examination is otherwise unremarkable. What does the image show?

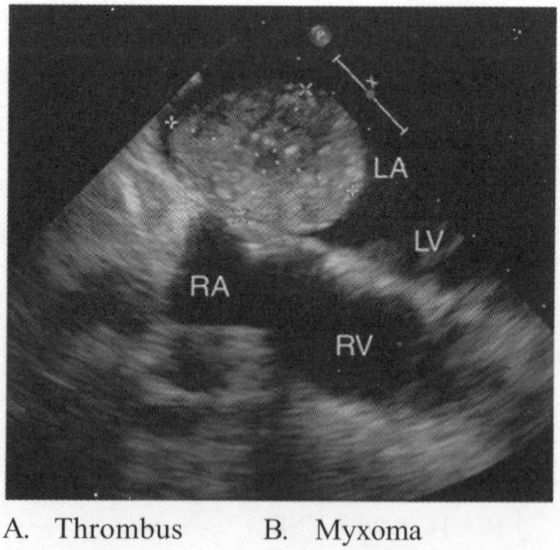

A. Thrombus B. Myxoma
C. Sarcoma D. Vegetation

47. A newborn baby was diagnosed with tuberous sclerosis. She has seizures. She had an echocardiogram. What does the image show?

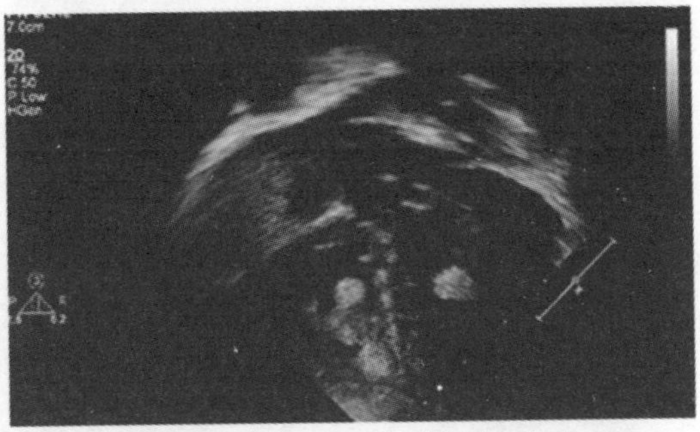

A. Multiple small tumors, likely rhabdomyoma
B. Lipomas
C. Sarcoma
D. Fibroma

48. What is the recommended management strategy for the patient?

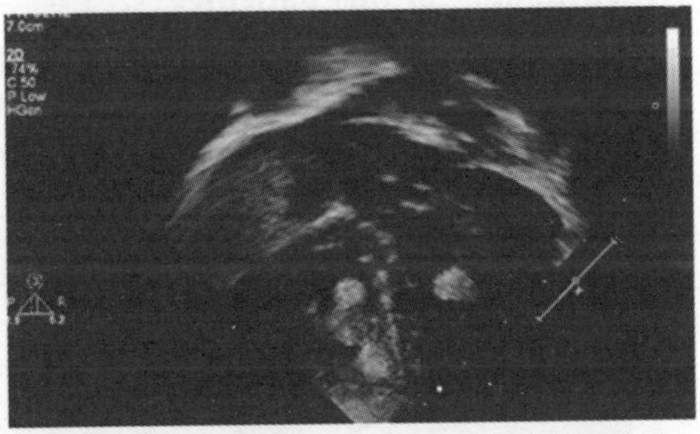

A. Refer for surgery
B. Chemotherapy
C. Observation
D. Radiation

49. 65 years old patient presented with acute anterior wall MI 5 days back which was not revascularized. At present, patient did not have any chest pain. Echo showed akinetic LAD territory. What should be the next line of management?

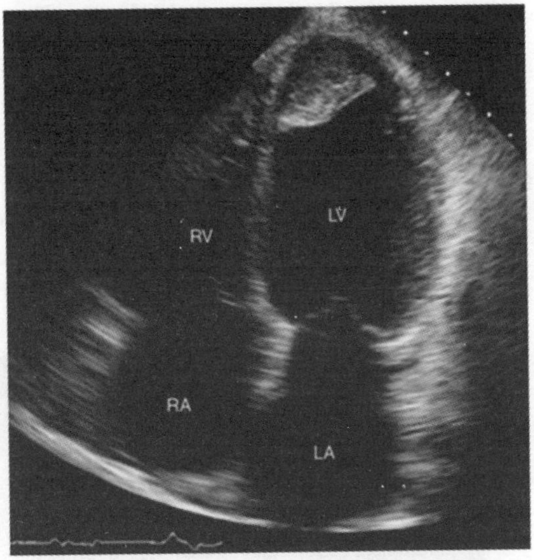

A. Urgent angiography and PCI of LAD
B. Dual antiplatelet therapy and anticoagulation
C. Coronary artery bypass grafting
D. Intravenous thrombolysis

50. 65 years old patient presented with acute anterior wall MI 5 days back which was not revascularized. At present, patient did not have any chest pain. Echo showed akinetic LAD territory. What should be the next line of management? What does the apical four chamber image show?

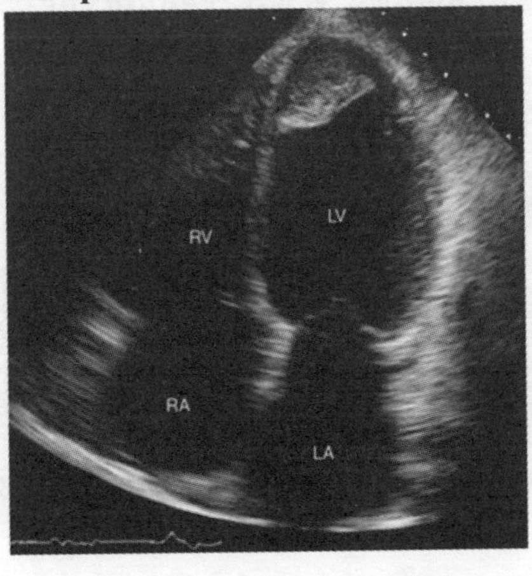

A. Tumor in the left ventricular apex
B. A thrombus in the left ventricular apex
C. Artifact from overlying ribs
D. Obliterative myocarditis

51. A 28-year-old male has a history of systemic lupus erythematosus and chronic kidney disease. He had a routine echocardiogram. What does the image demonstrate?

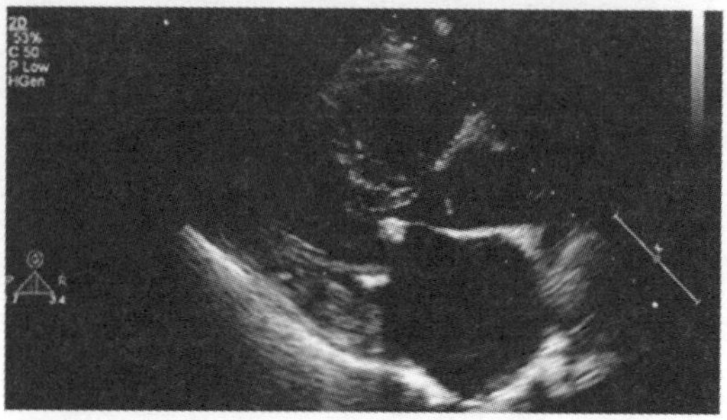

A. Normal looking mitral valve
B. Libman–Sacks endocarditis of mitral valve
C. Papillary fibroelastoma
D. Rheumatic changes of the mitral valve

52. 60 years old male patient presented with NYHA class II shortness of breath. On examination found to have grade 3 SEM at aortic area. Continuous wave doppler is shown below. What should be next approach?

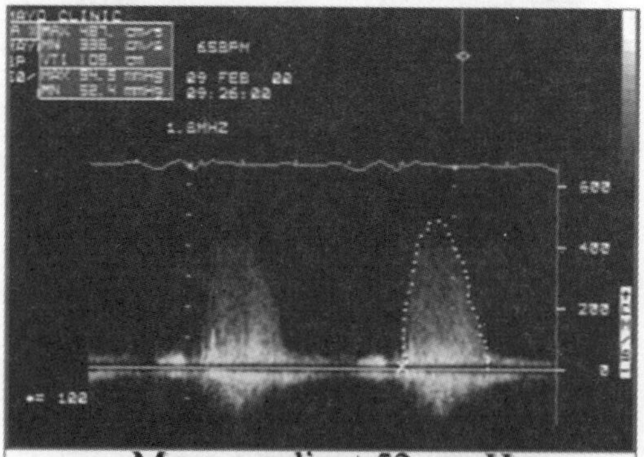

Mean gradient 52 mmHg
Peak vel. 4.8 m/sec

A. Surgical evaluation
B. Medical therapy
C. Stress Echocardiography
D. Observation

53. Which of the following is not associated with the following?

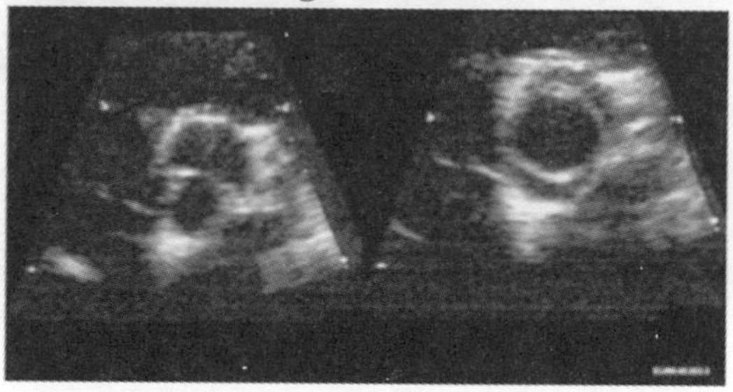

A. Coarctation of aorta
B. Mitral stenosis
C. Aortic dilatation
D. Patent ductus arteriosus

54. Which of the following may be an associated finding in this patient?

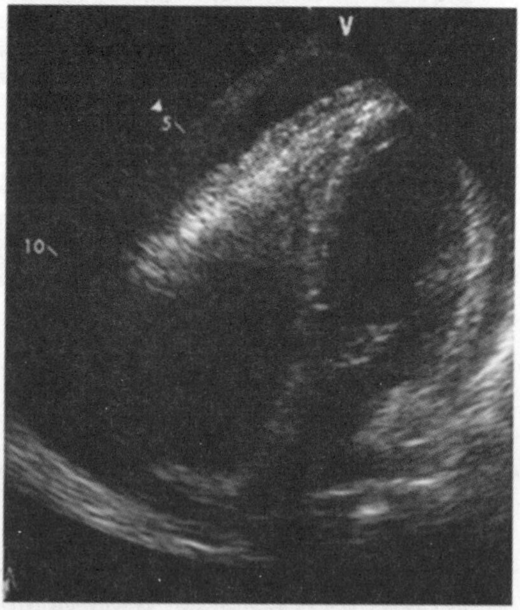

A. Anemia
B. Eosinophilia
C. Thymoma
D. Lymphoma

55. Doppler echo showing TR 4.80 m/s. This condition can be seen with all except:

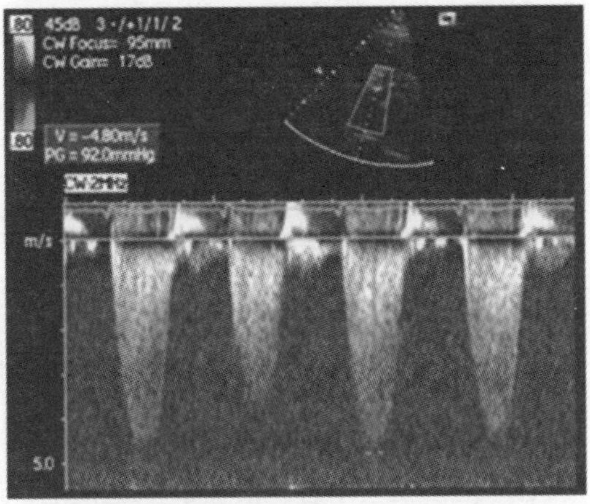

A. Ebstein's anomaly
B. ASD with Eisenmenger's
C. Primary pulmonary hypertension
D. Bilateral peripheral pulmonary stenosis

56. Image of PR jet, peak early diastolic velocity is 4 m/sec. Calculate mean pulmonary artery pressure if mean RA pressure is 6 mm Hg:

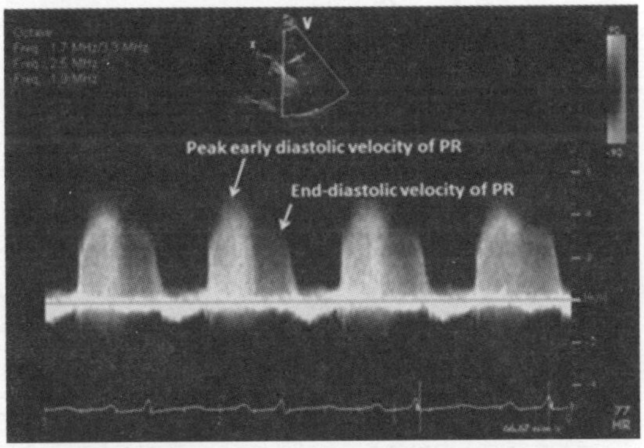

A. 58 mm Hg
B. 36 mm Hg
C. 70 mm Hg
D. 30 mm Hg

57. Echo of a 24 years old male patient is shown. Which of the following is not seen?

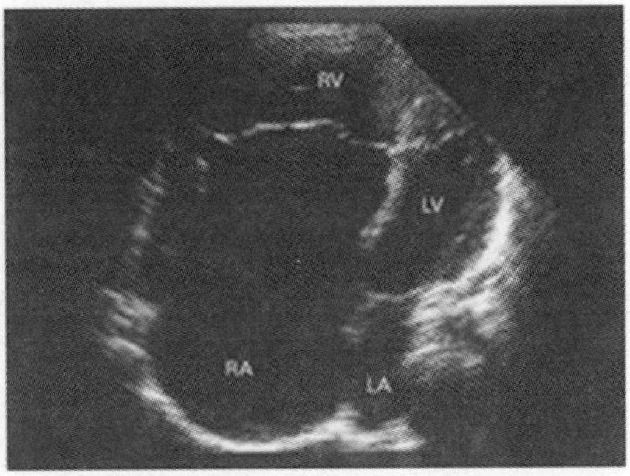

A. Multiple sounds
B. Cyanosis
C. Loud P2
D. Shunt at atrial level

58. 60-year-old hypertensive male presents with chest pain. ECG shows ST elevation in inferior leads. What is the diagnosis?

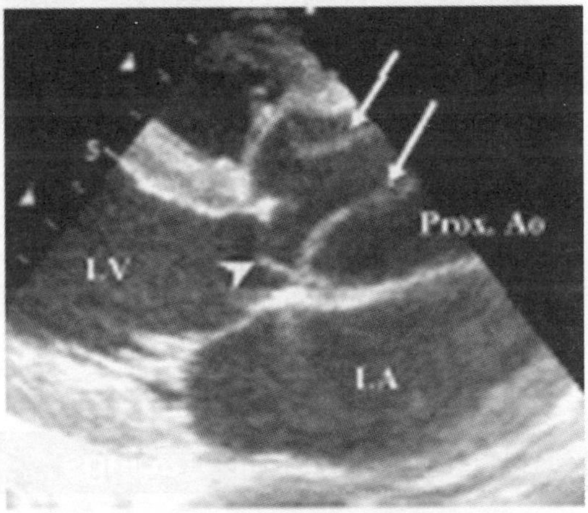

A. Acute aortic dissection with involvement of RCA
B. Left atrial thrombus
C. Infective endocarditis with RCA embolization
D. Intramural hematoma

59. Which of the following will not be seen in this patient?

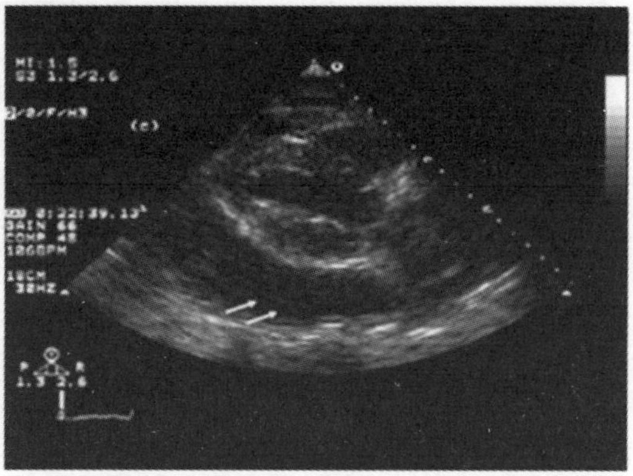

A. Equalization of diastolic pressures
B. Rapid y descent
C. Prominent X
D. Hypotension

60. True about rhabdomyomas all except:

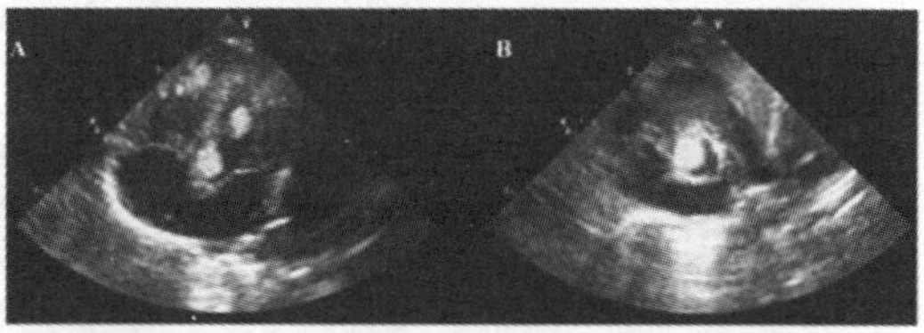

A. Cardiac rhabdomyomas are the most frequently encountered primary cardiac tumor in infants and children
B. Associated with tuberous sclerosis
C. Increase with age
D. Associated with cardiac conduction defects

Hemodynamic Tracings

61. The pull-back pressure recording from left ventricle apex to aorta of a 36-year-old patient is shown below. The likely treatment should be:

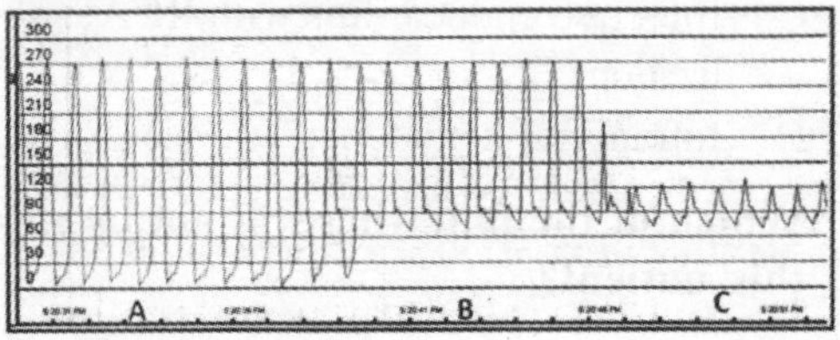

A. Aortic root replacement
B. Alcohol septal ablation
C. Aortic valve balloon dilatation
D. Aortic valve replacement

62. The likely diagnosis based on the hemodynamic trace shown below is:

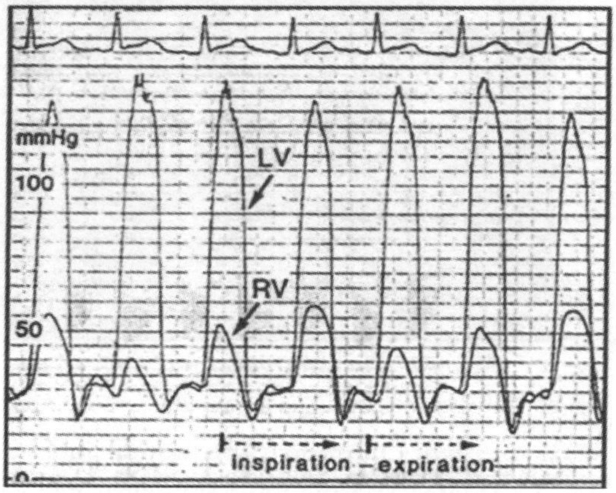

A. Restrictive cardiomyopathy
B. Cardiac tamponade
C. Chronic constrictive pericarditis
D. Hypertrophic obstructive cardiomyopathy

63. What is the diagnosis?

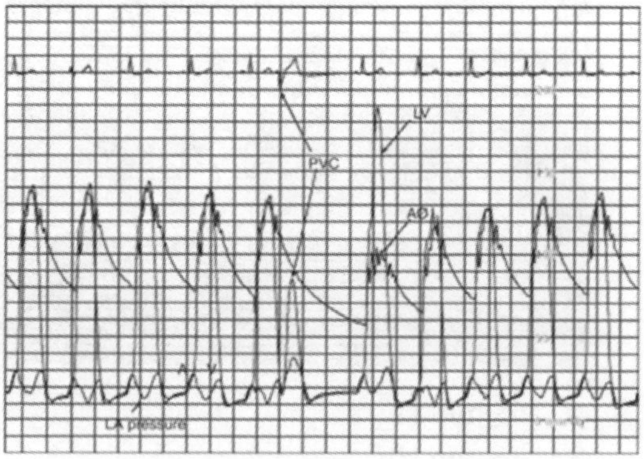

A. Valvular aortic stenosis
B. Supravalvular aortic stenosis
C. Hypertrophic obstructive cardiomyopathy
D. Coarctation of aorta

64. 16-year-old boy presents with chest pain and dyspnea. Pressure tracing given. Treatment of choice:

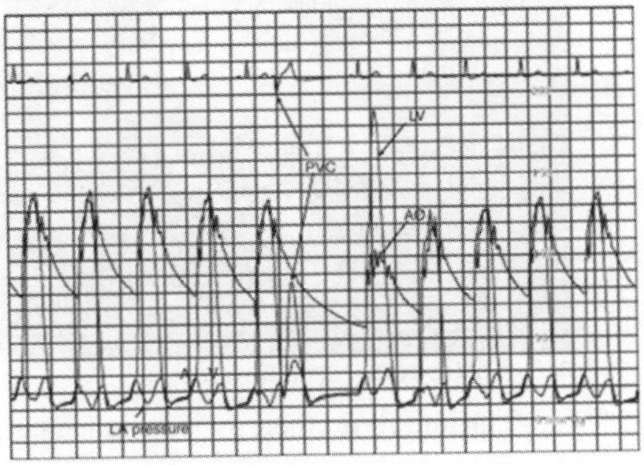

A. Mitral valve replacement
B. Aortic valve replacement
C. Surgical myomectomy
D. Aortic valvuloplasty

65. What is the diagnosis from the following trace?

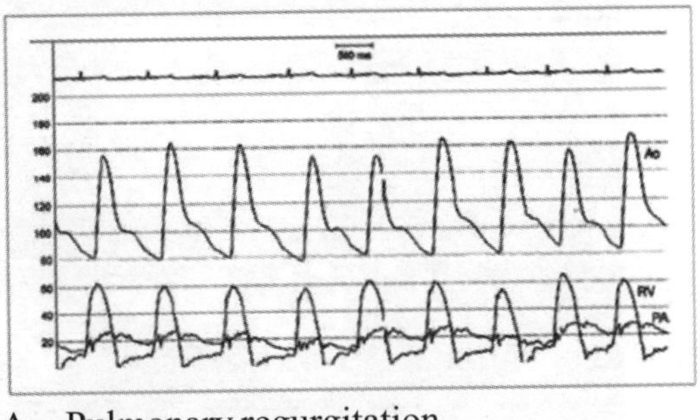

A. Pulmonary regurgitation
B. Pulmonic stenosis
C. Tricuspid regurgitation
D. Tricuspid stenosis

66. LV aortic catheter withdrawal shows following tracing:

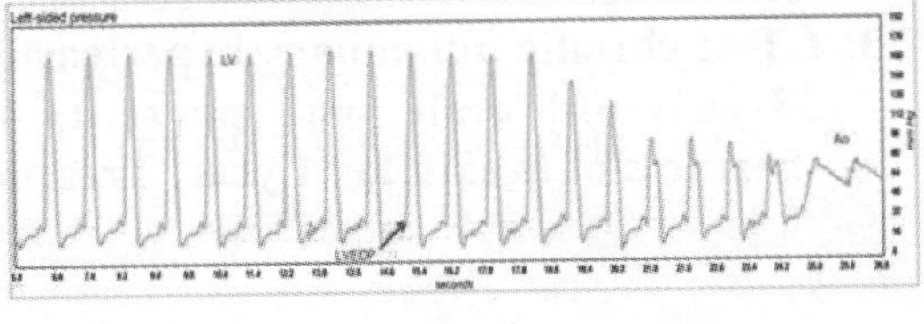

A. William's syndrome
B. Subaortic membrane
C. Coarctation of aorta
D. LV diverticulum

67. RV/LV pressure trace is given from a patient of tetralogy of Fallot:

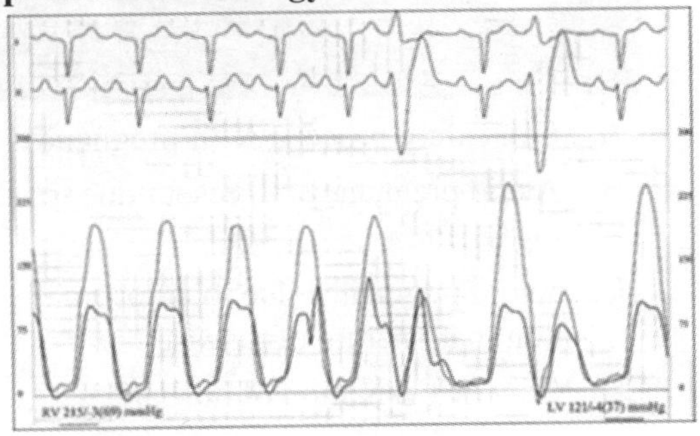

A. Valvular PS B. Restrictive VSD
C. Aortic stenosis D. LV dysfunction

68. LV to aorta pull back trace is shown. Which of the following may be seen in this patient?

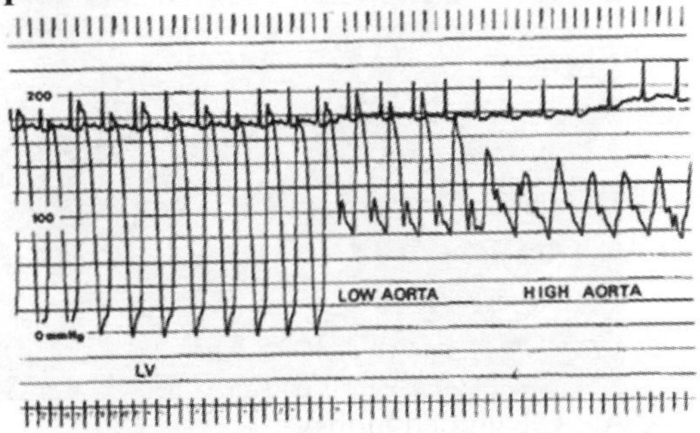

A. Elfin facies
B. BAV
C. Catch 22
D. Sub aortic membrane

Computed Tomography

69. 25 years old female, known case of Marfan syndrome came for pre-pregnancy counselling. What will be your advice after seeing the MRI?

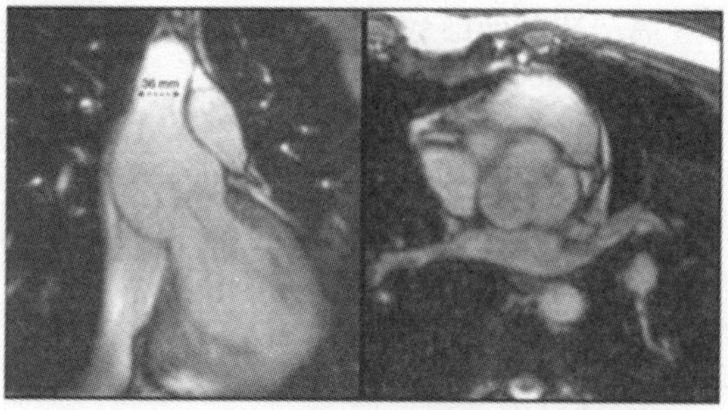

A. Can safely proceed with pregnancy
B. Avoid pregnancy at present due to size of the aorta
C. Avoid pregnancy due to autosomal dominant nature of disease
D. Genetic evaluation of husband

70. What procedure to be done?

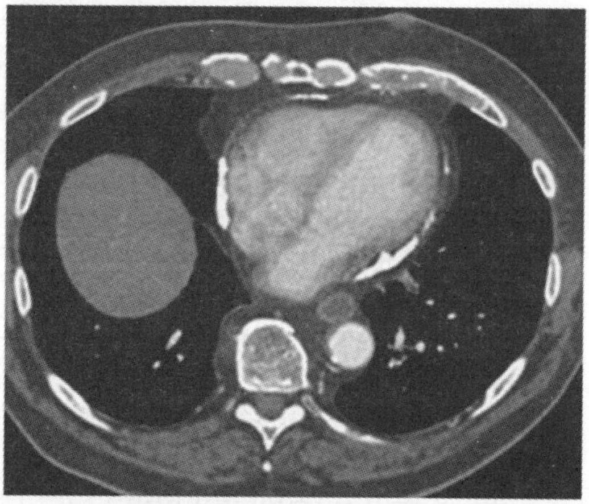

A. CT guided biopsy
B. Pericardiectomy
C. Stenting with Rotablation
D. Bentall procedure

71. A 45-year-old patient presents to medical emergency with chest pain and hypotension. CT angiography of the patient is shown below. The urgent treatment of this patient should include:

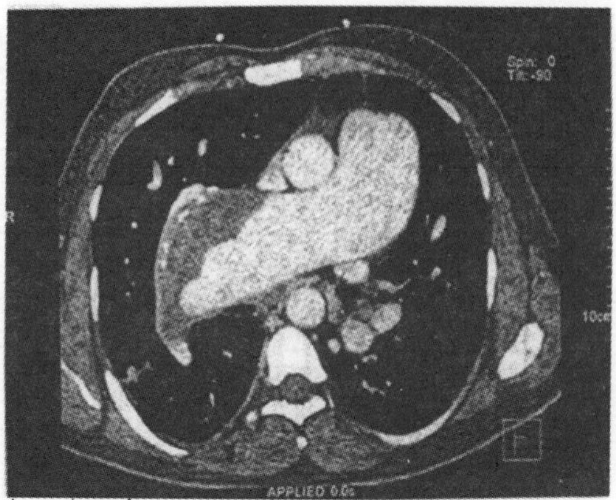

A. Aortic root replacement
B. Thrombolytic therapy with tenecteplase
C. Chest tube drainage
D. Percutaneous coronary intervention

72. CT scan image is given. Diagnosis:

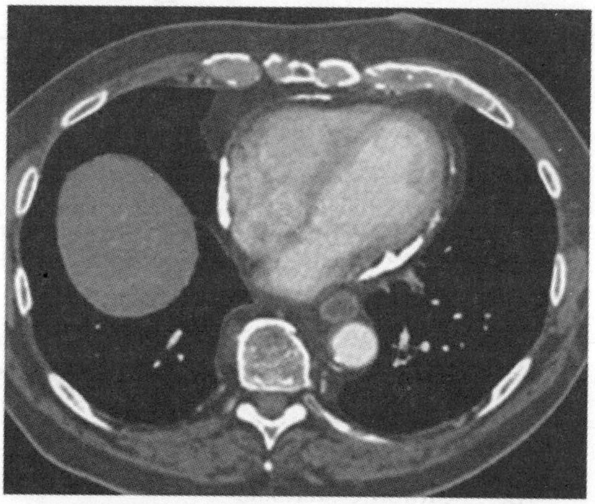

A. Pericardial effusion
B. Aortic dissection
C. Constrictive pericarditis
D. HCM

73. CT of chronic pulmonary hypertension in 58-year-old male who presents with shortness of breath for 1 year. Treatment:

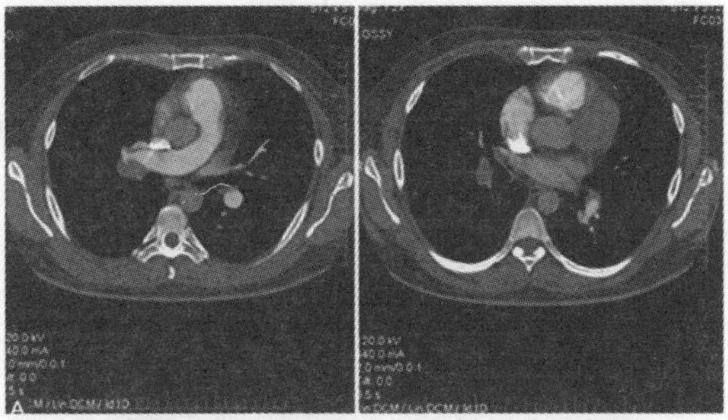

A. Surgery
B. Pulmonary artery stenting
C. IV prostacyclin
D. Pulmonary sympathectomy

Cardiac MRI

74. Which of the following abnormal structure is shown in this MRI?

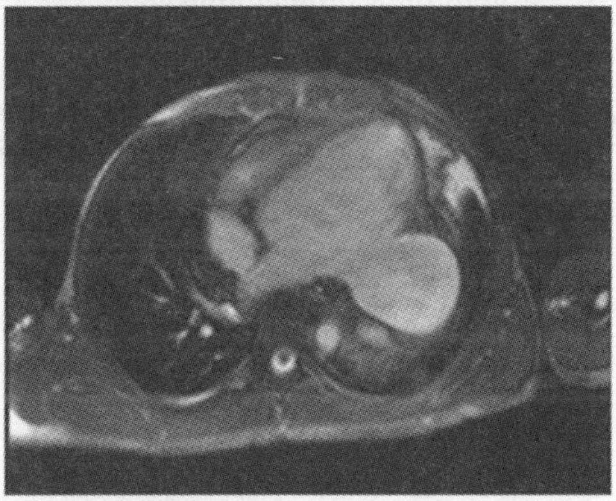

A. Pericardial cyst
B. Hydatid cyst
C. Unruptured sinus of valsalva aneurysm
D. Submitral aneurysm

75. Which of the following is likely diagnosis in this patient?

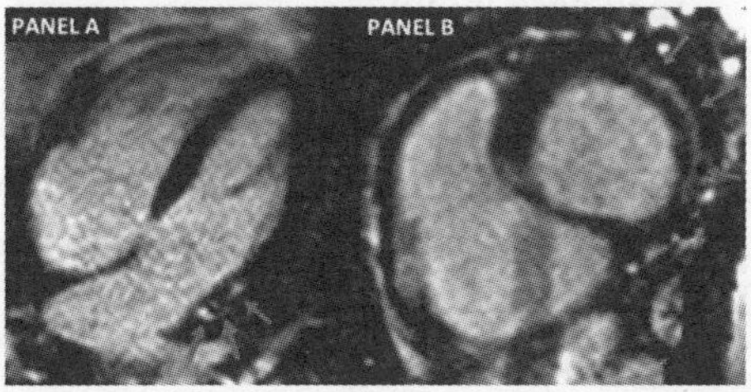

A. Endomyocardial fibrosis
B. Sarcoidosis
C. Amyloidosis
D. Tuberculosis

76. MRI image of late gadolinium enhancement is suggestive of:

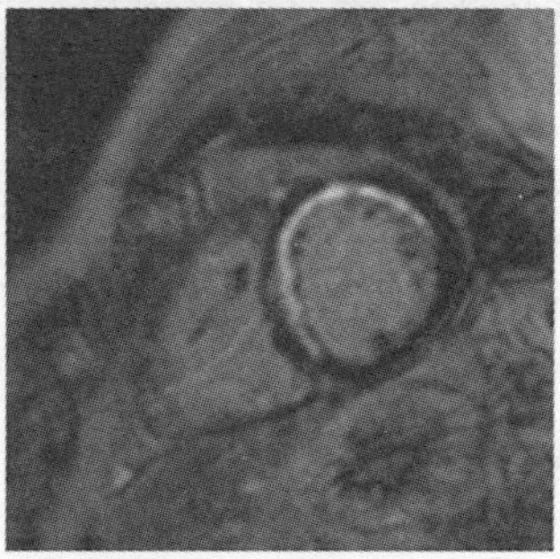

A. Amyloidosis
B. Subendocardial ischemia
C. Myocarditis
D. Infilterative cardiomyopathy

Angiography

77. Following images were obtained during systole and diastole at the time of coronary angiography. What is the likely cause of narrowing in left anterior descending artery?

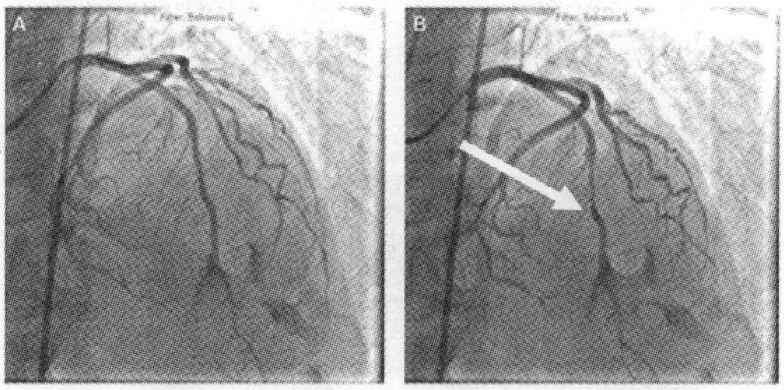

A. Myocardial bridge
B. Coronary spasm
C. Chronic total occlusion
D. Coronary dissection

78. Patient's angiogram in RAO caudal view is shown before and after percutaneous

intervention. Which coronary artery was involved?

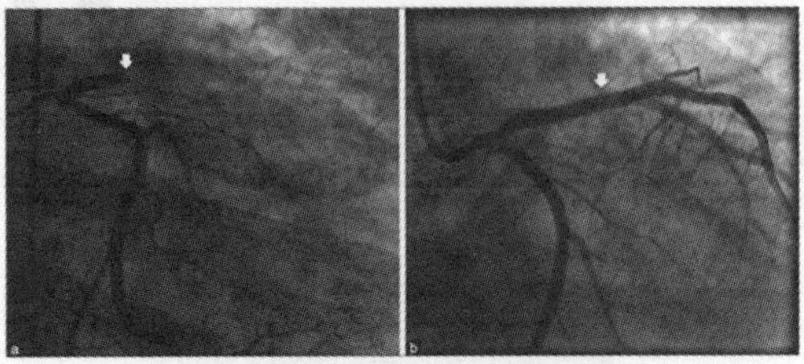

A. Left main coronary artery
B. Left anterior descending artery
C. Left circumflex artery
D. Right coronary artery

79. A 6-year-old boy presents with the following findings on Coronary angiogram given. What treatment should be given:

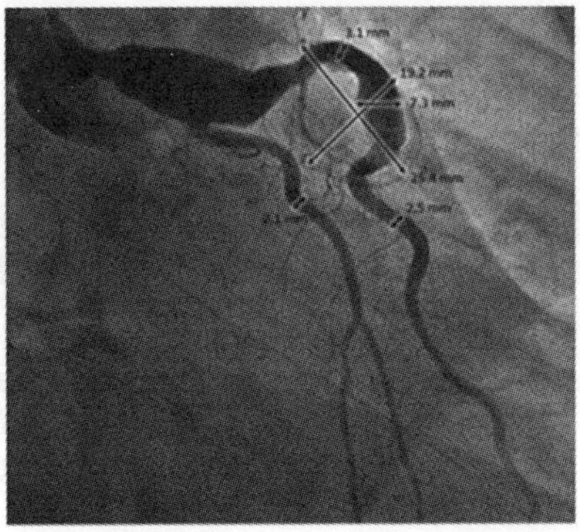

A. Aspirin
B. Methotrexate
C. Corticosteroids
D. Interferons

80. What is the diagnosis in this patient?

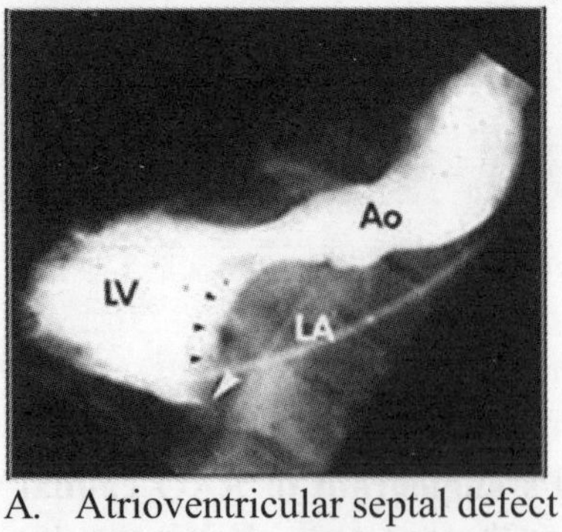

A. Atrioventricular septal defect
B. LV diverticulum
C. Supravalvular AS
D. HCM

81. Following abnormality may be seen in all except:

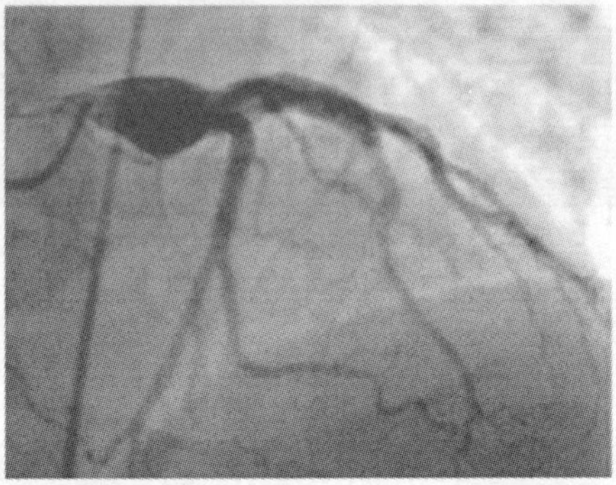

A. Kawasaki disease
B. Behcet's disease
C. Everolimus drug eluting stent
D. Acute rheumatic fever

82. 38 years old male patient being evaluated for hypertension. Which of the following is true about the condition?

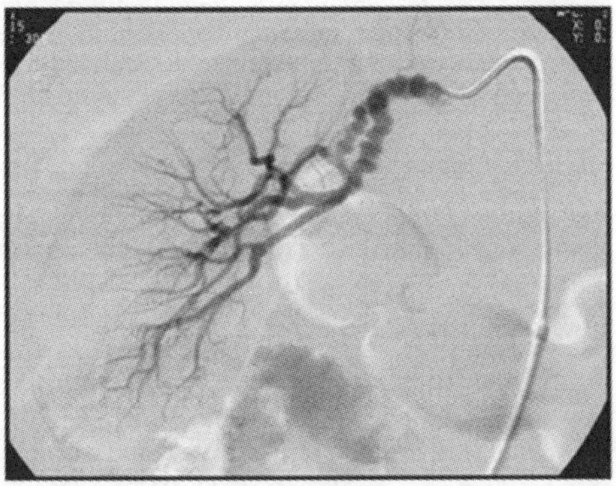

A. Aspirin, beta blockers and HMG CoA reductase inhibitors
B. Routine coronary angiography is indicated in all patients
C. Percutaneous renal artery intervention has little potential for cure of hypertension
D. More common in women than men

83. Right renal angiogram. Diagnosis:

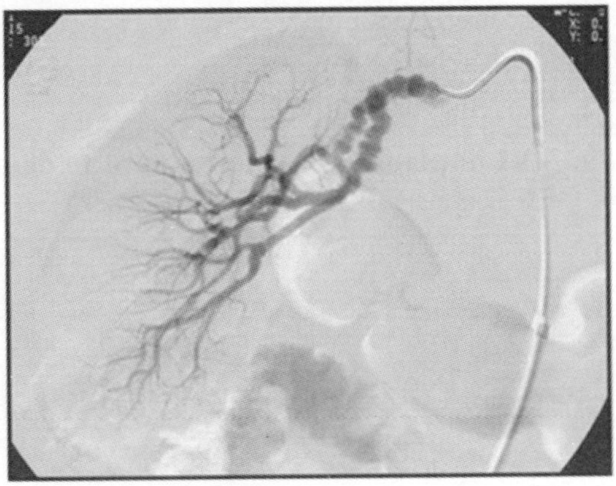

A. Atherosclerosis
B. Aortoarteritis
C. Fibromuscular dysplasia
D. Post sympathetic denervation

84. 60-year-old male patient presented with chest pain, BP 150/85, Mild RCA disease on coronary angiogram. Renal angiogram is given. First line treatment should include all except:

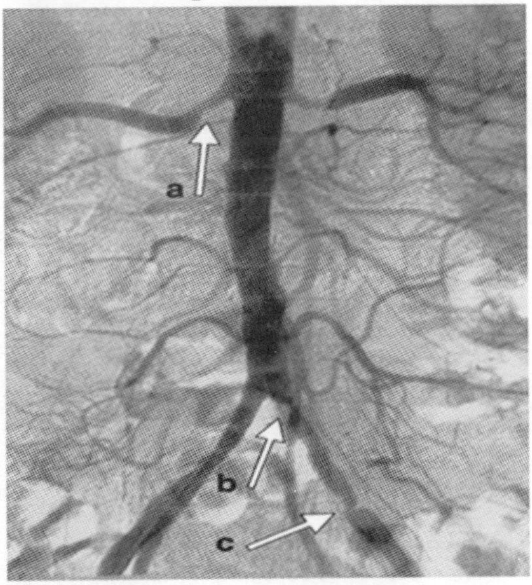

A. Aspirin
B. Atorvastatin
C. Amlodipine
D. Renal artery stenting

85. Diagnostic catheterization showing right ventricular angiography. What is the diagnosis?

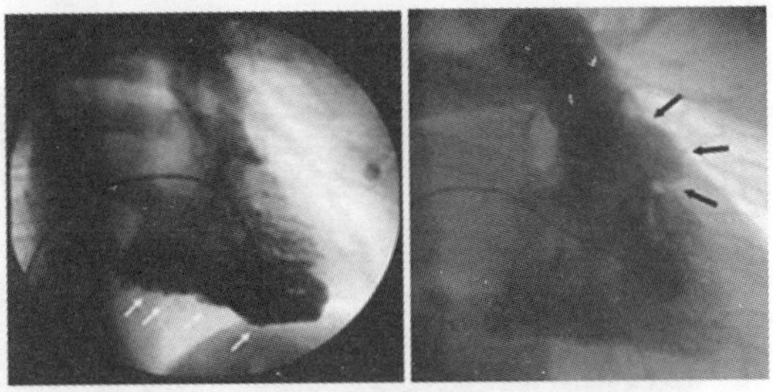

A. ARVC
B. Double chambered right ventricle
C. Endomyocardial fibrosis
D. LV non compaction

86. A 12-year-old presented with late peaking systolic murmur. All of the following are true except:

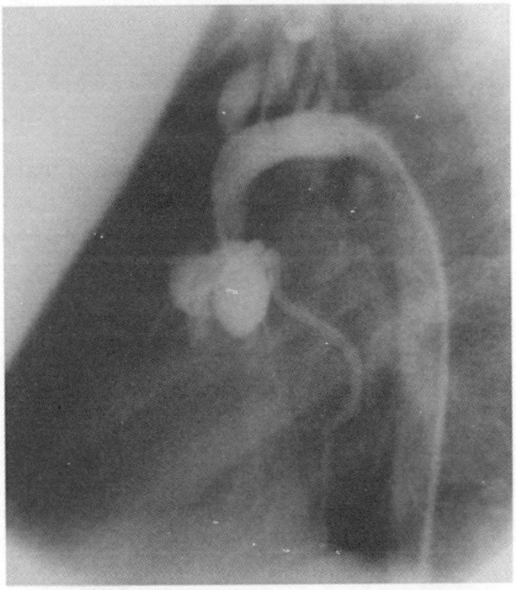

A. Right upper limb BP is more than left upper limb BP
B. There is increased predilection for CAD
C. Mutation in elastin gene
D. Treatment of choice is balloon dilatation

Miscellaneous

87. Which of the following is correct regarding following imaging modality?

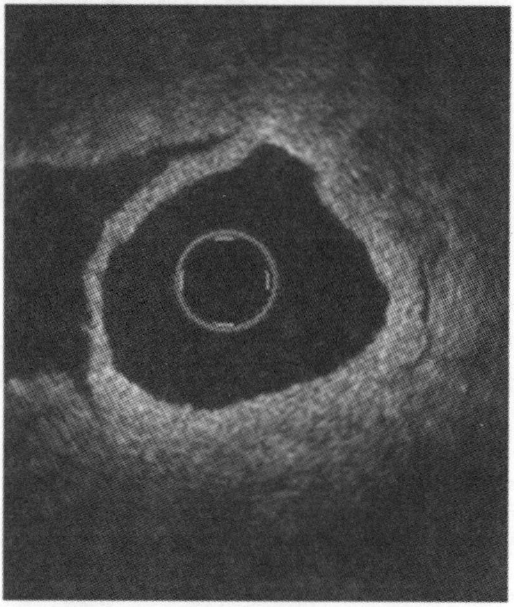

A. Some protrusion of wall present
B. Image resolution is higher than that of IVUS
C. It shows organized thrombus that has recanalised
D. Virtual histology

88. 1st automated external defibrillator is shown below, who invented this?

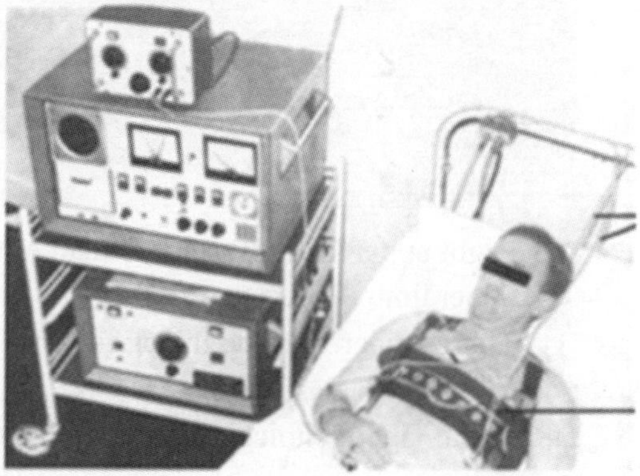

A. Levi Watkins
B. Fred Zacouto
C. Michel Mirowski
D. Wilson Greatbatch

89. VVI implant with rate reduced to 60/min. ECG is as follows shows:

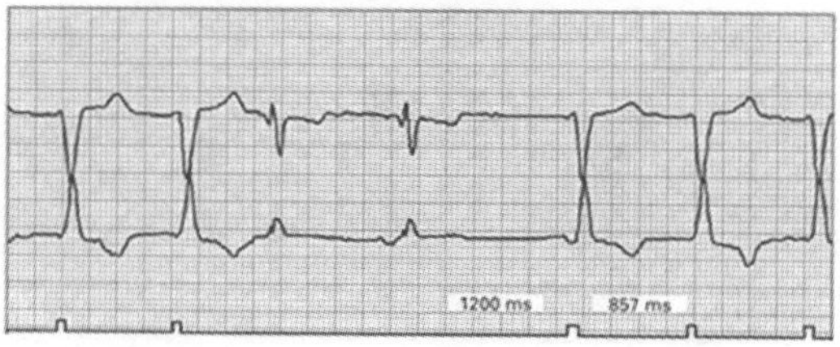

A. Oversensing
B. Undersensing
C. Hysteresis
D. Capture failure

90. Anti-hypertensive treatment of choice in patient with nuclear scan (approximate image given):

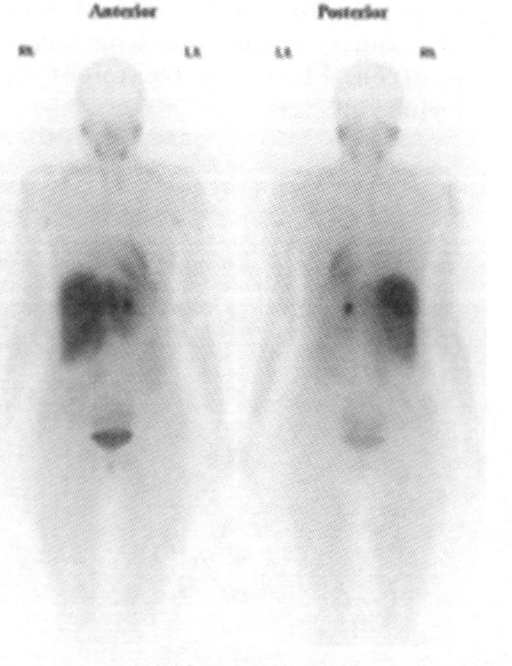

A. Prazosin/Propranolol
B. Spironolactone/Torsemide
C. Olmesartan/Amlodipine
D. Metoprolol/Spironolactone

91. What is the true statement regarding this image?

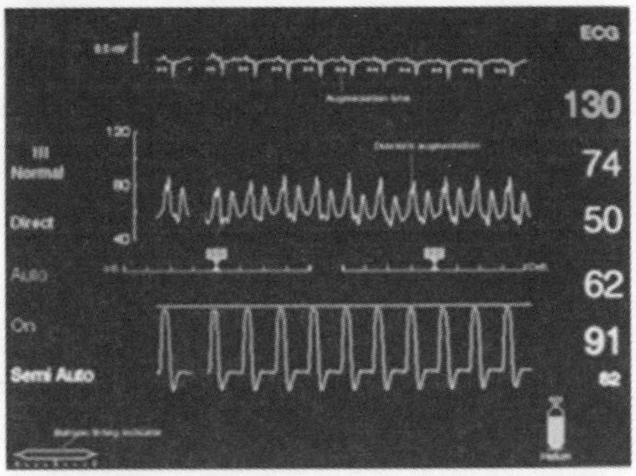

A. Randomised trial does not show any mortality benefit

B. It is best bridge to transplant

C. Increased cardiac output by 1.5-2 litres

D. It is used in respiratory failure

92. Following image can be present in all except:

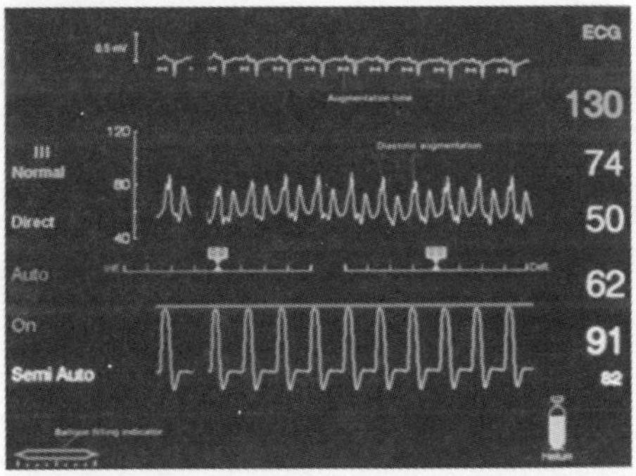

A. Acute MR

B. Acute AR

C. Post CABG

D. Acute MI with cardiogenic shock

93. Phonocardiogram, pansystolic murmur, wide splitting of s2, presence of s4. Diagnosis:

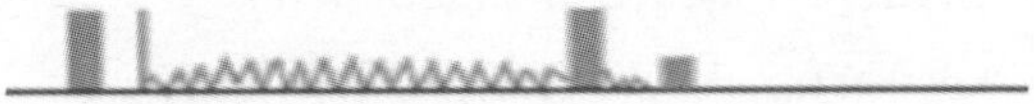

A. Aortic stenosis

B. Pulmonary stenosis

C. Supracristal VSD

D. TOF

94. Action potential trace given, wrong match:

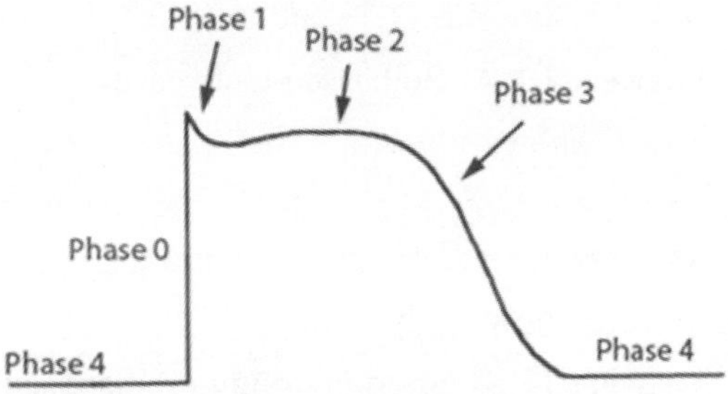

A. Phase 1- sodium channels

B. Phase 2- chloride channels

C. Phase 3- potassium channels

D. Phase 4- funny currents

ANSWERS

Electrocardiography

Answer: 1. B. Acute pericarditis

Answer: 2. C. Left ventricular outflow tract

Answer: 3. B. Long QT syndrome

Answer: 4. D. Right anterolateral

Answer: 5. A. OS-ASD

Answer: 6. A. Amyloid heart disease

Answer: 7. B. Hypertrophied interatrial septum

Answer: 8. B. Echocardiography

→ ECG shows LBBB, next patient should undergo echocardiography.

Answer: 9. A. Acute pulmonary embolism

→ ECG shows $S_1Q_3T_3$ pattern.

Answer: 10. A. Belhassen tachycardia

→ECG shows VT with RBBB pattern and right axis deviation; suggests anterior fascicle as origin of VT.

Answer: 11. A. DC cardioversion

→ ECG shows polymorphic VT.

Answer: 12. C. Short coupling predisposed to ventricular fibrillation

→ ECG shows Ashman's phenomenon in atrial fibrillation.

Answer: 13. A. MRI

→ ECG is suggestive of ARVC.

Answer: 14. D. LQTS

→ ECG shows bidirectional VT.

Answer: 15. A. Inferior wall MI with AV block

Answer: 16. A. Critical LAD stenosis

→ Wellen's pattern (Type B) is seen in ECG suggestive of proximal LAD involvement.

Answer: 17. A. AF with antidromic conduction over fast pathway

Answer: 18. D. Hypotension

→ Electrical alternans suggestive of hypotension.

Answer: 19. A. Hypotension

Answer: 20. A. Proximal LAD

→ ECG shows Wellen's pattern (Type A).

Answer: 21. B. RV outflow VT

Answer: 22. C. Nothing is to be done

→ ECG shows accelerated idioventricular rhythm after successful thrombolysis. But this pattern is not specific to thrombolysis only. Continuous observation and monitoring are required.

Answer: 23. A. Verapamil

→ ECG shows RVOT-VT.

Answer: 24. A. Atrial flutter

Answer: 25. A. Quinidine

→ ECG is suggestive of Brugada syndrome.

Answer: 26. C. LMCA

Answer: 27. A. DC shock

Answer: 28. B. Atrial fibrillation with antidromic AVRT.

Chest X-Ray

Answer: 29. C. Pulmonary embolism

→CXR shows pulmonary edema. Pulmonary embolism is unlikely to cause pulmonary edema, rest all can produce this condition.

Answer: 30. D. Tricuspid atresia

Answer: 31. C. CT chest and surgery consultation

→CXR shows constrictive pericarditis.

Answer: 32. D. Scimitar syndrome

Answer: 33. D. He is likely to have recurrent otitis media/sinusitis

→ Patient is likely to have Kartegener's syndrome.

Answer: 34. A. Dyspnea

→CXR shows pneumothorax.

Answer: 35. A. ICD insertion

→ Patient will require intercostal drainage tube insertion for pneumothorax.

Answer: 36. A. RVH with RAD

→ CXR is suggestive of TOF.

Answer: 37. A. Pacemaker lead

→Thin leads are pacing leads whereas thick one is ICD lead having shock coil.

Answer: 38. A. DLCO decreases very late in disease

→ Patient has amiodarone induced pulmonary fibrosis.

Answer: 39. A. RAD

→CXR is suggestive of tricuspid atresia.

Answer: 40. A. Obstructive TAPVC

Answer: 41. A. Tetralogy of Fallot

Answer: 42. C. Iatrogenic

→Pneumopericardium likely caused during central line insertion.

Answer: 43. A. Decreased pulmonary blood flow

→Snowman's heart which is suggestive of supracardiac TAPC.

Answer: 44. A. Supracardiac TAPVC

Answer: 45. A. IPAH

→Dilated PAs with pruning, RV enlargement is suggestive of severe PAH.

Echocardiography

Answer: 46. B. Myxoma

Answer: 47. A. Multiple small tumors, likely rhabdomyoma

Answer: 48. C. Observation

Answer: 49. B. Dual antiplatelet therapy and anticoagulation

Answer: 50. B. A thrombus in the left ventricular apex

Answer: 51. B. Libman–Sacks endocarditis of mitral valve

Answer: 52. A. Surgical evaluation

→ Patient has symptomatic severe aortic stenosis.

Answer: 53. B. Mitral stenosis

→ Patient has bicuspid aortic valve.

Answer: 54. B. Eosinophilia

Answer: 55. A. Ebstein's anomaly

→ Patient has high pressure tricuspid regurgitation. Ebstein anomaly is associated with low pressure TR.

Answer: 56. C. 70 mm Hg

→ Mean pulmonary artery pressure = $4v^2$ + right atrial pressure.

Where, v is peak early diastolic velocity across pulmonary valve.

Answer: 57. C. Loud P2

Answer: 58. A. Acute aortic dissection with involvement of RCA

Answer: 59. B. Rapid y descent

→ Patient has cardiac tamponade.

Answer: 60. C. Increase with age

Hemodynamic Tracings

Answer: 61. A. Aortic root replacement

→ Patient has supravalvular aortic stenosis as systolic pressure gradient is present within aorta.

Answer: 62. C. Chronic constrictive pericarditis

→ There is discordance in the ventricular pressures, which is suggestive of constrictive pericarditis.

Answer: 63. C. Hypertrophic obstructive cardiomyopathy

→ Brockenbrough-Braunwald sign is present in the trace. Post PVC, there is fall in pulse pressure.

Answer: 64. C. Surgical myomectomy

Answer: 65. B. Pulmonic stenosis

→ There is RV to PA gradient, which is suggestive of pulmonic stenosis.

Answer: 66. B. Subaortic membrane

→Trace shows there is intraventricular systolic gradient proximal to aortic valve, which may be seen in subaortic membrane.

Answer: 67. B. Restrictive VSD

→ In TOF physiology the VSD is non-restrictive, so LV and RV systolic pressures should be equal. Here, pressure difference between the LV and RV pressures is likely due to restrictive VSD.

Answer: 68. A. Elfin facies

→ Pressure trace shows systolic gradient at the level of aorta, hence there is supravalvular aortic stenosis, which is present in William's syndrome.

Computed Tomography

Answer: 69. B. Avoid pregnancy at present due to size of the aorta

Answer: 70. B. Pericardiectomy

Answer: 71. B. Thrombolytic therapy with tenecteplase

→ Patient has massive pulmonary thromboembolism with hemodynamic instability.

Answer: 72. C. Constrictive pericarditis

Answer: 73. A. Surgery

→ CT is suggestive of chronic thromboembolic pulmonary hypertension.

Cardiac MRI

Answer: 74. D. Submitral aneurysm

Answer: 75. B. Sarcoidosis

→ There is sub-epicardial LGE in the basal and lateral segments of the left ventricle, suggestive of sarcoidosis.

Cardiac amyloidosis appears as global subendocardial myocardial hyperenhancement on LGE.

Answer: 76. B. Subendocardial ischemia

Angiography

Answer: 77. A. Myocardial bridge

Answer: 78. B. Left anterior descending artery

Answer: 79. A. Aspirin

Answer: 80. A. Atrioventricular septal defect

→ There is goose-neck appearance on LV angiography which is seen in AV septal defects.

Answer: 81. D. Acute rheumatic fever

→ LMCA aneurysm may be seen in Kawasaki, Behcet's disease and iatrogenic after coronary stenting.

Answer: 82. D. More common in women than men

→ Image is suggestive of fibromuscular dysplasia.

Answer: 83. C. Fibromuscular dysplasia

Answer: 84. D. Renal artery stenting

Answer: 85. A. ARVC

Answer: 86. D. Treatment of choice is balloon dilatation

→Aortogram shows supravalvular aortic stenosis, likely diagnosis being William's syndrome.

Miscellaneous

Answer: 87. B. Image resolution is higher than that of IVUS

→ This is an OCT image, which has higher resolution than IVUS.

Answer: 88. B. Fred Zacouto

Answer: 89. C. Hysteresis

→ 5th QRS complex which is placed has relatively longer RR interval due to hysteresis.

Answer: 90. A. Prazosin/Propranolol

→ MIBG scan is suggestive of pheochromocytoma.

Answer: 91. A. Randomised trial does not show any mortality benefit

→ Image is of IABP.

Answer: 92. B. Acute AR

→ IABP is contraindicated in acute AR.

Answer: 93. C. Supracristal VSD

→ Pansystolic murmur is present.

Answer: 94. B. Phase 2–chloride channels

Important Images

1. **Pericardial calcification**

   Most common cause: Tuberculosis

   Treatment of choice: Pericardiectomy

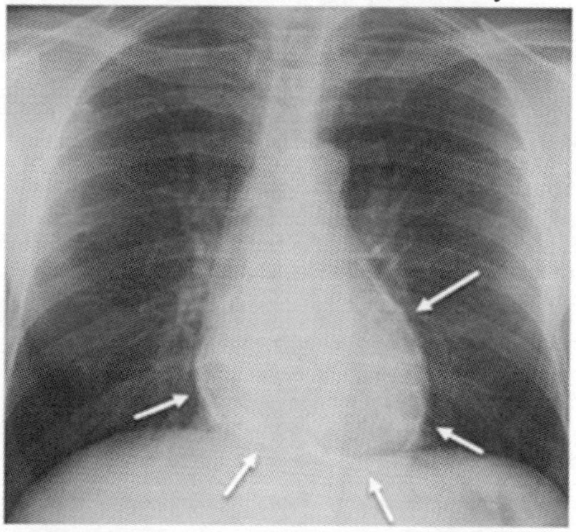

2. **Apical hypertrophic cardiomyopathy**
   - Also known as Yamaguchi Syndrome.
   - ECG shows repolarization changes and deep, inverted T waves in the antero-lateral leads (particularly in leads V4 and V5) with prominent R waves.

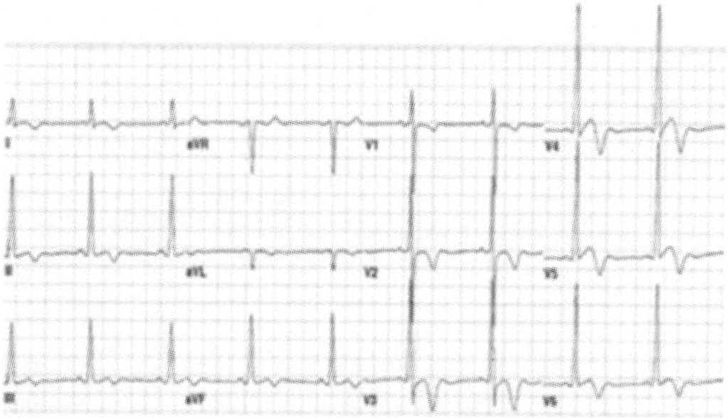

3. **Doppler of LVOTO gradient in HCM**
   - Doppler **dagger-shaped late-peaking signal** of the intracavitary gradient in hypertrophic cardiomyopathy.
   - LVOTO gradient is increased after Valsalva manoeuvre, characteristic of HCM.

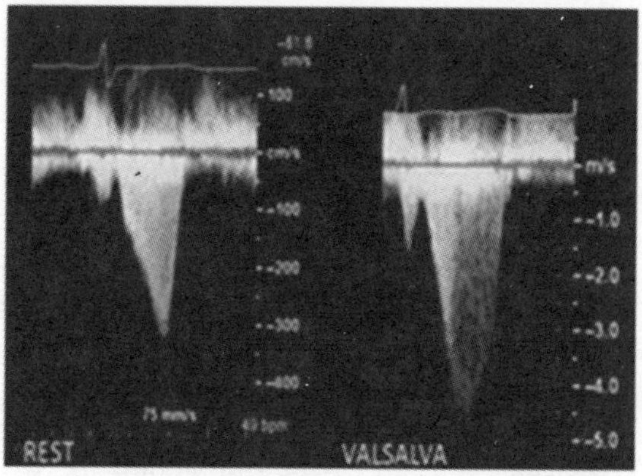

4. **Brockenbrough sign**

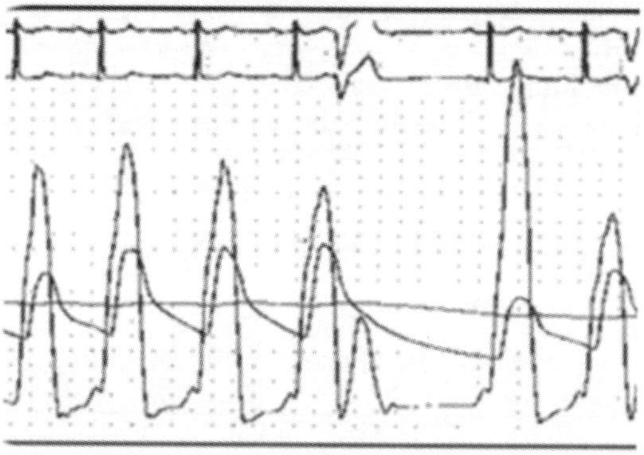

5. **Takotsubo cardiomyopathy**

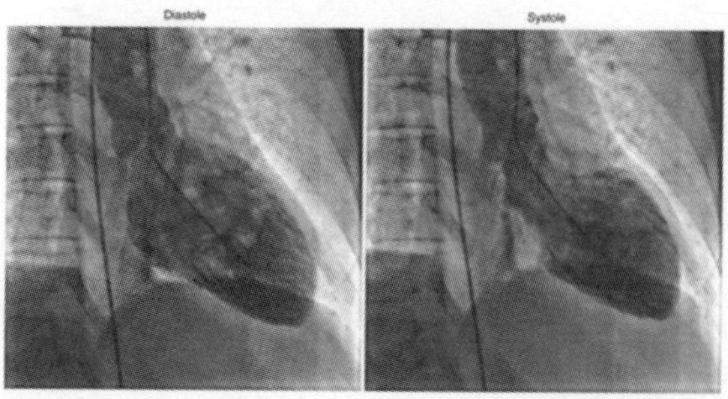

- Apical ballooning in systole is seen. Only basal part is contracting in systole whereas apical part of LV is dilated.
- Cause: Stressful condition.
- Coronary angiography: Normal coronaries.

6. **Aortic stenosis vs HCM**
   - Effect of VPC on Aortic stenosis and HCM.
   - There is increased LV peak systolic pressure as well as increased aortic systolic pressure in aortic stenosis.
   - Whereas, aortic systolic pressure is decreased in HCM, causing increase in pulse pressure after VPC. Also known as Brockenbrough-Braunwald phenomenon.

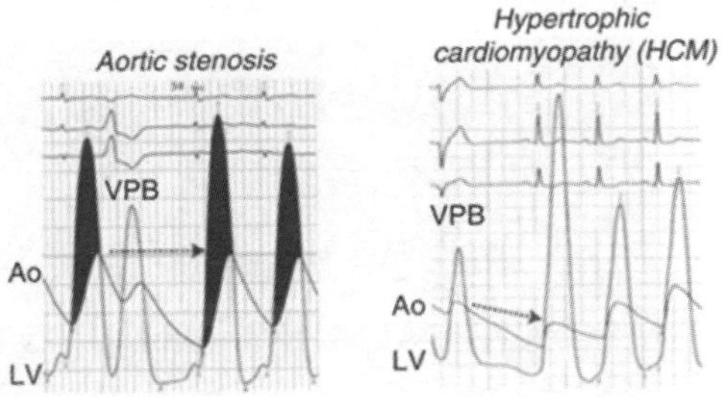

7. **Mitral stenosis**
   - There is significant transvalvular gradient between LA pressure and LV end diastolic pressure due to obstruction at mitral valve.

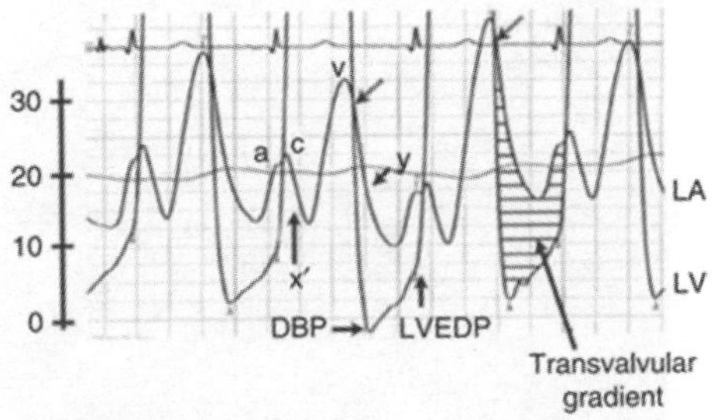

8. **Constriction versus Restriction**
   - There is discordance of pressures in LV and RV during respiration in constrictive pericarditis due to increased ventricular interdependence.
   - Whereas, there is concordance of pressures in LV and RV during respiration in Restrictive cardiomyopathy.

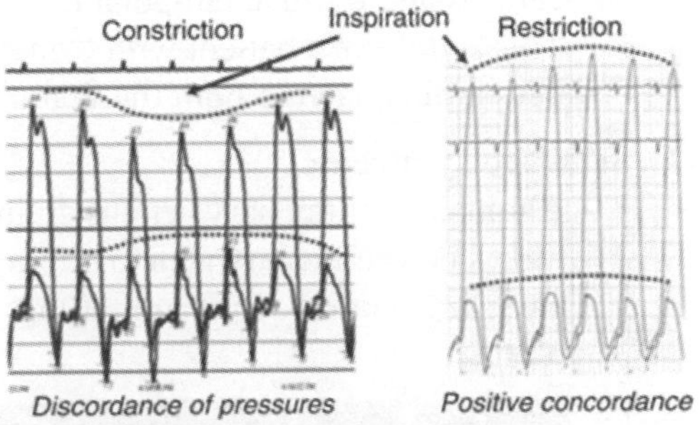

9. **Hypertrophic cardiomyopathy**
   - Asymmetric severe hypertrophy of IVS in HCM.

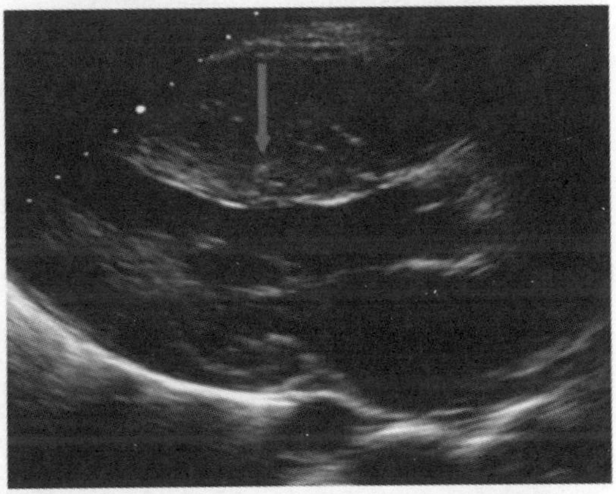

10. **Square root sign**
    - Dip and plateau in right ventricular diastolic pressure, known as square root sign.
    - Seen in Constrictive pericarditis as well as restrictive cardiomyopathy.

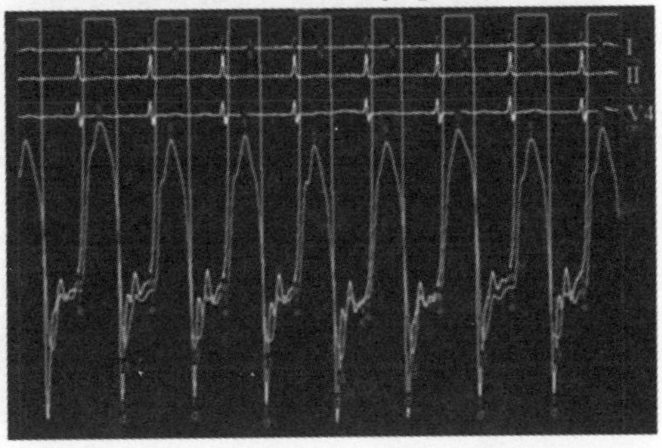

- Also seen in diastolic equalization of pressure in LV and RV (less than 5 mm Hg difference), feature of Constrictive pericarditis and Cardiac tamponade.
- This is trace of a patient with Constrictive pericarditis, having both the features.

11. Scimitar syndrome
- Anomalous pulmonary venous drainage of right sided pulmonary vein to inferior vena cava associated with right lung hypoplasia.

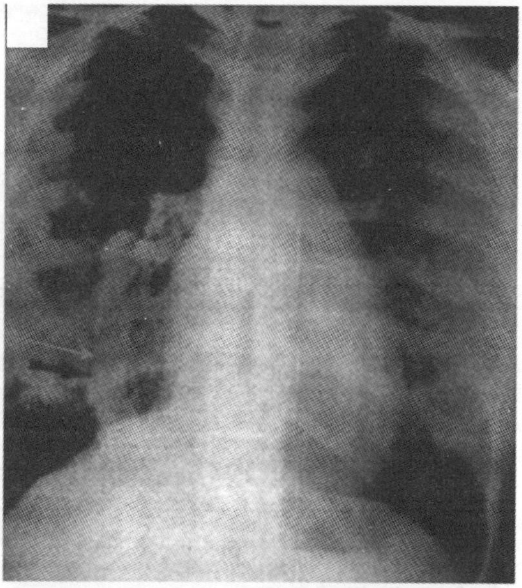

12. Ostium secundum ASD

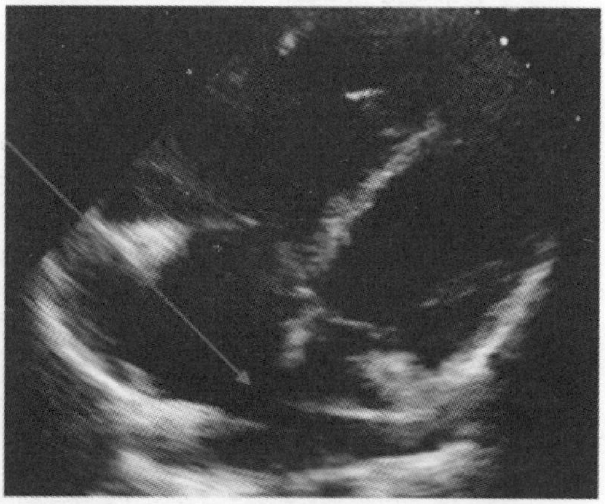

13. Cleft anterior mitral leaflet
- Associated with ostium primum ASD.

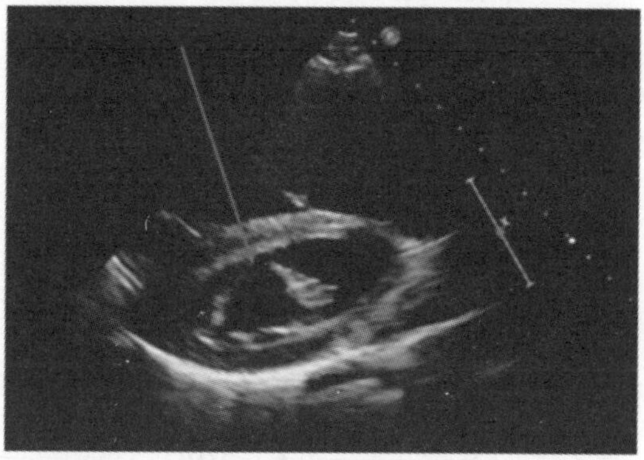

14. Peri-membranous VSD (parasternal short axis view)

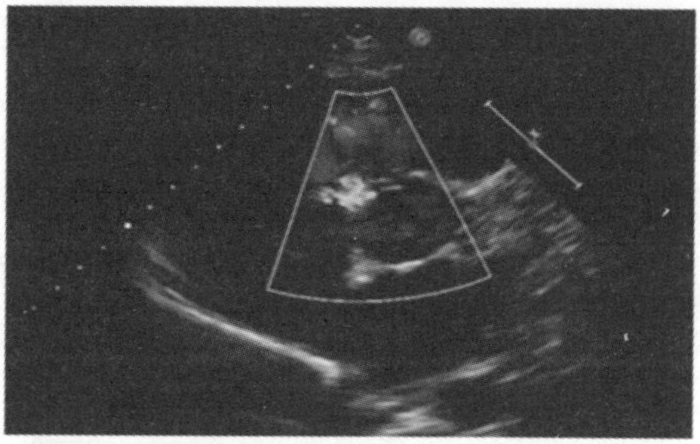

15. Patent ductus arteriosus

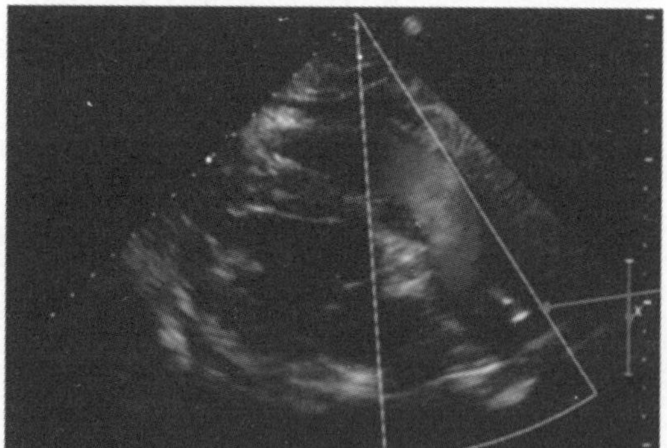

16. Ebstein's anomaly
- There is marked apical displacement of septal tricuspid leaflet causing atrialization of right ventricle.

- ECG might show wide and splintered QRS complex. Accessory pathways are common showing type B WPW syndrome.

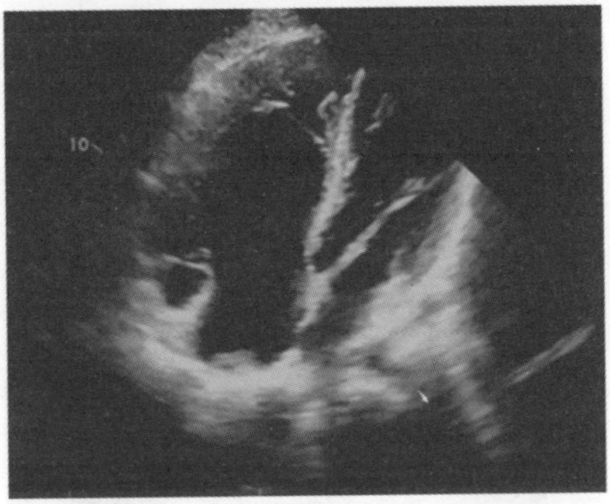

17. **Dextrocardia**
    - ECG shows poor precordial R wave progression with negative P waves in leads I, aVl and V1; and right axis deviation of QRS axis.
    - Other differential for negative p wave in lead 1 is right/left arm reversal but in that case R wave progression will be normal in chest leads.

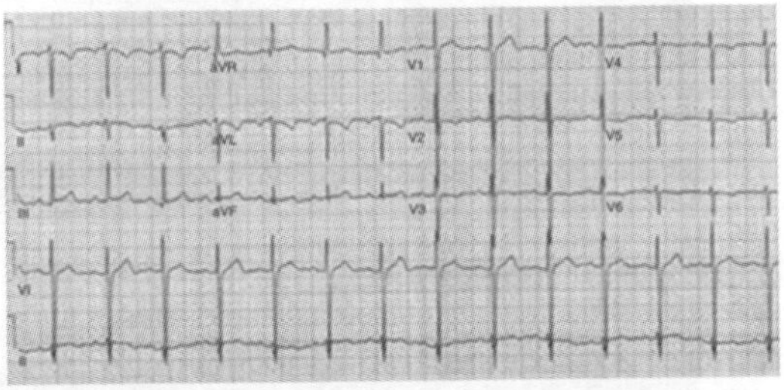

18. **Anomalous origin of coronary artery**
    - Reconstructed cardiac CT image showing RCA arising from left sinus along with left coronary artery. Note that all three coronary arteries arise from same left coronary sinus.

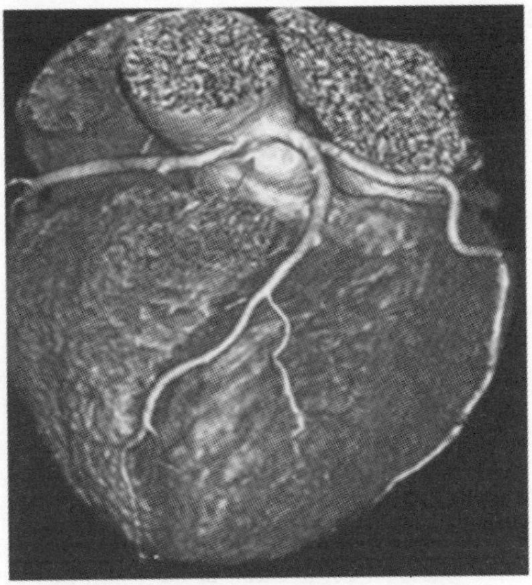

19. **Coarctation of aorta**
    - Suprasternal colour doppler echo image showing turbulence in DTA distal to origin of left subclavian artery. Continuous wave doppler at the same site shows increased gradient across the stenotic segment.

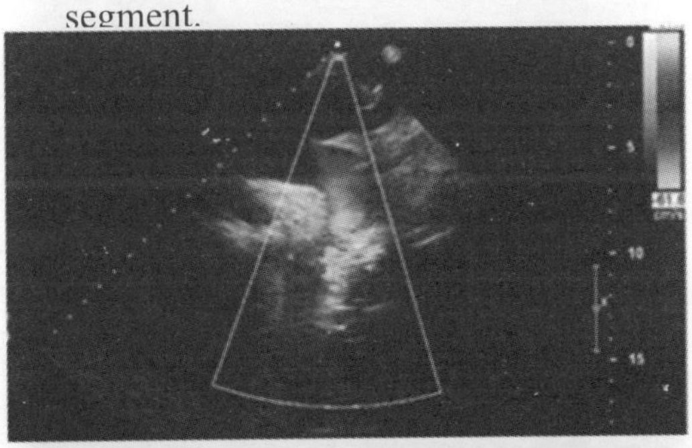

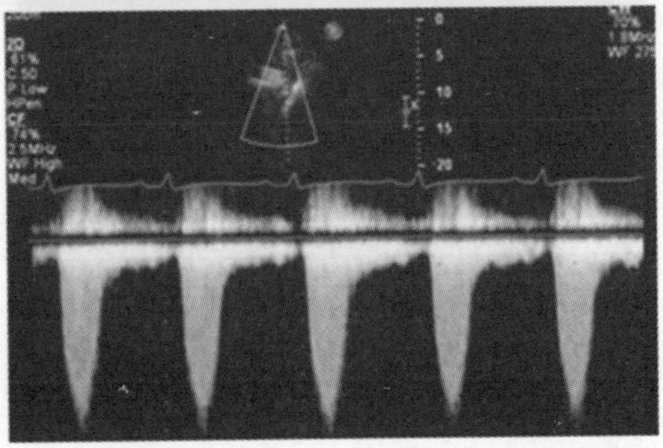

20. Systolic anterior motion of anterior mitral leaflet

- Diagnosis: Hypertrophic cardiomyopathy.

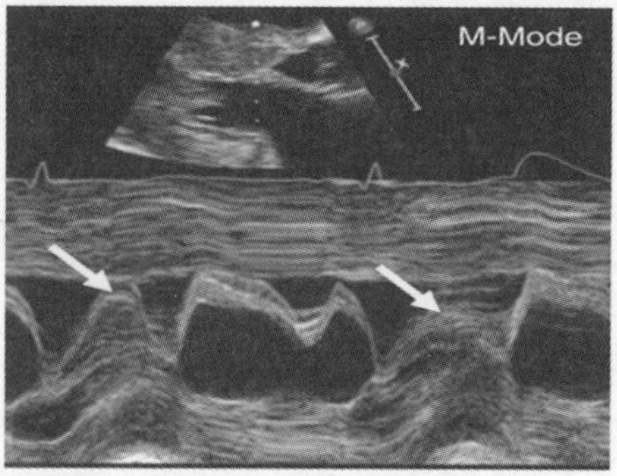

21. Takotsubo cardiomyopathy

- Apical hypokinesis and dilatation with preserved contraction at base can be seen in systole.

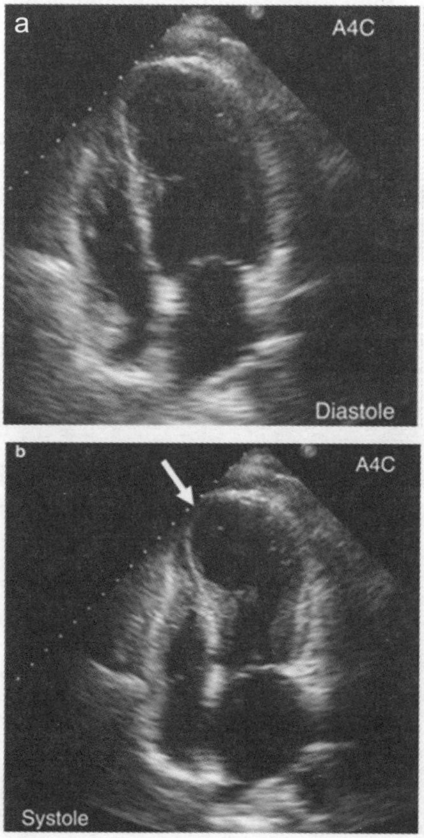

22. Rheumatic mitral stenosis

- Parasternal long axis view showing thickened mitral leaflets, hockey stick appearance of anterior mitral leaflet. Fishmouth appearance of mitral valve is seen in parasternal short axis.

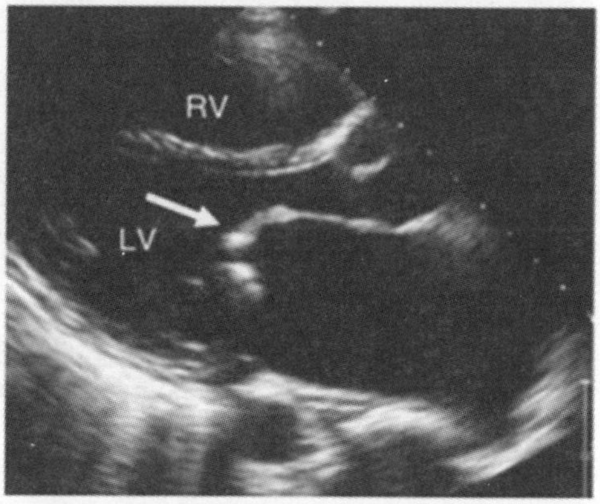

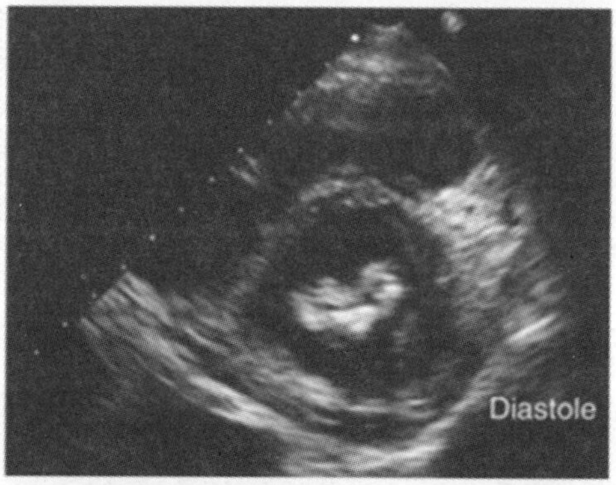

23. Coarctation of aorta

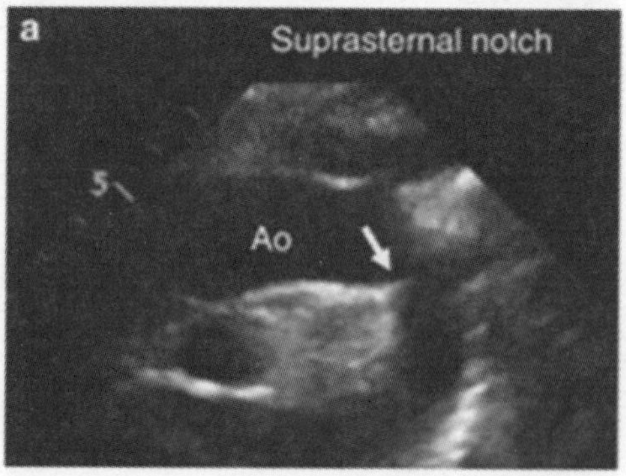

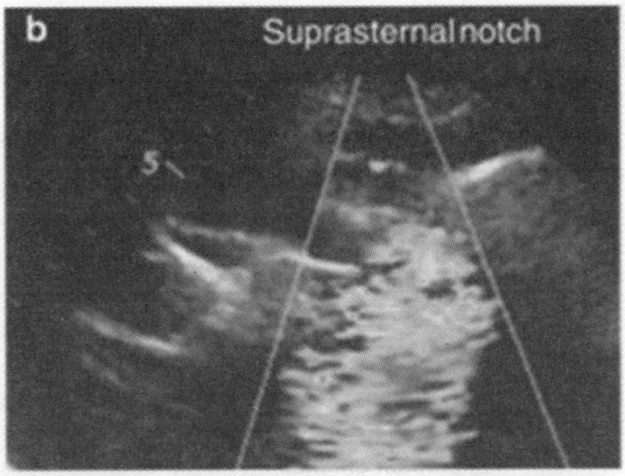

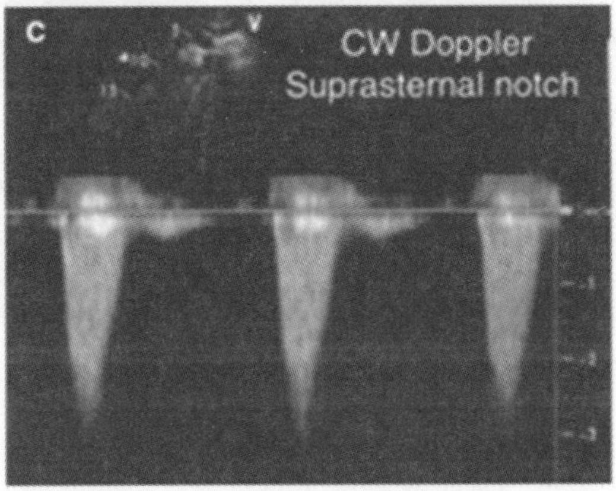

24. Atrial myxoma

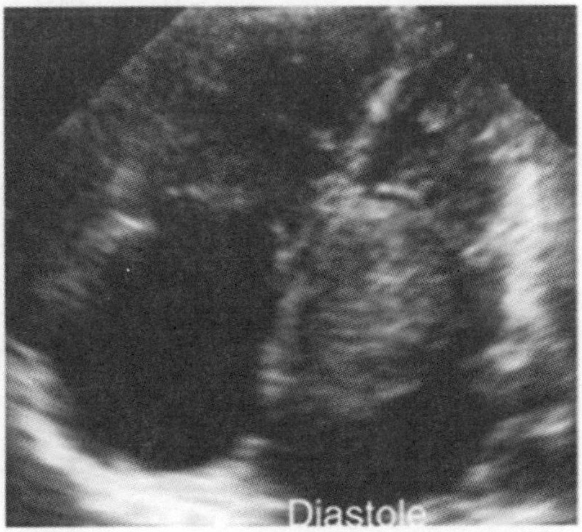

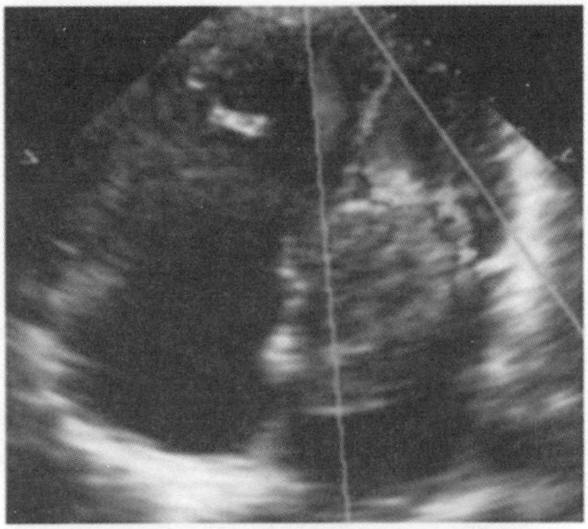

25. Ostium primum ASD

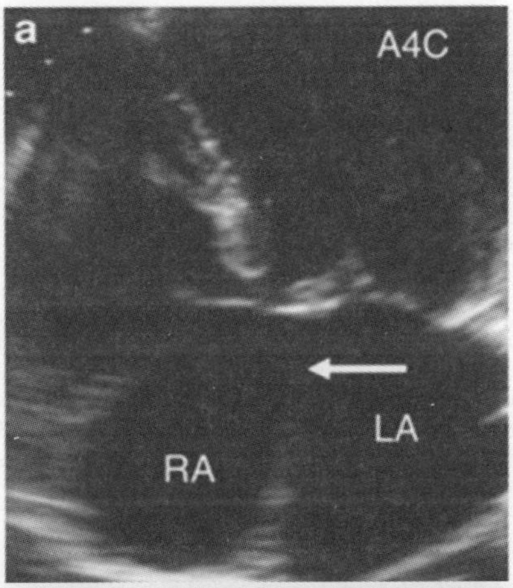

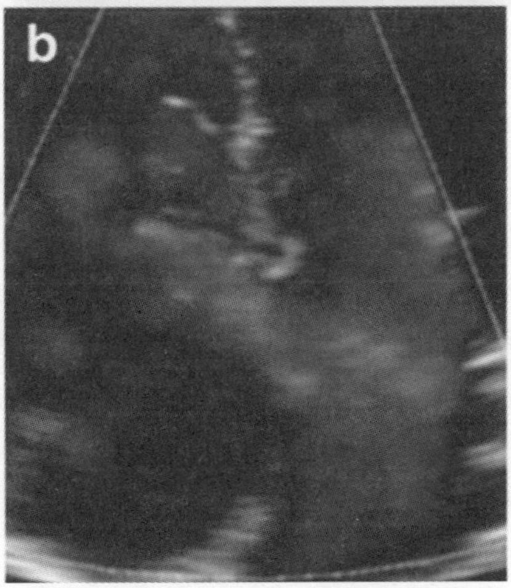

26. **Myocardial bridge**

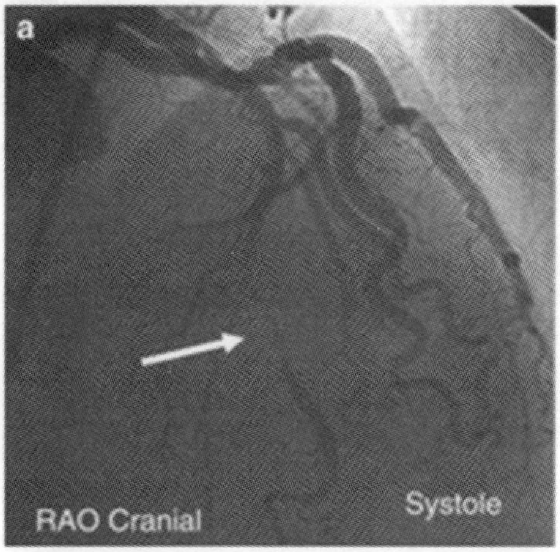

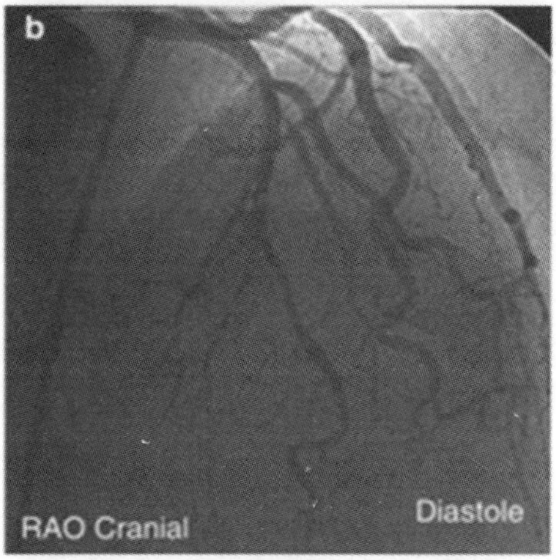

27. **Pulmonary embolism**
    - ECG–Sinus tachycardia, S1Q3T3 pattern, T wave inversion in V1 to V3.

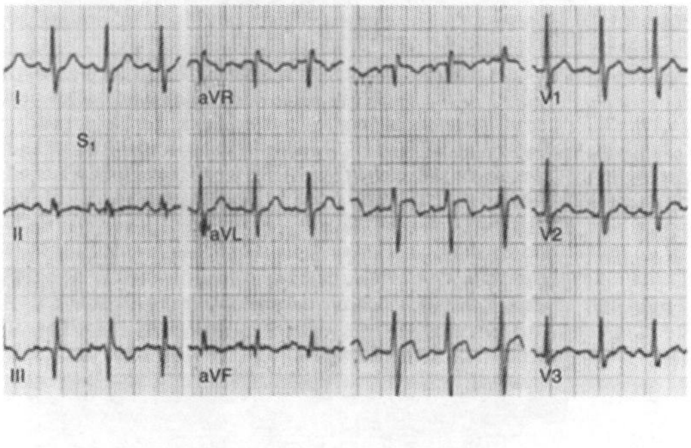

28. **Acute pulmonary embolism**
    - CT pulmonary angiography: Large thrombus in left pulmonary artery.

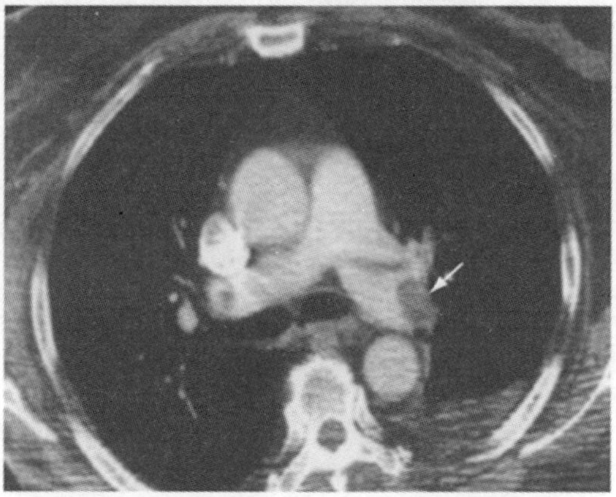

29. **Bidirectional VT**

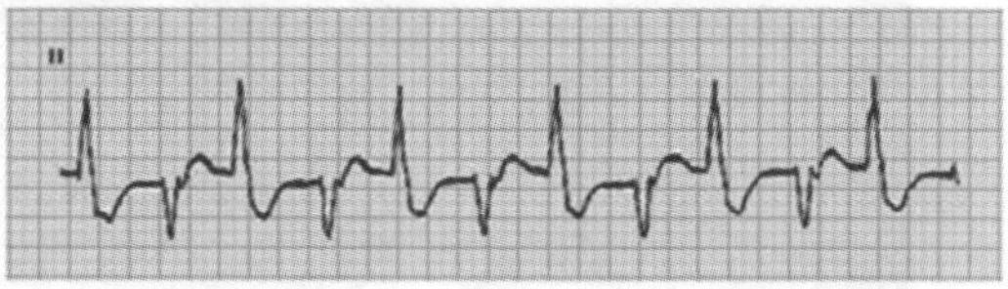

Causes:
1. Digoxin toxicity
2. Anderson syndrome
3. Aconite poisoning

30. **Patient with LV dysfunction**
    - Diagnosis–LV non-compaction.

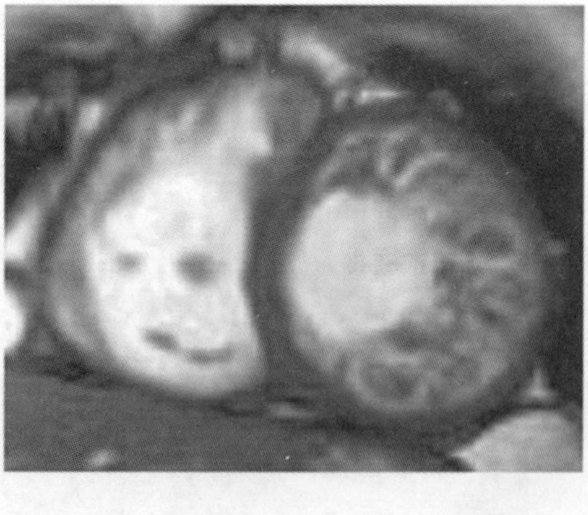

31. Anterior wall myocardial infarction

- Cardiac MRI following acute Anteroapical STEMI. There is thinning of anterior wall and apex and delayed gadolinium enhanced image shows infarcted tissue in anterior wall and at apex.

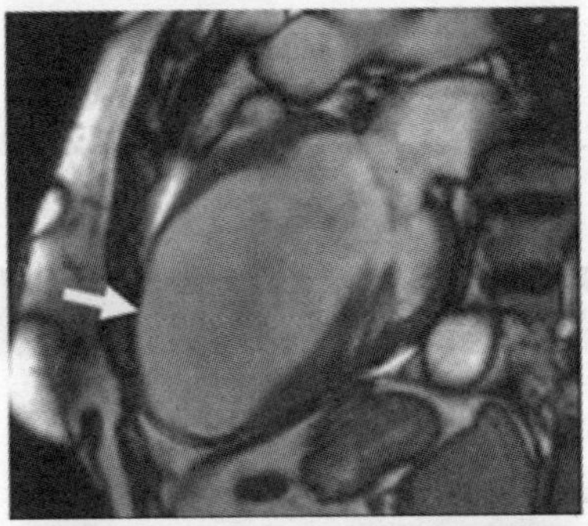

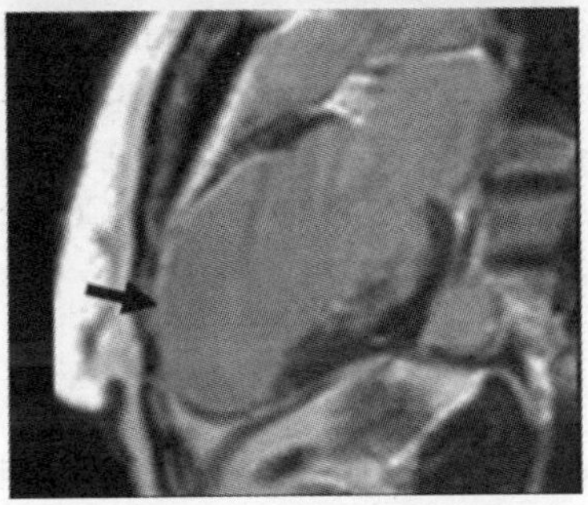

32. Brugada syndrome

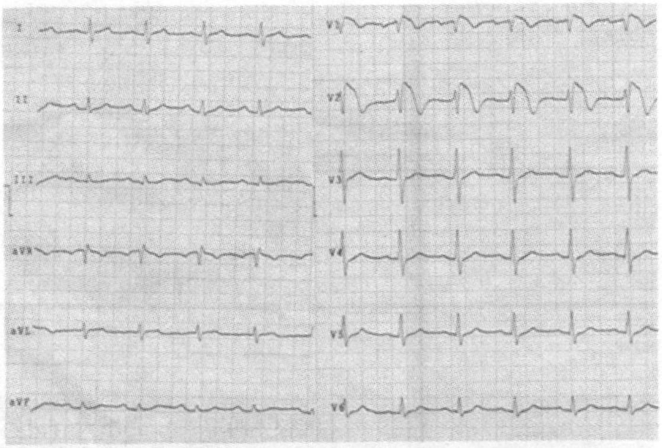

33. Type A WPW syndrome because of left sided accessory pathway

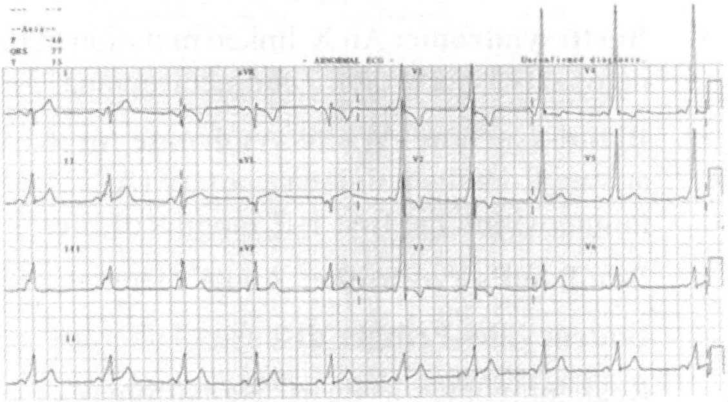

Appendices

1. Syndromes in Cardiology

- **Aase syndrome:** A clinical triad of congenital anaemia, triphalangeal thumbs and VSD.
- **Barlow's syndrome:** Myxomatous mitral valve prolapse, autosomal dominant trait.
- **Barth syndrome:** An X-linked mutation of the TAZ gene, leading to dilated cardiomyopathy, skeletal myopathy, short stature and neutropenia. 3-methylglutaconic acid excretion present in urine.
- **Bland–Garland–White syndrome (or ALCAPA):** Anomalous origin of the left coronary artery arising from the pulmonary artery (ALCAPA) resulting in myocardial ischaemia. Congestive heart failure within the first 1–2 months of life.
- **Bouillaud's syndrome:** Acute rheumatic fever.
- **Bourneville–Pringle disease:** Tuberous sclerosis.

  Rhabdomyomas in heart, Hamartomas of kidney associated with epilepsy, learning difficulties, cerebral cortical hamartomas, and adenoma sebaceum. Autosomal dominant trait.
- **Bradbury–Egglseton syndrome:** An idiopathic disorder of autonomic failure.

  Orthostatic hypotension; thermoregulatory, bowel, bladder, and sexual function disturbance.
- **Brugada's syndrome:** Mutation of the SCN5A gene on chromosome 3, results in malfunction of a sodium channel leading to initiation and perpetuation of ventricular arrhythmias; autosomal dominant trait.

  Clinically there is right bundle branch block, ST elevation in V1 to V3, and sudden death/syncope.
- **Carney syndrome:** Also known as the Carney complex; Autosomal dominant trait.

  Atrial myxomas with myxomas in other locations, e.g. breast or skin, spotty pigmentation, and endocrine overactivity, e.g. pituitary or testicular tumours.

  The mutation in the PRKAR1A gene on chromosome 17.
- **DiGeorge syndrome:** CATCH-22 syndrome, Velocardiofacial syndrome.

  Deletion of the TBX1 gene on chromosome 22q11.2

  Parathyroid hypoplasia (and hypocalcaemia), thymic hypoplasia (and low T-cell counts), and outflow tract defects of the heart, including tetralogy of Fallot, truncus arteriosus, interrupted aortic arch, right-sided aortic arch, and aberrant right subclavian artery.

- **Dressler syndrome:** A myocardial infarction-associated pericarditis, usually occurring one week after the onset of infarction, but may occur several months afterwards.

  Autoimmune aetiology, associated with pleuritis and pleural effusions, and response to non-steroidal drugs and steroids.
- **Duchenne muscular dystrophy:** An X-linked recessive disorder of the dystrophin gene. Severe skeletal muscle weakness, severe dilated cardiomyopathy. Supraventricular arrhythmias and heart blocks are also common.
- **Ebstein's anomaly:** Abnormal attachment of the tricuspid valve leaflets with apical displacement of the tricuspid valve, leading to atrialization of right ventricle. Tricuspid valve tissue is dysplastic.
- **Eisenmenger syndrome:** Any systemic-to-pulmonary circulation shunt that eventually leads to reversal or bidirectional flow of the shunt, with subsequent pulmonary hypertension and cyanosis.
- **Ellis–Van Creveld syndrome:** An autosomal recessive trait, characterized by short stature caused by metaphyseal dysplasia, polydactyly, dysplastic nails and teeth, and, most commonly, primum ASD.
- **Fabry disease:** A rare X-linked recessive lysosomal storage disorder, deficiency of the enzyme alpha galactosidase, accumulation of globotriasylceramide throughout the body.

  Cardiac manifestations include left and right ventricular hypertrophy and heart failure. Other systemic features include renal impairment, angiokeratomas, neuropathy, and corneal keratopathy.
- **Fallot's tetralogy:** The association of pulmonary stenosis, ventricular septal defect, overriding aorta, and right ventricular hypertrophy, causing cyanosis in the newborn.
- **Fallot's trilogy** comprises pulmonary stenosis, atrial septal defect, and intact ventricular septum.
- **Fallot's pentalogy** is the addition of an atrial septum defect or patent foramen ovale to the tetralogy.
- **Holt–Oram syndrome:** Autosomal dominant trait, dysplasia of the upper limbs associated with secundum ASD.
- **Heyde's syndrome:** The association of gastrointestinal bleeding due to angiodysplasia and calcific aortic stenosis. Bleeding occurs due to an acquired von Willebrands disease type 2a caused by high shear stress around the aortic valve. The bleeding abnormality ceases after replacement of the valve.
- **Jervell–Lange–Nielsen syndrome:** Sensorineural deafness associated with QT prolongation. Autosomal recessive condition, mutation in the KVLQT1 gene, or the KCNE1 gene, encoding delayed rectifier potassium channel.
- **Kartagener's syndrome:** A clinical triad of situs in versus, abnormal frontal sinuses, and immotile cilia. The patient has recurrent respiratory infections, sinusitis, bronchiectasis, and infertility. Inheritance is autosomal recessive.

  The defect lies in the genes encoding the dynein protein that contributes to the structure of cilia.
- **Kawasaki disease:** An acute vasculitis that affects children, which manifests with fever, cervical lymphadenopathy, bilateral conjunctivitis, erythema or desquamation of the palms and soles, and coronary artery aneurysms or ectasia. These may lead to myocardial infarction and sudden death.

- **Lenegre–Lev disease:** Accelerated degenerative process that primarily affecting conduction tissue. Leads to development of completed heart block. Autosomal dominant, chromosome 19.
- **Løffler's syndrome:** Hypereosinophilic condition (cause may be helminthic infection, leukemia or unknown) leads to fibrosis of endomyocardium leading to a clinical syndrome of restrictive cardiomyopathy.
- **Lown–Ganong–Levine syndrome:** A ventricular pre-excitation phenomenon characterized by a short PR interval (<120 ms) and normal QRS duration. It occurs due to intranodal or paranodal fibres that bypass the AV node.
- **Libman–Sacks syndrome:** A cardiac manifestation of systemic lupus erythematosus and antiphospholipid syndrome. Sterile, verrucous lesions on valve leaflets (Mostly mitral valve and aortic valve) and chordae consisting of fibrin, neutrophils, lymphocytes, and histiocytes.
- **Lutembacher's syndrome:** Combination of mitral stenosis (congenital or acquired) and ASD (congenital or iatrogenic), with left-to-right shunt.
- **Marfan syndrome:** Mutation in the `FBN1` gene on chromosome 15q21.1 encoding fibrillin-1. Features include tall stature, kyphosis, scoliosis, pectus excavatum, upwards lens dislocation, dural ectasia, retinal detachment, and a variety of cardiac abnormalities.

  These include mitral valve prolapse and regurgitation, dilated sinuses of Valsalva, aortic root dilatation with aortic regurgitation and increased risk of dissection. Autosomal dominant inheritance.
- **Noonan's syndrome:** A dysmorphic syndrome characterized by cardiac anomalies, short stature, low-set ears, hypertelorism and deafness. Autosomal dominant inheritance.

  Cardiac problems include valvular and supravalvular pulmonary stenosis. This syndrome has sometimes been called 'male Turner's syndrome', although it affects both sexes.
- **Ortner's syndrome:** First described as compression of the recurrent laryngeal nerve by a dilated left atrium in mitral valve stenosis, giving rise to a hoarse voice from vocal cord paresis. Sometimes used to describe any non-malignant cardiac or intrathoracic process that damages the recurrent laryngeal nerve. The left nerve is more commonly affected than the right, due to its longer course around the aortic arch.
- **Romano–Ward syndrome:** Genetic syndrome of QT interval prolongation without deafness.

  Autosomal dominant condition caused by mutation in genes encoding different components of both sodium and potassium channels. The QT interval is prolonged and there is a high risk of developing torsades de pointes and sudden cardiac death (SCD).
- **Stokes–Adams syndrome:** Syncope caused by cardiac arrhythmia.
- **Takotsubo cardiomyopathy:** Apical ballooning syndrome in response to stress with hypercontractile basal region of LV and normal coronaries on angiography.
- **Taussig–Bing syndrome:** Double outlet right ventricle with large subpulmonic VSD without pulmonic stenosis; behaves as transposed great arteries.

- **Turner's syndrome:** A disorder resulting from the absence of one of the X chromosomes, XO. Features include coarctation of the aorta, short stature, absence of secondary sexual characteristics, webbing of the neck, cubitus valgus, and lymphoedema.
- **Twiddler's syndrome:** The phenomenon of lead dislodgement from the cardiac attachment due to rotation of pulse generator in its subcutaneous pocket.
- **Wenkebach's heart:** A description of a heart located in the midline which is smaller than normal. Also known as mesocardia, or the 'hanging heart'.
- **Wenkebach's phenomenon:** A form of second-degree AV block characterized by progressive lengthening of the PR interval on the ECG until a P wave is not conducted to the ventricles.
- **Williams syndrome:** A congenital supravalvular aortic stenosis associated with peripheral pulmonary artery stenosis, hypercalcaemia, elfin facies, outgoing personality, learning difficulties, strabismus, and dental anomalies. The left ventricle may be hypertrophied, and the sinuses of Valsalva may be dilated. Autosomal dominant inheritance.
- **Wolff–Parkinson–White syndrome:** Tachyarrhythmias that occur as a result of an accessory atrioventricular pathway, typified by the ECG features in sinus rhythm of a PR interval less than 120 ms and QRS duration greater than 120 ms and presence of a delta wave, representing antegrade conduction through the accessory pathway.

2. Murmur Eponyms

- **Austin Flint murmur:** Mitral mid-diastolic murmur heard in severe AR.
- **Carey Coombs murmur:** Mid-diastolic mitral murmur due to mitral valvulitis in rheumatic fever. There is no mitral stenosis and it usually disappears over time as the valvulitis improves. It is usually associated with S3. It occurs because of increased blood flow across thickened mitral valve.
- **Cabot–Locke Murmur or Hemic murmur:** Early diastolic murmur seen in severe anemia, best heard at left sternal border.
- **Cecil Cole murmur:** Early diastolic aortic insufficiency murmur conducted to the apex and left axilla.
- **Cooing dove or Sea-gull's murmur:** The cooing dove murmur is a cardiac murmur with a musical quality, has been described in multiple conditions but commonly associated with aortic valve regurgitation (or mitral regurgitation before rupture of chordae). It is a diastolic murmur, heard over the mid-precordium.
- **Dock's murmur:** Continuous diastolic murmur seen in stenosis of left anterior descending artery.
- **Graham Steel murmur:** Early diastolic murmur of PR seen in severe pulmonary hypertension.
- **Gallavardin phenomenon:** A loud, harsh, blowing murmur at the apex associated with AS (easily confused with MR or HCM often and can be differentiated by maneuvers).
- **Gibsons murmur:** Continuous machinery murmur in PDA due to flow from the descending thoracic aorta to the pulmonary artery, with maximal intensity at S2.

- **Innocent murmur:** Functional murmurs.
- **Key–Hodgkin Murmur:** Diastolic murmur of AR due to retroversion of aortic valve leaflets in syphilitic aortitis.
- **Mill-wheel or Water-wheel murmur:** Usually associated with large intracardiac air embolism or pneumopericardium. It is a machinery-like, churning or splashing sound due to blood mixing with air, best heard over the precordium.
- **Roger's Murmur:** Harsh holosystolic murmur of small VSD, best heard at left upper sternal border.
- **Rytand's murmur:** Mid diastolic murmur in complete heart block.
- **Still's murmur:** Musical systolic ejection murmur seen in children which increases with fever, anxiety, or exercise. Exact cause is unknown, however, source may be vibration of chordae tendineae in left ventricle or sound of blood gushing into the aorta.

3. Surgical Procedures for Congenital Heart Diseases

- **Blalock Taussig Shunt:** Subclavian artery to branch PA connection.

  (Note: Reduced BP and pulse in affected arm)
- **Waterston Shunt:** Ascending aorta to right PA shunt.
- **Potts Shunt:** Descending aorta to left PA shunt.
- **Mustard/Senning:** Atrial switch for D TGA-redirects venous inflow (Mustard: pericardial or Gore-Tex patch, Senning: native atrial tissue).
- **Jatene arterial switch:** Arterial switch for D TGA (began in 1980s).
- **Glenn Shunt:** SVC to right PA shunt.
- **Fontan (total cavopulmonary anastomosis):** Redirecting systemic venous return to the lungs without a ventricular pump (RA to PA, lateral tunnel, extracardiac).
- **Rastelli operation:** Right ventricle to PA conduit, used in VSD with severe PS (Double outlet right ventricle and D-TGA morphology most commonly). LV patch directed to aorta by creating an intraventricular tunnel between VSD and aortic valve; RV conduit to PA.
- **REV procedure:** For D-TGA (or DORV) with VSD and severe PS, an alternative to Rastelli procedure.

  Infundibular resection to enlarge VSD, 2. Intraventricular baffle to direct LV output to aorta, 3. Aortic transection to perform the Lecompte maneuver (RPA is brought anterior to ascending aorta), 4. Direct RV to PA reconstruction by using an anterior patch.
- **Nikaidoh procedure:** For D-TGA (DORV) with VSD and severe PS, another alternative to Rastelli procedure.

  Harvesting aortic root from RV, 2. Relieving the LVOT by enlarging VSD, 3. Reconstructing the LVOT, 4. Reconstructing the RVOT with a pericardial patch.

- **Damus-Kaye-Stansel operation:** For VSD and significant subaortic stenosis (TGA or DORV with subaortic stenosis).

  1. Subaortic stenosis is bypassed by connecting the proximal PA trunk to ascending aorta, 2. VSD is closed, 3. Conduit is placed between RV and distal PA.
- **PA banding:** Surgically created stenosis of the main PA; palliative procedure to protect the lungs against high pulmonary blood flow when definitive repair is not immediately feasible
- **Warden procedure:** Baffle technique in SV-ASD with PAPVC in the SVC
- **Norwood operation:** Performed in neonatal period, initial palliative surgery for hypoplastic left heart syndrome. 1. Main PA is divided, distal stump is closed, 2. Proximal PA connected to hypoplastic ascending aorta, 3. Pulmonary blood flow is established by either modified BT shunt or RV to PA shunt (Sano modification).

  Norwood procedure is later followed by Glenn procedure and Fontan surgery for final palliation.
- **Danielson technique and Carpentier technique:** Both techniques used for reconstruction (repair) of tricuspid valve in Ebstein anomaly. Tricuspid valve repair is preferable to replacement.
- **Takeuchi repair and Tashiro repair:** Both used for repair of anomalous left coronary artery from pulmonary artery (ALCAPA).
- **Ross Procedure:** The autologous pulmonary valve is used to replace pulmonary valve, and pulmonary allograft is used for pulmonary valve.
- **Double Ross procedure:** When person's own aortic valve is used for pulmonary position in Ross procedure.

4. Channelopathies and Genetic Associations

Syndrome	**Gene**	**Protein/Channel affected**
LQTS 1	KCNQ1	I_{Ks} channel
LQTS 2	KCNH2 (HERG)	I_{Kr} channel
LQTS 3	SCN5A	I_{Na} channel
LQTS 4	ANK2	Ankyrin B
LQTS 5	KCNE1	I_{Ks}
LQTS 6	KCNE2	I_{Kr}
LQTS 7 (Anderson-Tawil syndrome)	KCNJ2	I_{K1}
LQTS 8 (Timothy syndrome)	CACNA1C	I_{Ca}
Jervell LN- 1	KCNQ1	I_{Ks}
Jervell LN -2	KCNE1	I_{Kr}
Romano-Ward syndrome	KCNQ1,KCNH2,SCN5A	I_{Ks}, I_{Kr}, I_{Na}

Brugada syndrome	SCN5A	I_{Na}
CPVT 1	RYR2	Ryanodine receptor
CPVT 2	CASQ2	Calsequestrin
CPVT 3	TECRL	Trans-2,3-enoyl-CoA reductase like protein
CPVT 4	CALM1	Calmodulin
CPVT 5	TRDN	Triadin
SQTS 1	KCNH2 (HERG)	I_{Kr}
SQTS 2	KCNQ1	I_{Ks}
SQTS 3	KCNJ2	I_{K1}

5. Major Clinical Trials (2019)

COACT trial: Coronary Angiography after Cardiac Arrest without ST-Segment Elevation

Among patients who have been successfully resuscitated after out-of-hospital cardiac arrest and have no signs of STEMI, a strategy of immediate angiography is not better than a strategy of delayed angiography with respect to overall survival at 90 days.

RACE 7 ACWAS trial: Early or Delayed Cardioversion in Recent-Onset Atrial Fibrillation

In patients presenting to the emergency department with recent-onset, symptomatic atrial fibrillation, a wait-and-see approach is noninferior to early cardioversion in achieving a return to sinus rhythm at 4 weeks.

CREOLE trial: Comparison of Dual Therapies for Lowering Blood Pressure in Black Africans

In black patients in sub-Saharan Africa, amlodipine plus either hydrochlorothiazide or perindopril is more effective than perindopril plus hydrochlorothiazide at lowering blood pressure at 6 months.

AUGUSTUS trial: Antithrombotic Therapy after Acute Coronary Syndrome or PCI in Atrial Fibrillation

In patients with atrial fibrillation and a recent acute coronary syndrome or PCI treated with a P2Y12 inhibitor, an antithrombotic regimen that includes apixaban, without aspirin, results in less bleeding and fewer hospitalizations without significant differences in the incidence of ischemic events than regimens that include a vitamin K antagonist, aspirin, or both.

MOMENTUM 3 trial: A Fully Magnetically Levitated Left Ventricular Assist Device

Among patients with advanced heart failure, a fully magnetically levitated centrifugal-flow left ventricular assist device is associated with less frequent need for pump replacement than an axial-flow device and is superior with respect to survival free of disabling stroke or reoperation to replace or remove a malfunctioning device.

WRAP-IT trial: Antibacterial Envelope to Prevent Cardiac Implantable Device Infection

Adjunctive use of an antibacterial envelope results in a significantly lower incidence of major CIED infections than standard-of-care infection-prevention strategies alone, without a higher incidence of complications.

PARTNER 3 trial: Transcatheter Aortic-Valve Replacement with a Balloon-Expandable Valve in Low-Risk Patients

Among patients with severe aortic stenosis who are at low surgical risk, the rate of the composite of death, stroke, or rehospitalization at 1 year is significantly lower with TAVR than with surgery.

Evolut Low Risk Trial: Transcatheter Aortic-Valve Replacement with a Self-Expanding Valve in Low-Risk Patients

In patients with severe aortic stenosis who are at low surgical risk, TAVR with a self-expanding supraannular bioprosthesis is noninferior to surgery with respect to the composite end point of death or disabling stroke at 24 months.

CLEAR Harmony Trial: Safety and Efficacy of Bempedoic Acid to Reduce LDL Cholesterol

Bempedoic acid when added to maximally tolerated statin therapy leads to significantly lower LDL cholesterol levels without increasing the adverse effects.

CIRT trial: Low-Dose Methotrexate for the Prevention of Atherosclerotic Events

Among patients with stable atherosclerosis, low-dose methotrexate does not reduce levels of interleukin-1â, interleukin-6, or C-reactive protein and does not result in fewer cardiovascular events than placebo.

PIONEER-HF: Angiotensin–Neprilysin Inhibition in Acute Decompensated Heart Failure

Among patients with heart failure with reduced ejection fraction who are hospitalized for acute decompensated heart failure, the initiation of sacubitril–valsartan therapy leads to a greater reduction in the NT-proBNP concentration than enalapril therapy. Rates of worsening renal function, hyperkalemia, symptomatic hypotension, and angioedema do not differ significantly between the two groups.

ANNEXA-4: Andexanet Alfa for Bleeding Associated with Factor Xa Inhibitors

In patients with acute major bleeding associated with the use of a factor Xa inhibitor, treatment with andexanet markedly reduces anti–factor Xa activity, and 82% of patients have excellent or good hemostatic efficacy at 12 hours.

POET trial: Partial Oral versus Intravenous Antibiotic Treatment of Endocarditis

In patients with endocarditis on the left side of the heart who are in stable condition, changing to oral antibiotic treatment after initial intravenous antibiotics for 10 days is noninferior to continued intravenous antibiotic treatment.

Arterial Revascularization Trial: Bilateral versus Single Internal-Thoracic-Artery Grafts at 10 Years

Among patients who are scheduled for CABG and have been randomly assigned to undergo bilateral or single internal-thoracic-artery grafting, there is no significant between-group difference in the rate of death from any cause at 10 years.

DECLARE–TIMI 58 trial: Dapagliflozin and Cardiovascular Outcomes in Type 2 Diabetes

In patients with type 2 diabetes who had or were at risk for atherosclerotic cardiovascular disease, treatment with dapagliflozin results in a lower rate of cardiovascular death or hospitalization for heart failure, a finding that reflects a lower rate of hospitalization for heart failure.

VITAL trial: Vitamin D Supplements and Prevention of Cancer and Cardiovascular Disease

Supplementation with vitamin D does not result in a lower incidence of invasive cancer or cardiovascular events than placebo.

CANTIC Study: Platelet Inhibition with Cangrelor and Crushed Ticagrelor in Patients with ST-Elevation Myocardial Infarction Undergoing Primary Percutaneous Coronary Intervention

In patients undergoing Primary PCI, cangrelor is an effective strategy to bridge the gap in platelet inhibition associated with the use of oral P2Y12 inhibition induced by ticagrelor. Ticagrelor can be administered as a crushed formulation concomitantly with cangrelor without any apparent drug-drug interactions.

DECISION-CTO Trial: Randomized Trial Evaluating Percutaneous Coronary Intervention for the Treatment of Chronic Total Occlusion

There was no difference in the incidence of major adverse cardiovascular events with CTO PCI vs. no CTO-PCI.

SAFARI-STEMI study:

There is no survival or bleeding advantage with radial over femoral access in STEMI.

PANACHE study:

Safety and efficacy of neladenoson bialanate for the treatment of patients with HF with preserved ejection fraction.

Neladenoson bialanate, a partial A1 receptor agonist in HFpEF patients, was safe at 20 weeks but no dose response relationship was demonstrated for any of the endpoints.

6. Major Clinical Trials (2018)

COAPT trial: Transcatheter Mitral-Valve Repair in Patients with Heart Failure

Among patients with heart failure and moderate-to-severe or severe secondary mitral regurgitation who remain symptomatic despite the use of maximal doses of guideline-directed medical therapy, transcatheter mitral-valve repair results in a lower rate of hospitalization for heart failure and lower all-cause mortality within 24 months of follow-up than medical therapy alone.

MITRA-FR trial: Percutaneous Repair or Medical Treatment for Secondary Mitral Regurgitation

Among patients with severe secondary mitral regurgitation, the rate of death or unplanned hospitalization for heart failure at 1 year do not differ significantly between patients who undergo percutaneous mitral-valve repair in addition to receiving medical therapy and those who receive medical therapy alone.

ODYSSEY OUTCOMES: Alirocumab and Cardiovascular Outcomes after Acute Coronary Syndrome

Among patients who had a previous acute coronary syndrome and who were receiving high-intensity statin therapy, the risk of recurrent ischemic cardiovascular events is lower among those who receive alirocumab when compared with placebo.

CULPRIT-SHOCK: One-Year Outcomes after PCI Strategies in Cardiogenic Shock

Among patients with acute myocardial infarction and cardiogenic shock, the risk of death or renal-replacement therapy at 30 days is lower with culprit-lesion-only PCI than with immediate multivessel PCI, and mortality does not differ significantly between the two groups at 1 year of follow-up.

ASCEND trial: Effects of Aspirin for Primary Prevention in Persons with Diabetes Mellitus

Aspirin use prevents serious vascular events in persons who have diabetes and no evident cardiovascular disease at trial entry, but it also causes major bleeding events. The absolute benefits are largely counterbalanced by the bleeding hazard.

ASPREE trial: Effect of Aspirin on Cardiovascular Events and Bleeding in the Healthy Elderly

The use of low-dose aspirin as a primary prevention strategy in older adults resulted in a significantly higher risk of major hemorrhage and did not result in a significantly lower risk of cardiovascular disease than placebo.

COMMANDER HF trial: Rivaroxaban in Patients with Heart Failure, Sinus Rhythm, and Coronary Disease

Rivaroxaban at a dose of 2.5 mg twice daily is not associated with a significantly lower rate of death, myocardial infarction, or stroke than placebo among patients with worsening chronic heart failure, reduced left ventricular ejection fraction, coronary artery disease, and no atrial fibrillation.

VEST trial: Wearable Cardioverter–Defibrillator after Myocardial Infarction

Among patients with a recent myocardial infarction and an ejection fraction of 35% or less, the wearable cardioverter–defibrillator does not lead to a significantly lower rate of the primary outcome of arrhythmic death than control.

ATTR-ACT Study: Tafamidis Treatment for Patients with Transthyretin Amyloid Cardiomyopathy

In patients with transthyretin amyloid cardiomyopathy, tafamidis is associated with reductions in all-cause mortality and cardiovascular-related hospitalizations and reduces the decline in functional capacity and quality of life as compared with placebo.

FAME 2 trial: Five-Year Outcomes with PCI Guided by Fractional Flow Reserve

In patients with stable coronary artery disease, an initial FFR-guided PCI strategy is associated with a significantly lower rate of the primary composite end point of death, myocardial infarction, or urgent revascularization at 5 years than medical therapy alone. Patients without hemodynamically significant stenoses had a favorable long-term outcome with medical therapy alone.

RADIAL trial: Radial-Artery or Saphenous-Vein Grafts in Coronary-Artery Bypass Surgery

As compared with the use of saphenous-vein grafts, the use of radial-artery grafts for CABG results in a lower rate of adverse cardiac events and a higher rate of patency at 5 years of follow-up.

PRESERVE Trial: Outcomes after Angiography with Sodium Bicarbonate and Acetylcysteine

Among patients at high risk for renal complications who undergo angiography, there is no benefit of intravenous sodium bicarbonate over intravenous sodium chloride or of oral acetylcysteine over placebo for the prevention of death, need for dialysis, or persistent decline in kidney function at 90 days or for the prevention of contrast-associated acute kidney injury.

CASTLE-AF trial: Catheter Ablation for Atrial Fibrillation with Heart Failure

Catheter ablation for atrial fibrillation in patients with heart failure is associated with a significantly lower rate of a composite end point of death from any cause or hospitalization for worsening heart failure than medical therapy.

TRANSIENT study: Timing of revascularization in patients with transient ST-segment elevation myocardial infarction

Overall, infarct size in transient STEMI is small and is not influenced by an immediate or delayed invasive strategy. Outcomes in terms of MACEs are similar in both immediate PCI and delayed invasive PCI groups.

ULTIMATE Trial: Intravascular Ultrasound Versus Angiography-Guided Drug-Eluting Stent Implantation

IVUS-guided DES implantation significantly improves clinical outcomes and was associated with lower frequency of target vessel failure, compared with angiography guidance.

IABP-SHOCK II Trial: Intraaortic Balloon Pump in Cardiogenic Shock Complicating Acute Myocardial Infarction (6 years outcomes)

IABP has no effect on all-cause mortality at 6-year long-term follow-up. Mortality is still very high, with two thirds of patients with cardiogenic shock dying despite contemporary treatment with revascularization therapy.

ISAR-TEST 4 trial: Biodegradable Polymer Versus Permanent Polymer Drug-Eluting Stents and Everolimus- Versus Sirolimus-Eluting Stents in Patients With Coronary Artery Disease (10 years outcomes)

PCI with a biodegradable polymer DES was noninferior to PCI with a permanent polymer-based DES with regard to the composite endpoint of cardiac death, MI related to the target vessel, or TLR at 12 months. Results were sustained over 10 years of follow-up

TRED-HF trial: Withdrawal of pharmacological treatment for heart failure in patients with recovered dilated cardiomyopathy

Withdrawal of HF medications among patients with DCM who had recovered their LV function results in relapse of HF.

ABSORB IV trial: Absorb BVS is noninferior to cobalt-chromium-based Xience DES up to 1 year for cardiovascular outcomes in fairly simple lesion types.

CHAMPION PHOENIX trial:

In patients with stable or unstable coronary artery disease undergoing PCI, the use of cangrelor reduced early ischemic events, including stent thrombosis and MI, compared with clopidogrel.

DETO2X-AMI trial: Determination of the Role of Oxygen in Suspected Acute Myocardial Infarction

Routine use of supplemental oxygen in normoxemic patients with suspected myocardial infarction does not reduce the composite of all-cause mortality and hospitalization for heart failure, or cardiovascular death within 1 year or during long-term follow-up.

CABANA trial: Catheter Ablation vs Antiarrhythmic Drug Therapy in Atrial Fibrillation

Ablation is not superior to drug therapy for CV outcomes at 5 years among patients with new-onset or untreated AF that required therapy. Catheter ablation is associated with a significant reduction in recurrent AF compared with drug therapy.

ARRIVE trial: Aspirin to reduce risk of initial vascular events in patients at moderate risk of cardiovascular disease

Aspirin was not associated with a reduction in adverse cardiovascular events. Bleeding events were low and similar between treatment arms.

TOPCAT trial:

Spironolactone is not superior to placebo in improving CV outcomes in patients with HFpEF.

ORBITA trial: Percutaneous coronary intervention in stable angina

In patients with medically treated angina and severe coronary stenosis, PCI did not increase exercise time by more than the effect of a sham procedure.

EUROCTO trial: A randomized multicentre trial to compare revascularization with optimal medical therapy for the treatment of chronic total coronary occlusions

Percutaneous coronary intervention leads to a significant improvement of the health status in patients with stable angina and a CTO as compared with OMT alone.

VANISH trial: Ventricular tachycardia ablation versus escalation of antiarrhythmic drugs

Among individuals with prior myocardial infarction and ischemic cardiomyopathy with persistent episodes of VT, catheter ablation of VT was superior to escalation of antiarrhythmic drug therapy.

PRAGUE-18: Comparison of Prasugrel and Ticagrelor in the Treatment of Acute Myocardial Infarction

Among patients with STEMI undergoing primary PCI, similar efficacy and bleeding was observed for either prasugrel or ticagrelor.

7. Major Clinical Trials (2017)

COMPASS trial: Rivaroxaban with or without Aspirin in Stable Cardiovascular Disease

Among patients with stable atherosclerotic vascular disease, those assigned to rivaroxaban (2.5 mg twice daily) plus aspirin had better cardiovascular outcomes and more major bleeding events than those assigned to aspirin alone.

DETO2X–SWEDEHEART trial: Oxygen Therapy in Suspected Acute Myocardial Infarction

Routine use of supplemental oxygen in patients with suspected myocardial infarction who do not have hypoxemia is not found to reduce 1-year all-cause mortality.

CANTOS Trial: Antiinflammatory Therapy with Canakinumab for Atherosclerotic Disease

Antiinflammatory therapy targeting the interleukin-1β innate immunity pathway with canakinumab at a dose of 150 mg every 3 months leads to a significantly lower rate of recurrent cardiovascular events than placebo, independent of lipid-level lowering.

CANVAS trial: Canagliflozin and Cardiovascular and Renal Events in Type 2 Diabetes

In two trials involving patients with type 2 diabetes and an elevated risk of cardiovascular disease, patients treated with canagliflozin had a lower risk of cardiovascular events than those who received placebo but a greater risk of amputation, primarily at the level of the toe or metatarsal.

ROOBY-FS trial: Five-Year Outcomes after On-Pump and Off-Pump Coronary-Artery Bypass

Off-pump CABG leads to lower rates of 5-year survival and event-free survival than on-pump CABG.

ATHOS-3: Angiotensin II for the Treatment of Vasodilatory Shock

Angiotensin II effectively increases blood pressure in patients with vasodilatory shock that do not respond to high doses of conventional vasopressors.

AIDA trial: Bioresorbable Scaffolds versus Metallic Stents in Routine PCI

There is no significant difference in the rate of target-vessel failure between the patients who receive a bioresorbable scaffold and the patients who receive a metallic stent. The bioresorbable scaffold is associated with a higher incidence of device thrombosis than the metallic stent through 2 years of follow-up.

DEFINE-FLAIR trial: Use of the Instantaneous Wave-free Ratio or Fractional Flow Reserve in PCI

Coronary revascularization guided by iFR is noninferior to revascularization guided by FFR with respect to the risk of major adverse cardiac events at 1 year. The rate of adverse procedural signs and symptoms is lower and the procedural time is shorter with iFR than with FFR.

SURTAVI trial: Surgical or Transcatheter Aortic-Valve Replacement in Intermediate-Risk Patients

TAVR is a noninferior alternative to surgery in patients with severe aortic stenosis at intermediate surgical risk.

CORONARY trial: Five-Year Outcomes after Off-Pump or On-Pump Coronary-Artery Bypass Grafting

The rate of the composite outcome of death, stroke, myocardial infarction, renal failure, or repeat revascularization at 5 years of follow-up is similar among patients who undergo off-pump CABG and those who undergo on-pump CABG.

EXCEL Trial: Everolimus-Eluting Stents or Bypass Surgery for Left Main Coronary Artery Disease

In patients with left main coronary artery disease and low or intermediate SYNTAX scores by site assessment, PCI with everolimus-eluting stents was noninferior to CABG with respect to the rate of the composite end point of death, stroke, or myocardial infarction at 3 years.

NOBLE Trial: Percutaneous coronary angioplasty versus coronary artery bypass grafting in treatment of unprotected left main stenosis

In patients with left main coronary artery disease, CABG was better than PCI in terms of MACEs at 5 years.

EMPA-REG OUTCOME trial: Empagliflozin, Cardiovascular Outcomes, and Mortality in Type 2 Diabetes

Patients with type 2 diabetes at high risk for cardiovascular events who receive empagliflozin, as compared with placebo, have a lower rate of the primary composite cardiovascular outcome and of death from any cause.

SPRINT trial: A Randomized Trial of Intensive versus Standard Blood-Pressure Control

Among patients at high risk for cardiovascular events but without diabetes, targeting a systolic blood pressure of less than 120 mm Hg, as compared with less than 140 mm Hg, results in lower rates of fatal and nonfatal major cardiovascular events and death from any cause, although significantly higher rates of some adverse events are observed in the intensive-treatment group.

DKCRUSH-V trial: Double Kissing Crush Technique Versus Provisional Stenting Technique for Coronary Artery Bifurcation Lesions

Two-stent DK crush strategy was superior to provisional stenting (with a need for bailout stenting in nearly 50% of patients) for clinical outcomes at 12 months for unprotected distal LMT PCI, driven by a reduction in TLR and target vessel MI; stent thrombosis rates were also better with the DK crush strategy.

CHAMPION trial: CardioMEMS Heart Sensor Allows Monitoring of Pressure to Improve Outcomes in NYHA Class III Heart Failure Patients

Among individuals with recent hospitalization for heart failure with reduced ejection fraction, the use of an implantable device to provide daily pulmonary artery hemodynamic information was beneficial. This device also resulted in decreased hospitalizations for heart failure.

ENABLE trial: Effects of the Endothelin Receptor Antagonist Bosentan on the Morbidity and Mortality in Patients With Chronic Heart Failure

Treatment with bosentan among patients with severe congestive heart failure was not associated with a reduction in death or rehospitalization for heart failure. It caused fluid retention in some patients, which was associated with a higher risk of adverse clinical outcomes.

TACTICS-HF trial: Targeting Acute Congestion With Tolvaptan in Congestive Heart Failure

Among patients hospitalized with acute heart failure and treated with standard intravenous diuretic therapy, the addition of tolvaptan versus placebo did not improve dyspnea symptoms.